How to Use
Your Pie-Hole

How to Use Your Pie-Hole

An Uncensored Food Guide for the
Nutritionally Challenged

Learn to Safely and Naturally Rid Yourself
of Disease, Return to a Healthy Weight,
and F*cking Stay That Way Forever

Jennifer M. Babich

with contributions from
Jeffrey A. Rosenblatt, M.D., F.A.C.C.

This book is educational in nature. Nothing herewith should be viewed or taken as medical advice or be used to self-diagnose. Changes in diet or lifestyle are to be made at your own risk. You have a brain for a reason—make educated decisions and don't come crawling to me with a lawsuit if you fuck up.

Wellness & Health In Motion (WHIM)
Copyright © Jennifer M. Babich, 2016
All rights reserved. Published 2016.
Printed in the United States of America by WHIM Press

ISBN-13: 978-0692676097
ISBN-10: 0692676090

Jennifer M. Babich gratefully acknowledges the generous support of the following contributors, all of whom spent substantial hours assisting with this work:

Cover Design: Sarah Murdoch

Interior Artwork: Karen E. Dies

Assisting Editors: Jill M. Leduc, Lyn Taggart, Marissa M. Barber, Michele Morris

Contributing Author: Jeffrey A. Rosenblatt

To my courageous mother

The first wealth is health.
—Ralph Waldo Emerson

If diet is wrong, medicine is of no use.
If diet is correct, medicine is of no need.
—Ancient Ayurvedic proverb

Let food be thy medicine, and medicine be thy food.
—Hippocrates

Mainstream medicine would be way different if they focused on
prevention even half as much as they focused on intervention.
—Unknown

The doctor of the future will give no medicine, but [instead] will instruct his
patient in the care of the human frame, in diet and in the cause
and prevention of disease.
—Thomas Edison

People are fed by the food industry, which pays no attention to health,
and are treated by the health industry, which pays no attention to food.
—Wendell Berry

Any food that requires enhancing by the use of chemical
substances should in no way be considered a food.
—John H. Tobe

The best and most efficient pharmacy is
within your own system.
—Robert C. Peale

Pie-Hole (n): The facial orifice into which one shoves pie and other food and beverage items (i.e. the mouth).

Contents

Section IV: *Variety* is the Fuckin' Keystone of Nutrition

Section V: Suits on! Shields up! Balls to the Wall!

Foreword

*There is something noble in publishing the truth,
though it condemns oneself.*
—Dr Samuel Johnson

I am privileged to have worked in one of the top medical centers in the US, and alongside some of the brightest and most talented cardiovascular specialists in the world. Thousands upon thousands of sick individuals have sat in front of me, desperately searching for answers to their painful, debilitating ailments. Sadly, they could have saved themselves thousands upon thousands of dollars in medications, procedures, and doctor visits, had they been educated about what occurs between their mouth and their rear end.

As a cardiologist, and with heart disease being the number one cause of death in the western world, I have seen a heck of a lot of sick hearts in my time. Over the years, advances in technology and drug therapy have dramatically improved the outcomes for patients diagnosed with advanced heart disease. And because of those advances, we healthcare providers are highly sought out for assistance. Frankly though, we are not "healthcare providers." We are simply *disease managers*. You see, by the time a patient reaches our doors, they have already developed disease far too advanced to be *cured* by any drug or technology. Instead, we prescribe drastic (and highly expensive) measures to provide stabilization and palliation. We relieve their pain without fixing the underlying problem. We then usually continue to see them for the rest of their "managed" lives, as this system provides customers, not cures.

What's even more disconcerting, are the guidelines now in place to evaluate and reward doctors for dispensing and monitoring the use of expensive medications. Yet, the ability of any of these medications to halt progression, or to cause disease reversal or regression, is abysmal. As an example, when a patient presents with heart disease, we often prescribe the so-called statin miracle drug. However, this go-to pill exerts only a dreadful 20% chance on preventing future heart events.[1-9] This means there's still an *80% chance* we haven't eliminated your risk of having another serious heart event. We haven't cured you, and I don't think there is a colleague of mine out there that would disagree that—despite having these medications and procedures—patients keep coming back with recurrent events. We all wind up scratching our heads, trying to come up with an explanation as to why the medications and procedures didn't work. But hey, I'm sure most healthcare providers are grateful to be able to work under an ideal business model where you're always getting new customers and old ones keep coming back.

The worst part about all of this is that, while billions of your health care dollars are being spent on mainly unsuccessful treatments and research on how to remedy advanced disease, little has been accomplished in the area that would actually *prevent* the development or progression of disease from ever occurring. In fact, less than 5% of the American health care dollar is spent on prevention.[10] This backwards system has left us with an ever-growing population of sick people who are dependent on a myriad of costly medications, with a multitude of side effects and potential long term complications. In fact, we are now seeing an expansion of this trend to our children as the overall state of wellness deteriorates.

What you don't usually hear about is the robust data that supports nutritional intervention as being highly effective—more effective than any drug or procedure. And without side effects!

The Lyon heart study demonstrated a 40% reduction in recurrences of heart attacks and death by adherence to a Mediterranean type diet.[11] More recently, a Cleveland Clinic study showed impressive reversal of coronary artery disease by switching to a plant-based diet.[12] Yet, dietary prescriptions are nearly unheard of. Instead, when patients leave the hospital after an acute or recurrent event, they are given a list of instructions— the most emphasized instruction being a list of necessary *medications* to help manage (not cure) disease.

You know what the average number of medications listed is? *Eight*. Now guess how many instructions are given on nutrition— the key to their success. Generally, none. Or, perhaps a few simple words like, "low fat diet" are scribbled down, which on their own are meaningless if someone has minimal nutrition knowledge. This lack of nutrition prescription happens because, we, as disease care managers, have little or no insight into the fact that appropriate nutrition is more powerful than any medication or intervention. We simply write a vague diet recommendation and hope that our patients figure it out themselves.

It's sickening to see this lack of nutrition knowledge infiltrating the very establishments meant to improve the health of society. I'm referring to hospitals. Recently, while making rounds on a patient in the ICU being treated for a heart attack, I noticed their cardiac diet consisted of a coca cola, cheese burger, and potato chips. How does that make sense? Do we really believe they will heal if he eats that way? Maybe if we write a few more prescriptions.

Coincidentally, a recent study looked at how a Macdonald-type meal affected the ability of blood vessels to constrict and dilate—a vital component of circulatory system function. The results were as follows: there was an *immediate* blood vessel narrowing and decreased blood flow following ingestion.[13] Immediate! What a way to start your day! But patients eat the horrible fast-food-like hospital food, because it because it was given to them in a hospital: a place that's supposed to be helping them heal.

We doctors are not the only ones who are uneducated. This lack of nutrition-can-heal insight extends to many nutritionists as well, who would have you believe that our body is nothing more than a human furnace that needs to be stocked with a controlled number of calories, not taking into account the powerful effects of the ingredients and chemical makeup of foods.

Thus, I have concluded that our disease managers and conventional institutional nutritionists—often referred to as your health care providers—should not be your go-to people for helping you achieve wellness. And they should certainly not be your first choice to alleviate or eliminate the need for costly medications, medical procedures, or recurrent visits. You see, it was actually shown that routine follow up appointments with your doctor don't actually reduce your risk of death, or the amount you spend on health care.[14] In fact, it was shown that these visits simply *increased* the amount of diagnoses, which leads to more medications and treatments. Basically, your visits improve business for us, and don't do much for you.

Don't get discouraged though, there's still hope. Who can you turn to? Yourself! What can you do? Read (and digest) *this* book! Educate yourself, become accountable, and refer to the lists in the final chapter of this book for ways to further your education.

Learn to control your future as you become the master of your own wellness.

—Jeffrey A. Rosenblatt, M.D., F.A.C.C.

Preface

For those of you who know me, you know that publishing a book has been on my bucket list for donkey's years. I was five when I started writing my first novel in a little tattered notepad. The masterpiece was called "The Kid," and explored the life of Alfred Klard—a boy with "sticking up hair." Sadly, by the sixth chapter, the content disappears. The only words that remain are random chapter titles jotted on abandoned pages, eager to be filled in some day. I can only hope this endeavor is slightly more successful, and actually makes it off my desk. If you're reading this, then high-five to me.

I would like to believe I've matured substantially since the days of worrying about Alfred's hair issue, and also that the message here is little more significant than how to deal with a bad hair day. The motivation behind the message here evolved for several reasons—the main one being that for years I've been slammed with nutrition questions. I finally realized I needed a "quick" solution to the barrage—not only because there are so many people struggling with nutrition, but because I became completely overwhelmed by the questions (which rarely have simple answers). Therefore, this book isn't exclusively for you. It's also for me—to shove in front of someone when they ask me a "simple" nutrition question that has a lengthy and extremely complicated answer. Halle-frickin'-lujah.

While this guide is well over five hundred pages (welcome to the 'War and Peace' of nutrition books), the words within it still only chronicle the *tip* of the nutrition iceberg. There are topics such as the type of pans you cook with, as well as the soil in your garden, which also play a role in what ultimately ends up in your pie-hole. I tried to address the topics I get bombarded by the most, and I therefore hope this guide will answer the majority of your questions.

Furthermore, while the statistics and information scattered throughout these pages are heavily based on American data, it's important to understand that these topics and issues are widespread throughout the developed, or "western," world (often because people follow America's lead, assuming we have our shit together. Well, WE DON'T). Therefore, almost all of the information can be translated to anyone reading this, in whatever corner of the world you may be in—especially if your country likes to emulate America.

Lastly, my intent is not to use scare tactics to make you feel hopeless in the big steaming mound of confusion our food system has become. However, I *do* want to help turn the tables, and therefore, I write with brutal honesty. I don't care who I call out, or how deep their pockets are. Your health is my first priority, and this book will change your life . . . if you let it.

Introduction

After years of working with numerous clients around the globe, I have come to the conclusion that 99% of the population has no fucking clue how to eat. That's right—*eat*.

It may sound completely absurd, but "knowing how to eat" has become a talent only a small percentage of the population seems to possess. This innate task has become a complex, foreign chore to the rest. They spend their lives slowly eating themselves to death, by routinely consume shit that shouldn't be considered edible, and are six feet under before they can shout, "Help! I have nofuckingcluehowtousemypie-hole!"

It also seems most people don't even realize that what they put in their mouth has any relation to the state of their body, or how it functions or develops. You could take a baby, clone them, feed each one different foods and you would wind up with two vastly different people (both physically and mentally)—even though they started out identical. Because of this misunderstanding, disease is on the rise, and we're not only killing *ourselves*, but we're destroying generations that follow. Pat on the fucking back to us.

Thankfully, someone stepped up to the plate and wrote an actual guide on how to eat, right? And here you are reading it! What's even more exciting, is that you'll be able to use this guide to improve your nutrition habits—regardless of your nutrition

1

beliefs. I don't care if you're a vegetarian, vegan, carnivore, or cannibal. The biggest lesson I hope you will pull out of this, is that no two people should ever attempt to have the exact same nutrition habits. If all goes well, you will learn how to find *your* particular habits, will stop continually trying to follow fad diets and other peoples' habits, will ignore marketing ploys and misleading labels, and will take a giant leap towards feeling fucking awesome.

It's important to first understanding why two people (or millions of people) shouldn't attempt to follow the same diet. For starters:

- We are all genetically different. Identical twins out there are now shouting, "not us!" But you all know what I mean, so shut your pie-holes. Besides, if we're going to get nit-picky, then not all identical twins are actually genetically the same, so stick that in your pipe and smoke it.[15] My point is that different genes mean that we all function differently and therefore burn energy at different rates.
- We all have different stress levels. This includes mental *and* physical stress—both of which change the way we metabolize food. Furthermore, stress levels fluctuate daily based on our distinct thoughts and actions. For instance, right now I'm thinking about how fucking ridiculous it is that I have to write a guide on how to *eat*, and it's stressing me the fuck out.
- Some people have religious or ethical reasons for not eating certain foods.
- Some people have food allergies.
- People live in different climates where different fresh foods are available.
- People *prefer* different foods.

Could we *be* any more different? Thus, with all of those differences (and there are plenty more), how laughable is it that people try to preach *one* diet, follow the same diet, or believe there's *one* right way to eat?! It's completely irrational, and has gotten WAY out of control. Down with the diets! Who the fuck wants to diet for eternity? This is *not* a diet book, in case you haven't figured that out yet.

This guide will assist you in beginning to understand your relationship with nutrients, and how to choose the best foods for you. It will help you form habits. It will teach you. It's a *lifestyle* change. And while that may sound daunting and treacherous, it's what you need. So quit your bitchin' and saddle up. In the end, you will, beyond a doubt, begin to transform into a healthier version of yourself. After all, *health* is the gold medal at stake here; we're not simply trying to fit into skinnier caskets. Thus, if you're merely looking for a weight loss tool, please feel free to head outside, find a brick wall, and keep banging your head against it. I hope you enjoy your skinny-ass casket.

For the rest of us who want to achieve optimal *health* (which includes our bodies returning to their intended sizes), each of us must find the magic nutrition equation that supports *our own* nutritional needs. It will be based on how *our own* body functions, what *our own* activity levels are, the climate in which *we each* live, and what *our own* food preferences are. With any luck you will have found your way by the end of this guide. If not, well screw it, you can eat the fucking book.

Moral of the Story:

Chances are you're confused as fuck about what you should be putting in your pie-hole. This guide will help you find the specific nutrients *you* need in order to achieve optimal health, eliminate disease, and return to your natural weight. Fist pumps all around.

SECTION I

The Shit We Need to Discuss Before We Get to the Juicy Stuff

Chapter 1

Preaching Versus Teaching

If you give a man a fish he is hungry again in an hour.
If you teach him to catch a fish you do him a good turn.
— Anne Isabella Thackeray Ritchie

Give someone a specific diet plan, recipe, or menu, and they will most likely eat that same shit until they get bored out of their minds and fall back to their unhealthy ways. As much fun as that sounds, it is far more beneficial to *teach* someone about nutrition. Ah hell, being taught probably doesn't sound like much fun either. But, once you figure this shit out, you can fly your beautiful ass into the sunset, sprinkling nutritional fairy dust on the rest of mankind — and *that* sounds amazing.

My point is, it is far more beneficial for someone to *learn* about nutrients, and which ones to choose based on what *their* body needs, than to listen to someone else preach beliefs to them (or even worse: have someone else do it for them). People need to *understand* nutrition in order to find value in it and go the distance. Unfortunately, most people don't want to sacrifice the amount of time this teaching route takes. They're more inclined to reach for "simple" meal plans, programs, concepts, and diets — all of which usually dictate the specific food types or amounts they can or can't eat. How's that workin' for ya? I'm guessing, if you're reading this, it's not. This is why I want to punch every diet plan in the throat. Nobody should *tell* you what to put in your mouth. Instead, they should *teach* you about the nutrients you need, and where the fuck to find them.

The common "preaching" approach does not create a lifetime of healthy eating. Instead, it creates a confused customer that keeps coming back for help (great moneymaker, not-so-great health maker). That, my fellow readers, is never my goal. My goal is always to *teach* people about how to find the right nutrients for their body (and their partner's body, and their children's bodies), so they can do it on their own and NEVER COME BACK. I often joke with clients during our last meeting by saying, "I hope I never see you again!" Meaning, I hope they have learned enough that they can carry on being healthy on their own, teach their kids how to be healthy, and create a long line of healthy people for generations to come. It's not about the money for me. It's about getting people to figure this shit out for themselves.

Thus, I'm not going to dish out menus or meal plans that will get me repeat customers—even if that's what the majority of you are looking for. If I give you a menu and tell you point-blank what to eat, you're either going to eat that same menu for the rest of your life (holy boring, Batman), or you're going to fall back to your unhealthy ways as soon as you get fed up with the menu. You will feel frustrated and convince yourself that "eating healthy is hard." This method won't *teach* you anything, and then we both would have failed. Similarly, if I provide you with a shopping list of healthy foods, it won't teach you anything either. You're just going to wind up with a bunch of healthy foods in your kitchen, and wind up pulling your hair out as you wonder what the fuck you should do with them.

But, if I *teach* you about food (real food!), how to recognize whether or not it does your body good, where to find it, how to cook it, and how to come up with fantastic recipes so you can CONTINUE TO DO SO FOR THE REST OF YOUR LIFE, you will have infinite possibilities of dishes to create, and will *understand* foods and the nutrients they provide. Hip hop hurray!

Does all of this make sense? Of course it does! Yet, this is why most people choose to *not* go the learning route.

"Holy shit what a rigmarole that sounds like! You mean I have to actually use my brain and make an effort?!"

Yes.

"You mean I have to spend more than a week making an effort?"

Yes.

"You mean I have to continue to make an effort until it becomes a habit, and therefore no longer an effort?"

YES.

Initially this may seem like an impossible challenge. Don't worry though—it's only because your brain is mostly likely working at partial-capacity due to the nutrient-depleted "food" it's being fueled with. Take my word for it—put the effort in now, and the lifetime of health and wellness you (and generations to come) will experience will be *more* than rewarding. Healthy eating will become easy and enjoyable. I promise.

Sadly, most nutrition-touters put their desire to fill their pockets above their desire to sincerely help people. This is one of the chief underlying issue of why people don't know how to eat. Not a day goes by where I don't see some news article or social media post about the "Top 10 Foods to Avoid," or "*This* Food will Melt Away Your Belly Fat," or "Everyone must eat like a Caveman." I won't even get into the slogans that are placed right on consumer products these days. What's sad about this, is that people are so desperate for a solution that they'll follow all of the money-hungry, preachy shit. If it were up to me, it would be illegal for someone to make specific nutrition claims and put them out to the general public *telling* them what foods they specifically should or shouldn't eat—especially when they know nothing about their followers. Shit, that gets my blood boiling. Oh, and for the record, the only way you're going to "melt away your belly fat" is by lighting yourself on fire. Good luck with that.

Unfortunately, there's a fine line between obnoxious preaching and helpful teaching. I've tried my darndest to stay on the "teaching" side of things. However, I also feel it is my duty to warn people about harmful foods, ingredients, and chemicals. If something is high on the fuck-you-up scale, I will shout it to the world. Hence, there may be times when you feel I may be preaching my beliefs. Please realize I'm instead trying to lay down a framework of (unfortunately terrifying) facts so you're able to make your own educated decisions afterward.

Side note: I just mentioned "chemicals" above. I'm not a fucking idiot. I realize everything in this world is technically made up of "chemicals." For Christ's sake, water is a chemical. So let's get this straight before we go any further: when I refer to "chemicals" throughout this guide, I'm talking about the harsh, toxic, fuck-you-up chemicals. Generally the ones that are man-made.

Carrying on. I have chosen my own eating habits based on many years of experimentation and research. Does that make me an expert? Who knows. Does that give me the right to tell you that you should eat like me? Of course not. However, it *will* make me write and talk about all of the research I've uncovered, which ultimately led to my diet decisions. Only *you* can determine the foods that make you feel fantastic, and which ones you're therefore going to incorporate into your diet. If you take in all of the information and decide to make the same decisions as me, great! If not, great! As long as you're making educated decisions on your own, based on how *you* feel and what makes *you* happy, *that's* what's important.

How do you know if you're eating the wrong foods? Simple. If your body is anything but its intended shape, or if you have ailments of any kind, then you're probably eating the wrong foods. Yes, there are also genetic and extrinsic factors that may affect you and make you feel like shit, but if you have a kick-ass immune system (fueled by the foods you eat) you should be able to combat the majority of them.

Finding the nutrition equation that makes you happy *and* makes your body thrive is a trial and error process that takes time, but is 100% doable. I'm not here to blow smoke up your ass, so I'm not going to promise it's going to be easy. If there were an easy solution, everyone would have bloody done it already. And, because it's *not* easy, most people usually run screaming for **the** hills when they realize it's going to take longer than a week-long, eat-a-bunch-of-cabbage-and-lemons detox. Nutrition is not an alternative, hippy fad with a following of half-baked tree huggers. Nutrition is a *science*.

Once you make the commitment to yourself and begin to put in the effort, you will stumble upon what I like to call your "magical nutrition equation." This magic nutrition equation consists of the right nutrients for *your* body and will leave you looking and feeling kick-ass. It will have your body running like a well-oiled machine, and will fight off ailments like a sharp-shooter. The science world calls this "homeostasis," but if that word isn't long and annoying, I don't know what is. Do we want to find our "*homeostasis*," or do we want to find our *magic*?! Magic it is!

Once you discover the magic equation that your body has been waiting for, you just need to make sure you don't go around boasting this incredible new "diet" you're on to everyone else. It's *your* nutrition equation, for *your* body, that *you're* going to maintain for the rest of *your* life. It has nothing to do with anyone else (other than the fact that they might take your advice and go find *their* magical nutrition equation). Basically, what makes *you* thrive could make someone else miserable. Keep that magic equation to yourself, enjoy not feeling like crap, and motivate others to do the same.

Moral of the Story:

Following someone else's diet plan will get you nowhere. It's imperative to learn about *your* body and what nutrients it needs. If you have no aliments to speak of, and you can pull a tractor with your eyelids, you've nailed it.

Chapter 2

Me and My Pie-Hole

All truths are easy to understand once they are discovered;
the point is to discover them.
—Galileo Galilei

L et's talk about me for a second. I'm not a narcissist—I merely
need you to understand a bit about my background so you
actually believe half of this shit.

For starters, I'm an optimist *and* a realist (talk about a fun
internal battle):

Me: "I'm going to save the *world!*"

Me: "What the fuck are you talking about, you over-zealous
hippie!?"

Me: "Okaaaay . . . I'll just stick to saving a few lives."

Me: "Welcome back to reality. Now go save lives!"

Besides having voices in my head, I'm also an athlete, an
exercise physiologist, a personal trainer, and a nutrition specialist.
And let's not forget I'm a wife, mother, rump shaker and green
smoothie maker. I love the outdoors, I love chocolate, I hate
ironing, and I can't golf for shit. If you haven't yet figured it out,
I'm also a tell-it-like-it-is, don't-beat-around-the-bush kind of
person. I often stick my nose "where it doesn't belong," because
I'd rather make someone aware of the fact that they're killing

themselves, than potentially have them die a slow, miserable death.

Some people get my approach, some people don't. Some people take offense by it, some people don't. It's ultimately someone else's decision on how they take my advice, but I'd rather raise the flag than turn a blind eye. It makes me live without regret. Why ignore someone's problems if I know I can help? If they don't want my help, they can tell me to piss off. It's like letting someone walk around with a big, crusty booger dangling from their nose without telling them—except on a much larger, and much more serious scale. I'm the type of person that will always tell you about your dangly boogers.

This approach sometimes comes across as harsh and abrasive, but I see it as simply being brutally honest. I will never apologize for trying to improve someone's life, especially when it comes to disease and suffering. I'd rather cut to the chase and **solve** an issue *quickly* so whoever is facing the problem can improve their quality of life and live ailment-free for the rest of their days. Anyone who responds with, "I don't care that I'm like this," "I'm fine being fat," or "I'm okay being miserable," is purely pointing out how unwell and miserable they actually are.

You *should* care. It's *natural* to care. If you don't, then you're even further gone than most. And enough of this "life is too short" bullshit. You are actually *shortening* your life every time you decide to consume something harmful. If you *don't* want your life to be short, make it *longer* by fueling your body as intended.

Watching people trudge through life year after year battling certain goals or ailments and complaining about the same recurring pains makes me incredibly sad. People deserve better. What saddens me even more is when people simply lose weight or buff up and become disillusioned that they're suddenly healthy and "done" with their journey. Yet, they still get sick, still have low energy, still sprout acne, still fight headaches—heck, *any* sort of ailment—and they assume that's normal. It is *not* normal to be sick. You have an immune system for a reason, and if it's not working, well then Houston, WE HAVE A FUCKING PROBLEM.

Sadly, my don't-waste-time attitude came because I lost several family members (including my mother, father, step-mother, aunt and all grandparents) by the time I was of drinking age. I witnessed years of unnecessary suffering, and it was HORRIBLE. By my early twenties I had made it my goal to find a way to educate the public on how to steer clear of avoidable agony and death. I was sure there was a way. It took me almost a decade to ascertain what I was looking for, but I did. And now I present my findings to you in one fabulous ginormo-guide.

Initially, I assumed I had to get people active and exercising more. I grabbed a sports medicine degree in exercise physiology and became a personal trainer. Unfortunately, after years of working in those fields, a certain trend emerged: I realized I could exercise the pants off someone (disclaimer: I didn't literally take the pants off of my clients), and it *still* wouldn't make them healthy or even necessarily lose any weight. They usually just became exhausted versions of their unhealthy selves. Or, sometimes they'd lose weight, but would still be riddled with injury and disease. It finally occurred to me that other factors such as stress, sleep habits, and most importantly nutrition, were *way* more important than exercise was when it came to whole-body health and wellness.

Lucky for me, I had a slight advantage when it came to pie-hole knowledge. I grew up in idyllic rural Vermont, surrounded by organic farms, maple syrup sugarhouses, farmer's markets, chicken coops, and vegetable gardens. I grew up eating "healthy." We never had soda or sugary cereals in the house and we frequently made foods from scratch (like homemade buckwheat pancakes, instead of the chemical-infested buttermilk pancakes from a box). Growing up, most of what I ate was organically grown, and much of it came from our own garden. This set the tone for my nutrition intake later on in life. Add that to the motivation of "finding an answer" after losing so many family members, and I had the foundation and drive I needed.

Before I started barking at everyone about nutrition, I wanted to first make sure I did my research and had *my* nutrition where it needed to be. I read scientific research articles, I watched documentaries, and I read books until I had carrots growing out of my eyes. For shits and giggles, I also became a fitness nutrition specialist and obtained a certificate in plant-based nutrition. What I purposely *didn't* do was go spend a million dollars banking a PhD in Dietetics. I wanted to prove that anyone can, and should be able to, figure this shit out. You shouldn't have to drop your life savings to become a specialist to discover how to fucking eat. You just need to be able to talk, listen, or read. That's it.

It didn't take me long to realize what was wrong with the food system, and it took me even less time to determine which magical nutrition equation made *my* body thrive. I simply focused on the foods that made me feel like I could take on the Galactic Empire, and eliminated the foods that made my insides revolt. I cut out whatever few processed foods I was consuming, and steered myself towards a wide variety of whole, organically grown foods.

The foods that made me thrive turned out to be unprocessed plant foods. This means that almost all of the nutrients I consume come from whole, organically grown plants (e.g. fruits, veggies, beans, lentils, grains, herbs, nuts, seeds). I rarely eat meat, eggs, or dairy, because I feel like a bloated manatee when I do. In other words, my immune system breaks down, and my body floods with ailments. Those, my friends, are called "red flags," and you will hopefully learn how to recognize yours.

Having a whole-food, plant-based diet made me energized. It made all of my body's processes fall into line, made me function like a well-oiled machine, and allowed me to run two businesses, be a wife and a mother, work out, be a competitive athlete, write a book, and *still* have energy left over. I poop at the same time every day, menstruate at the same time every four weeks, and don't have any ailments to speak of—including menstrual symptoms. I only get sick when I become extremely sleep deprived (which I can generally thank my three-year-old for). In the rare instance I *do* get sick, it's mild, only lasts a day or two, and then I send that shit packin'. I have become the definition of healthy, and I'm often mistaken for much younger than I actually am (sometimes a *decade* younger). I'm not bragging, I'm justifying my choices.

Rest assured though, I'm not going to point-blank tell everyone to go eat a plant-based diet. That was *my* magic nutrition equation. You're going to be the one to figure out what yours will be. I'm here to simply give you the tools you need to help you find your way. Whatever equation makes your body thrive and feel fan-friggin'-tastic is "right," and no one can tell you otherwise. Unless, of course, you determine that you should predominantly eat cupcakes. Then I will most definitely show up at your door and tell you otherwise. And by "tell you otherwise," I mean smack some sense into you—by high-fiving your face.

Moral of the Story:
You don't need to be a professional, and you don't need a professional's help, to fucking figure out how to *eat*.
You just need to know how to read (or be read to).
Hey! I know a good book!

Chapter 3

I Screwed the Pooch

Let's get something straight before we go any further: I'm *not* skinny, and I'm *not* lucky. I'm goddamn HEALTHY, and I work my fucking ass off to stay that way (even though it may not feel like I'm working at it anymore). Thus, if you use the word "skinny" when describing me, I will likely drop some f-bombs and tell you there's a big difference between being "skinny" and "healthy." That is to say, do NOT put me in the same category as people who simply lose weight or grow some biceps and believe that's all it takes. It takes much more to actually be *healthy*.

Additionally, by telling me I'm "lucky" for looking a certain way, you're devaluing all of the time and energy I've put into being healthy year after year. Think about that the next time you tell someone they're "lucky" and have no idea what work went into their success.

Here's what usually happens: People look at me (and everyone else who has their shit figured out), resent me, think I'm "lucky" for being "skinny," and then assume that I "could never gain an ounce, even if I tried." They also assume I've never been overweight or unhealthy. Ah-ha! False. I've been both, you overly-judging mo-fos! While it *is* difficult for me to gain weight because I'm like an overactive tachyon (Google that shit) who would rather run around doing a million tasks at once than sit still, there have been a few times in my life I have "slipped" from my healthy

19

ways. I'm telling you this so you don't assume I'm simply an annoying, scrawny bitch who is preaching out of her descending colon (it would be a clean one though). I want you to find *value* in my words. I've seen the other side; I know how it works. I have screwed the pooch many-a-time. Thank goodness for the screw-ups though—I wouldn't be where I am without them.

The first fuckup came in college. I was seventeen, living on my own for the first time, and was no longer surrounded by organically grown, healthy foods. I was surrounded by cheap beer and fried meat. Lots of it. Heck, there was even a cafe on campus (dubbed the "crack shack") that delivered endless shitty food straight to my door! And it was *free* if you were on the meal plan! Score!

Lucky for me, I was a multi-sport athlete who trained year-round, so the weight gain was kept to a minimum. Don't be fooled though—my insides were screaming. For the first time in my life I had horrible menstrual symptoms. I constantly felt like shit, I seemed to sprout a sporting injury on a weekly basis, I was absolutely exhausted, my academic and athletic achievements suffered, and I was nowhere near a walking health advertisement. The athletic trainers at my alma mater even used to joke about my injury file and how it was "record-thick." I laughed it off and thought, "sweet—I'm so hardcore!" At the time I didn't put two-and-two together: my nutrition was fucked, and my health and body were crumbling before my eyes.

The second blunder occurred in New Zealand when I lived with my then-boyfriend's family for a short period during grad school. They were incredibly kind to provide meals for me, but this meant that I took on their very foreign eating habits. Never had I ever seen so much food on a plate before—yet I packed it in. Desserts aren't just for birthdays?! Score! Looking back at the photos from that time, I definitely had one more chin and a couple more boobs than I should have had. My face was puffy and I had acne for the first time in forever. I looked like crap rolled up in more crap. I felt like crap, and I probably smelled like crap. I remember feeling like I was in a constant mental fog, completely void of energy, and frequently wanting to nap. I didn't want to offend my boyfriend's family though, so instead of doing what I knew was right for my health, I did what was right to impress them. Lesson learned.

Side note: My boyfriend's mother (who eventually became my mother-in-law) passed away four years later from colon cancer (and *her* parents soon wound up with cancer as well). The loss was extremely tragic; mainly because I believe her death was 100% avoidable.

The third shit-show occurred when I moved back to America and took on a job with a supervisor from hell who bullied me into submission. I never realized how bad the situation was until I looked back in hindsight. My eating habits completely sunk down the shitter as I became exhausted and defeated. Comfort food flew into my mouth. Couple that with a gnarly, "you may never run again" blow-out knee injury, and I became beaten and lazy. I totally skewed from my "norm." Get this though—I was managing a large *gym*. I worked out regularly, and was surrounded by fitness, fitness, and more fitness. IT DIDN'T MATTER. I still put on weight, had the memory of a fish, enjoyed weekly migraines, and developed kidney infections. I looked and felt like Satan's anus.

The fourth and final hiccup—which was simply a weight gain, and not necessarily a nutrition "slip"—was when I gained forty-nine (*not* fifty) pounds during my pregnancy (a normal weight gain for someone with my height and body fat percentage, by the way). After my son was born, I, like every other child-sprouting woman, was left with a lot of extra weight. For the first time I felt what it was like to have my stomach sit on my legs and my thighs cuddle with each other. YUCK. However, I refused to believe that simply because I had birthed a child it meant my pre-pregnancy body was gone forever. I knew it was buried in there somewhere, and it was my full intention to let it resurface.

Ready for the magic? Each of these slip ups or weight gains was easily (and *quickly*) corrected by simply returning to my normal eating habits (or continuing them in the case of my pregnancy). In fact, after my pregnancy, I easily shed my extra flab within roughly six weeks. If you account for the weight I lost during delivery, that's about seven pounds per week GONE, without any special diet, diet pill, fat suction, stomach stapling, or other ridiculous approach. And I ate like a queen (my calorie consumption was upwards of 3,000 per day)! Granted, I was breastfeeding which certainly helps (please don't try this at home if you didn't just have a baby), but get this—I hardly did *any* exercise. At the time, I would have rather put a pillow over my head and hibernate than hit the gym—and we owned one that was attached to our house! I returned to regular exercise when my son was about six months old, and wound up *gaining* weight because I needed to add muscle to my slim frame. I didn't diet. I simply continued with my magical nutrition equation and my body shrunk back to its intended size. SHAZAM! Magic.

This isn't purely about weight loss though. During the other instances where I fell off the nutrition wagon, I felt like I was being slowly exterminated by some unseen force. My ripped-apart-and-then-pieced-back-together-knee would be so painful, that while driving I'd have to physically lift my left leg with my hand in order to get my foot on and off the clutch *every* time I shifted (I was too stubborn to drive an automatic). That alone brought tears of frustration to my eyes, but I assumed that's how it was always going to be. I also wanted to sleep all of the time, and started acquiring a list of ailments I had never heard of (what the heck is a chilblain?!). As soon as I returned to my healthy eating habits, not only did my body return to its intended *size*, but I *felt* amazing as well. My debilitating knee pain *disappeared.* I shit you not, something that had been crippling was 100% gone, and I eventually returned to being a competitive athlete again. Fuck yeah! To help understand this concept, I have come up with an equation for you. No explanation needed.

Equation 3.1: How to obtain optimal health

$$\frac{\text{NOT A HINT OF A CRAZY EXERCISE PLAN} + \text{MAGICAL NUTRITION EQUATION}}{\text{A BODY OF OPTIMAL SIZE AND HEALTH}}$$

You don't need to be a math whiz to understand that equation. And guess what?! This equation works for *everyone*! This will pertain to *you* — assuming you don't currently have anything extreme going on in your body, your **environment**, or with your lifestyle (i.e. if you're a meth addict who turns tricks on the streets of Chernobyl and you only sleep two hours per night, this probably *won't* be relevant to you, but thanks for buying my book). If you don't have any other crazy shit going on, and you use your pie-hole correctly, your body will *magically* return to its intended size and function the way it is supposed to function. Most people get the equation backwards though, and try something similar to what's found in equation 3.2.

Equation 3.2: Typical health plan

$$\frac{\text{ENDLESS HOURS IN THE GYM "BURNING CALORIES"} + \text{FAD DIETS, CALORIE COUNTING, SUPPLEMENTS, POWDERS, AND HIGHLY-PROCESSED, LOW-FAT FOODS}}{\text{A LIFE OF STRUGGLE, FRUSTRATION, RESENTMENT OF FIT PEOPLE, DISEASE, AND YEARS OF YO-YOING UP AND DOWN}}$$

As much fun as that second equation sounds, I'm going to stick with the first one. It's all about how you use your pie-hole, folks. Don't get me wrong, being active certainly has its health benefits and is important to round off the "general health" title. However, exercise should be considered a *supplement* to health, whereas nutrition *is* health—not the other way around.

On a side note, next time you see an athlete wind up with a life-threatening disease and say, "but they're so active and healthy," please realize their health has little to do with their activity level. If you don't know what they're putting in their mouth, you don't know how healthy they are. I know plenty of athletes who eat shit 24/7 and still manage to get their body through the motions. And I constantly wonder how good they'd *actually* be if they fueled their body properly.

I'm sure you've heard the phrase, "you can't out-train a bad diet" (and if you haven't, well there you go). Exercise is *not* the sole solution when it comes to weight loss or health. You can't put shit in your pie-hole and then expect your body to turn around and answer with "health"—even if you spend four hours at the gym every day. Yet, when someone realizes their health has gone down the crapper, they immediately buy a gym membership and start snorting protein powders. They buy into the madness that you *need* those things to be healthy. You don't. You *need* food.

Exercise isn't even "needed" to lose weight. Exercise isn't even "needed" to lose weight. Yes, I wrote that sentence twice. I wanted to make sure it sunk in. Say it with me: "EXERCISE ISN'T EVEN NEEDED TO LOSE WEIGHT." Go on, take a moment to celebrate. Shout from the hilltops. Then go construct a bonfire of the thigh masters and shake weights you have scattered around your house. Burn that shit to the ground!

This doesn't mean you never have to exercise again. Nice try. Realistically, once you discover how to use your pie-hole and begin to approach optimal health, the more active, happy, and motivated you will be. Your quality of life will skyrocket. The desire to spend your time engaging in regular physical activities you actually *enjoy* doing will explode from you like a calorie-burning orgasm. Activities that perhaps you haven't enjoyed for years—like gardening, biking, hiking, skiing, and dancing. You know, as opposed to counting calories and pounding out hours on the treadmill next to the guy that smells like rotting tuna. In effect, you will lead an active, healthy, enjoyable lifestyle (by choice!), rather than wasting away your days trying to sweat for the sake of burning off the shit you keep shoving down your pie-hole.

Once I figured that concept out, and learned what my body needed, I went on to teaching others about nutrition. And whenever you get degrees or certifications in health-related fields, you're reminded an obnoxious amount of times that "you are not a doctor, and you cannot diagnose or make health claims." Well, here I am making health claims, so clearly my stubborn ass didn't get the picture.

Nutrition heals. Here's why I'm comfortable making that claim: Over the years of working with people on their diets, I have seen cholesterol problems disappear. I have seen high blood pressure return to normal. I have seen fibromyalgia disappear. I have seen joint pains and arthritis disappear. I have seen body odor and insomnia disappear. I have seen fertility issues disappear. I have seen skin and hair become commercial-worthy. I have seen energy levels skyrocket and smiles from people who once seemed broken. All from improvements in nutrition—and that's merely the tip of the iceberg. Here's the "funny" part: many of those people had been to multiple conventional doctors first . . . and *none* of them had gotten the results they had seen with me (you'll soon understand why).

Eating properly allows the body to heal itself in a million ways you would never imagine, from the inside out. I'm talking everything from acne to cancer. You *can* cure yourself.

Moral of the Story:
Nutrition trumps exercise. End of story.

Chapter 4

Trust Me, You're Malnourished

Symptoms are not enemies to be destroyed, but sacred messengers who encourage us to take better care of ourselves.
—Food Matters documentary

Let's move on to you. I'm guessing you've picked up this guide because you've either hit a wall, or after years of trying you've finally realized you're at a complete loss of what to do with your pie-hole. Or, perhaps you *think* you're consuming the right foods but aren't seeing the results you'd expect. Regardless, I'm stoked you're here. Good for you, high five, step one DONE!

Most people come to me looking for personal training. They tell me over and over that "they feel great," "don't need help with nutrition," and "just need help with losing weight" (and clearly believe that losing weight exclusively correlates with how much time they put in the gym). I initially bite my tongue, because I *know* they feel like shit. Unfortunately, *they* don't know they feel like shit. Additionally, they usually don't realize that weight loss is simply a *side effect* of being healthy—it's not something that needs to be intently focused on. It's something that should just happen if all the health stars align.

After coercing these people into nutrition counseling and putting in some long hours, I regularly get the following response: "Holy *shit*! I had no idea what it was like to feel like this!" It's crazy—they *thought* they felt great, but in reality they had no idea what it was like to feel great because they had literally never felt great before.

This happens all the time. This could be you. Regardless of what you currently feel like, I can guarantee you can feel better. Most people are walking around with their bodies running at partial capacity. That's all they know, and therefore that's what they imagine is the norm. Their symptoms and ailments become a way of life. As soon as I help get their bodies functioning as intended . . . POW! They're like super-ninjas and are ready to take on the world!

I don't give a shit if you're an obese diabetic or an Olympic athlete; if your eating is "off," there is *zero* chance you are functioning at your optimal capacity. Imagine what would happen if all Olympic athletes cleaned up their nutrition! Wowza. Hey athletes—give me a ring! Let's break some records!

Alright, let's cut to the chase. We need to listen to our bodies, plain and simple. Signs, symptoms, ailments, disease . . . whatever you want to call them—they should all be considered messengers that are there to let us know that something is awry. In other words, they're signs you're experiencing malnutrition. By the way, the word "malnutrition" simply means "shitty nutrition." It isn't a word used to define starving children in different corners of the world. Most of the world's population is malnourished, and chances are, you're included in that statistic.[16]

Going off what I've encountered in the past decade, I'm guessing you have some, if not many of the following side effects of malnutrition. Go ahead and make note of the ones you experience on a regular basis, or have permanently acquired. That way you can come back later—after you've made nutrition changes—and reminisce about how shitty you originally felt. I'm serious, go get a pen and start checking them off.

Side Effects of Malnutrition

abnormally heavy or
   painful periods
acne or greasy skin
ADD/ADHD
Alzheimer's
anemia
anxiety/panic attacks
aneurysm
arthritis
asthma
atherosclerosis
autism spectrum
   disorder
bloating or gas
blood clots
blood in urine
blurred vision/loss of
   vision
body odor
brain fog/confusion
brittle or discolored
   nails
Buerger's disease
burning eyes
burning when
   urinating
cancer
cataracts
chilblains
chronic bad breath
chronic fatigue or
   lethargy

cold sensitivity
constipation
cracked lips
Crohn's disease
dark circles under eyes
dark yellow or cloudy
   urine
decreased sex drive
deep vein thrombosis
deformities in your
   offspring
depression
diabetes (type 1 or 2)
diarrhea
diverticulitis
dry/scaly skin
early onset of puberty
endometriosis
excessive bruising
excessive weight loss
   or gain
frequent cold or flu
frothy or foamy urine
gall stones
gestational diabetes
gout
grey or pale skin
gum disease
headaches or
   migraines
heart attack
heart failure

hemorrhoids
high blood pressure
high blood sugar
high cholesterol
hormone imbalance
inability to perspire
inadequate blood
   clotting
infertility
insomnia
intense food cravings
irregular periods
irritable bowel
   syndrome
itchy skin, eczema,
   psoriasis
kidney failure
kidney stones
lack of menstruation
light sensitivity
loss of appetite
loss of height
lupus
macular degeneration
memory loss or
   confusion
mood swings or
   irritability
mouth sores/ulcers
multiple sclerosis
night time urination
nose bleeds

osteomalacia or rickets

peripheral vascular
   disease

poor growth or
   development

poor or broken sleep

poor or slow healing

pre-eclampsia

Raynaud's
   phenomenon

reduced ability to
   taste, hear, or smell

respiratory infections

severe pre-menstrual
   symptoms

sleep apnea

sore tongue

sound sensitivity

swelling in the feet or
   ankles

thinning or loss of hair

thyroid disorders

tooth decay or enamel
   erosion

transient ischemic
   attack (TIA)

tremors (e.g. hands,
   voice)

ulcerative colitis

varicose veins

vomiting (randomly)

That list could go on forever. If you have ailments or symptoms other than what are listed (regardless if you think they're insignificant), add them to the list. I left space for a reason, so use it. *Any* ailment out there could be linked to malnutrition, and when you come back to this list in the future, you'll want to remember all of the crap you were experiencing.

Now you're saying, "Well everyone has some of these ailments!" Guess what, Einstein? You're absolutely right! Herein lies the problem. All of these horrible ailments (and the thousands that aren't listed) are signs that "something is wrong" within your body. One or more of your body's systems are screaming profanities at you, and you need to recognize the signs and make changes so they don't get worse.

The body was never meant to be overweight, in pain, or symptomatic. The body is a kick-ass machine that is perfectly capable of functioning brilliantly, 100% of the time—if provided with the right fuel. Furthermore, you're either sick or you're not. Just because you didn't circle 75% of that list, doesn't mean you should be high-fiving yourself. Even *one* symptom means something is "off."

Charlotte Gerson, the daughter of the famous Dr. Max Gerson (founder of the Gerson Institute) put it perfectly: "You can't keep one disease and heal two others—when the body heals, it heals everything." Get it? If you truly achieve optimal health, you won't have *any* signs of breakdown. It is black and white. Any ailment—big or small—is a sign of breakdown. You could have one symptom, or one hundred symptoms—you're still going to wind up on the "malnourished" list.

For those of you who are blaming your ailments on genetics, I'm willing to bet that almost all of you are wrong. More often than not, someone simply has the same diet or lifestyle as their parents and grandparents, and therefore wind up with the same malnutrition issues. It usually has nothing to do with genetics and has everything to do with bad habits. Either that, or I've solved many genetic disorders over the last decade. Do yourself a favor: stop using "genetics" as a scapegoat, and see what happens.

Back to the list. All of those ailments can be caused by the wrong combination of nutrients. Riddle me this then: If someone is severely lacking in, let's say, three nutrients that are causing several of the mentioned ailments, wouldn't it seem logical to find out what those nutrients are, give them a top-up, and then find a solution for long-term intake? DING DING DING! You would think that would be the logical solution, but unfortunately instead of saying "let's eat this food with this nutrient in it," we say, "let's concoct this less optimal product that makes money and shove it down our throats." The majority of society has decided that little pills, with a long list of horrible side effects, somehow make more sense when it comes to solving our malnutrition issues.

We have become pill-poppers. We consistently reach for pills that will treat the symptoms of an issue that was, in fact, caused by a lack of nutrients. And the issue never really goes away. If you're still eating the same shit, you're still malnourished. You've simply managed to temporarily mask the symptoms with a little, nasty pill. God-forbid we get to the root of the problem and combat the shit out of it.

Actually, that's exactly what we intend to do. Your goal should be to find out what nutrients may be lacking in your diet, where to find the best versions of them, how to incorporate them into your diet regularly, and how to live a life free of ailments, disease, *and* prescription medications. I'm here to help you get started. Here's to all of us feeling like kick-ass super ninjas!! Heee-yaahh!

Moral of the Story:
Being "skinny" or "buff" does *not* mean you're "healthy." Malnourishment comes in many forms, and if you have any ailments of any kind, chances are you're malnourished. Nutrients, and not pills, should be used to heal malnourishment. Duh.

Chapter 5

Health, Not Hobby

Every time you eat or drink, you are either feeding disease or fighting it.
—Heather Morgan

You've probably heard the term "everything in moderation" at some point in your life. People seem to use that line so they can go out and consume shit they know they shouldn't be eating, as long as they don't eat "too much of it." Let's hop off the denial train for a second. You obviously can't go around eating light bulbs and arsenic in moderation, so we have to draw the line somewhere (and some foods and beverages are not far off from having the same nutritional value as a light bulb or arsenic).

If you go around eating tons of different types of shitty food "in moderation," you are *still* eating tons of shitty food, regardless of how you look at it. That ton of shitty food (or even *some* shitty food) winds up taking the place of the health-promoting foods you *should* be eating. Thus, I hate to break it to you (no I don't), but eating isn't about consuming everything you *want* in moderation. Eating is about fueling and nourishing your body with the nutrients it *needs*.

This is the very concept you must comprehend before even attempting to learn about different foods and beverages (which ones are good, which ones will slowly poison you to your death, and why you can't go around eating everything "in moderation"). The concept is that eating was never meant to be a hobby, a means for social gatherings, or even an indicator of social status. Eating was meant to be the way in which we provide our bodies with the fuels needed to run and regulate the millions of processes within them effectively and efficiently. SAY WHAT!? Food is fuel.

What a bizarre, boring concept, right? We need to *fuel* ourselves with the proper gas, just like we fuel our vehicles with the proper gas. I don't see anyone dumping sand and popsicles (clearly the wrong fuels) into their car's tank. But I do see a heck of a lot of people dumping the wrong fuels into their pie-holes. If you're looking for a hobby, eating isn't it.

Everything we shove down our pie-holes potentially becomes our fuel. Every time we consume something (even a light bulb!), our body will attempt to break it down into little pieces, and then distribute and use those pieces wherever they're needed as fuel. Or, in the case of the light bulb, the body will just waste precious time and energy trying to get rid of the shitty fuel, and will wind up harming itself in the process.

The *good* fuel we consume regulates everything in our bodies, from the more simple processes like picking our nose (don't pretend you don't), to the more complex ones like pumping blood around our vascular system while we run a marathon. Eating is NOT a cool talent we possess in which we see how much shit we can shove down our throats at any given time purely because we *feel* like it (unless you're one of those stupid fuckers on ESPN who eats a thousand hotdogs in three minutes). To truly obtain optimal health (proper weight, skin tone, hair quality, nail quality, energy level, sleep state, no disease, etc.), we have to eat what our bodies *need*, not what we *want* "in moderation."Have I made that clear yet?

Guess what happens when we eat the wrong fuel? Let's go back to the car example. Imagine putting cat piss into your car's gas tank and then trying to drive it to Columbia. You won't get far, and you'll no doubt damage the shit out of your ride. And let's face it, you should feel like an absolute ding-dong for even attempting something so ridiculous. See where I'm going with this? We should feel like idiots for shoving anything but the right fuel down our pie-holes, and in the same breath expecting our bodies run as intended, stay at an ideal weight, and remain disease-free.

The wrong fuel, regardless of how much, means you're on your way down destruction lane faster than you can say "everything in moderation." You *will* wind up tired and cranky, your skin *will* become dull or greasy, and you *will* get dark circles under your eyes. You *will* feel bloated and your bowel movements *will* become irregular. You *will* get the flu. You *will* start to fall apart from the inside out, and that long list of ailments in the previous chapter will start to sound like an autobiography.

Realistically though, how often do you go to eat something and think, "hmmm, what specific fuels might my body be lacking and therefore needing at the moment?" Never? Don't worry—you're not alone! If you're in the 99% mentioned in the introduction, you probably say something more along the lines of, "what do I feel like eating," or "what can I grab that's quick and easy," right? Or maybe—just maybe—you *do* decide to have a "healthy" meal, but in actuality it's not as healthy as you think *or* what your body needs. We'll soon find out.

But first you must wrap your head around the fact that when you eat you should be concerned with what fuels your body *needs*, and not what shit you have an immense desire to masticate. If you can do that, you're ready to make changes. This is when things start to get exciting. Balls OUT, I say!

I have developed a tool for my clients in order to help them understand the importance of eating for health. It's extremely complex (not at all), and took years (minutes) to formulate. I call it my Nutrition Spectrum. It's pretty rad, pretty self explanatory, and I'll be referring to it throughout this guide. Wait—pictures?! This book just got even *more* awesome!

In the following illustration, you will see that individuals who have their shit figured out are hanging around the top of the spectrum and spend their days frolicking with bountiful energy in lycra superhero suits. Becoming Captain America is the ultimate goal. I'm more of a Batman fan myself, but hear me out. Captain

America is a super-human. His strength, speed, endurance, agility, reflexes, resilience, and healing are unsurpassed. He is the epitome of how a human should be able to function when fueled properly (okay, perhaps he had a little help from some serum, but you get my point). Go print out a photo of Captain America and tape it to your mirror, so every time you look into it you'll be reminded of the ultimate goal here: become a superhero.

The malnourished zombies I have previously mentioned live at the bottom of the spectrum and get to bathe in diseases like cancer, diabetes and heart disease (along with all other shitty illnesses). Alternatively, they're six feet under. Rest in Peace, zombies.

Everyone else is scattered in between, still malnourished, but without the serious disease (yet). They experience their daily dose of minor ailments like colds, the flu, acne, dark eye circles, joint pain, menstrual symptoms, headaches, fatigue, etc.

If you haven't figured it out, the goal is to shimmy up that Nutrition Spectrum as high as you are able. By the end of this guide, you should be on your way. Grab your shield and spandex ensemble and get ready to fuckin' suit up, soldier.

The Nutrition Spectrum

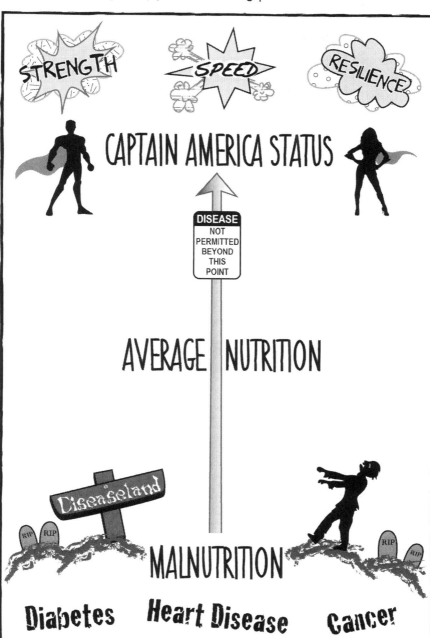

Moral of the Story:

Everything you consume becomes your fuel. Don't shove shit down your pie-hole and then act surprised when you feel or look like Turd McShitty. Grab your cape and haul your ass up that Nutrition Spectrum.

Chapter 6

You *Should* Be Fucking Confused

If you can't convince them, confuse them.
—Harry S. Truman

Can you honestly say that the food industry doesn't confuse the fuck out of you? Of course it does. We're constantly being conned because there's no other option for the food industry—they *have* to confuse us in order to sell their toxic products. They're sure as shit not going to profit by declaring, "there's a good chance this crap will cause you to die a slow, painful death." Instead, they mislead us by telling us little white lies about how their product *may* be healthy or contain *one* good component. This puzzling system is working because people will forever want to hear good news about their bad habits:

"Chocolate has antioxidants?! Yessss! Chocolate for days!"

"This soda is sugar-free?! Must be good!"

"Cheese is high in protein? Melt that shit over everything!"

"These hot dogs are low-sodium?! I'll take twelve!"

Let's face it, we get sucked into advertising. If we're confused about a delicious-looking product, and it comes bearing a big, bold statement boasting its awesomeness, we're most likely going to celebrate and then consume it. We certainly don't research whether or not those marketing statements hold water.

Unfortunately, sometimes those advertisements or marketing statements contradict each other. Now what? Who do we believe? How do we overcome the confusion? Well, now that you've (hopefully) wrapped your head around the fact that eating is actually the way we ward off disease and make our bodies function properly—and that ailments of any magnitude can be a sign that we are malnourished—let's back up a bit. We first need to understand where the confusion comes from. Get ready, I'm about to start pointing (middle) fingers.

Parental Guidance

This is one of the obvious reasons for some of the confusion. Everyone trusts their mother. Whatever she says or does, goes. Not so much their father, but definitely their mother. I'm joking! Jeesh dads, loosen up, we're just getting started!

You grow up eating delicious home-cooked meals, and you most likely have the notion that the food your loving parents gave you is *good for you.* I mean, heck—why would they ever feed you anything harmful? Unfortunately, chances are if *you're* clueless about nourishment, then your parents probably lacked substantial nutrition knowledge as well—or else they would have educated you, right? I'm not taking a stab at your folks here, so take a breather (just like it's not your fault, it's not theirs either). This is where the cycle of death starts. Everyone trusts their parents, and therefore usually builds their personal nutrition habits in a similar manner—and then sends that info on to *their* children. Just because your parents ate it or served it does *not* give it the healthy stamp of approval.

The 100% Accurate World Wide Web

The second obvious reason for the confusion actually creates a butt-load of business for me. Enter the age of technology. The Internet is *fantastic!* It will tell you in 0.03 seconds that you're going to get morbidly obese if you eat bread, and that a brain tumor is the cause of your headaches. The answers to everything are at your fingertips—even the incorrect and misleading ones!

Everyone turns to the Internet to find the solutions to their problems. Check this out: a 2011 survey showed that even physicians—almost 50% of them—admit to frequently using websites like Google and Yahoo to treat, diagnose, and care for their patients rather than using other tools such as medical reference books.[17]

Hopefully, the physicians out there find it easy to sort through the copious amounts of information in order to find the trustworthy sources they're looking for. For us "average folk" though, it's one big cesspool of contradictory information. People come to me all of the time because they're so confused over what they read on the Internet. I literally want to find the Internet and punch it in the boner. It is a festering sea of confusion, and causes more harm than good (when it comes to health advice anyway). If you want health advice, you either need to learn how to source out reputable websites, or find a health *professional* who knows their ass from their elbow. Do not simply follow "Christie's Top 10 Diet Tips" on Facebook and adhere to it like it's your sole purpose in life. If that's a real thing, my apologies to Christie.

Beyond parents and interwebs, there are many more reasons why someone may be completely puzzled about the role of nutrition in their life. Here's where the money-hungry jerks come into play and my blood begins to boil.

Diets

As far as I'm concerned, all diets can go to hell in gasoline underwear. They are nothing but money-making schemes that provide temporary "fixes" and false hope, and suck money out of uneducated people (I don't mean that in a belittling way).

Let's start by stating the obvious: if diets worked, they would have worked. Thus, we can pretty much conclude that diets are a sham. Obesity and other ailments would have been smothered in the 1930s by the popular grapefruit diet, or in the 1950s by the cabbage soup diet. Surely Weight Watchers—which has been around since 1963—would have solved the health crisis by now, right? Wrong. All they have solved is their lack-of-money issue.

Over the years we have discovered the Sleeping Beauty diet, the Cookie Diet, Slim-Fast, diet pills such as Dexatrim, the Atkins diet, the Zone diet, Macrobiotic Diet, South Beach Diet, Master Cleanse, the HCG diet, and the Paleo diet, to name a few. *Surely*, with all of those promising options, we would have our shit together, right?! Well we don't, and in actuality we look back on most of those and say, "what the heck were we thinking?!" Yet at the time, everyone jumped in line in order to become the next diet success story. Diets are marketing tools which attract incredible attention because they promise results—usually quickly—and come with clear-cut instructions. Sweet jubilation!

Alas, even with all of those wonderful, "results proven" diet options listed above, we are still sicker than ever, still fatter than ever, and *still* chasing after the next diet craze. I know people who hop from one diet to the next, convinced the next one will work. Their weight fluctuates up and down faster than a honeymooner's pants, and they never take a step back to reflect on how many years they've spent unsuccessfully dieting. If this sounds like you, for fuck's sake, STOP IT.

Here's the funny part about all of this: most diets throughout history tout extremely similar "requirements" (they just seem to get recycled and polished up a bit before they get renamed and spit back out). Meet the low-carbohydrate, high-protein diet.

That being said, here's a high-protein diet statistic to tickle your pickle: as dietary protein increases, so does the incidence of cancer.[18-22] On the contrary, as dietary protein is reduced, cancer occurrence is reduced (even if already present). There are similar results for other diseases (e.g. diabetes, heart disease, autoimmune diseases). Hmmm . . . interesting. It shouldn't be surprising then that we are being ravished by these very diseases as people continue to search out high-protein diets. Side note: it is extremely important to mention that this correlation specifically pertains to protein obtained from *animals,* and not plants. We will discuss this much more in depth later on.

While these high-protein diets can often show rapid weight loss or muscle gain, they also bat one thousand with long-term sickness (if you're not a baseball fan, that's another way of saying, "you're going to fucking get sick if you consume a high-protein diet"). The sad thing is, I know many people out there who will choose a quick-fix weight loss or muscle gain plan over long-term health because they care more about what they look like NOW, than whether or not they're going to be around in another thirty years. MUST GET "BIKINI BODY" READY FOR SUMMER!

In fact, did you know that the word "diet" actually means "devil" in Latin? I totally made that up, but it should. Diets are a waste of time and suck people further away from actually learning how to permanently and properly nutritionalize themselves (yes, I made that word up too). Diets foster a belief that eliminating or restricting *one* component of nutrition is the magic answer, and they usually focus on *eliminating* foods, rather than *adding* highly nutritious foods. This is probably why typical diet companies also often have side "supplement" businesses where they insist you have to take certain vitamins or powders in order to fulfill your diet requirement (an impressive marketing scheme, and total trickery). Take the popular Beachbody programs (P90X, Insanity, PiYo). They start and end every workout telling you that you should use Shakeology supplement shakes to enhance your results—a totally unnecessary, yet fantastic way for them to make more money. If they're assuming that most people are malnourished and need more nutrients, then they're right—but those people should learn to get those needed nutrients from *real* food. Go away, friggin' supplement pushers.

In reality, nutrition is a complex science that cannot be looked at or approached in a simple, one-dimensional way. It is a multi-faceted system, in which all sides need to be addressed and understood so they can work together in synergy. If you purely focus on one aspect—like limiting calories or cutting carbs—it will not work. You don't need to diet. EVER. You simply need to educate yourself and start making permanent changes so you can step away from malnutrition and into your Captain America suit. Have you purchased yours yet?

It's My Product, I can Label it Whatever the Fuck I Like! Screw marketing tactics. Just because a food or beverage item sits on a shelf, is available to the public, boasts one redeeming quality, or *looks* healthy, does not mean it *is* healthy or should wind up anywhere near your pie-hole. Most food and beverage companies want to make money first and foremost, and that usually means sourcing the easiest, cheapest ingredients and hiding them in highly attractive, misleading packages. Whether or not their product is going to fuel you or fuck you up is generally of little-to-no concern. Marketing strategies (e.g. deceitful brand names, slogans, advertisements, packaging) are your worst enemy.

Let me paint a scenario for you:

- I invented a cookie.
- I named it "Nature's Pure Best Natural Cookies." *Wow! That has GOT to be the healthiest cookie EVER!*
- This is a CHOCOLATE cookie. *Yumm-o! EVERYONE loves chocolate!*
- This cookie is pre-made! Therefore, there's no need to actually use your own kitchen *or* your brain to make it! *Right on! My kitchen is purely for looks, and let's face it, my inadequately-fueled brain isn't functioning well enough to follow instructions anyway!*
- This cookie is low-fat! *Yay! I heard that fat is B-A-D, BAD!*
- This cookie is reduced-calorie! *Sweet! I can't actually define what a calorie is, but I know for certain they're the devil!*
- This cookie has been pumped full of vitamin A—1,000% of your daily allowance to be exact! *Wow! I really haven't got a*

friggin' clue what vitamin A does, but dude, it's FANTASTIC that there's so much in there!

- This cookie has 30% more antioxidants! *30% more than WHAT? I don't care, that sounds AMAZING!*
- This cookie is packaged in a brightly-colored, kid-friendly, puppy-covered wrapper, and has the word "NATURAL" in big letters before the word "Cookies." *Puppies?? Yay! And, if it says "natural" it HAS to be good for me! And, did I mention PUPPIES?!*
- This cookie is marketed worldwide because I spent a billion dollars doing so. This cookie now shows up everywhere—in commercials, radio ads, magazines, billboards, sides of buses, you name it. It's even endorsed by Olympic athletes. Beautiful chocolaty-puppy goodness in all its glory.

Guess what? Suddenly my cookie is on the plate of every child across the planet due to my awesome marketing skills. I marketed it as being natural, healthy, and full of vitamins and antioxidants, without giving any care to the "other" ingredients—because *that* sells. Now I'm filthy RICH!! YESSSS! Now I can go invent more shitty food and market it as healthy to make *more* money! Muuahh haaa haaaa! I'm the devil in disguise!! And I don't care! Because, BENJAMINS!!

This is how most "foods" and "beverages" are marketed today. I put "foods" and "beverages" in quotation marks because most of the products marketed today are food-*like*, or beverage-*imitations*, and do not actually contain many (or any) natural ingredients. That issue will be explained in more detail later.

As mentioned previously, most "food" and "beverage" companies first and foremost want to make money (of course they do, that's the purpose of a business). Unfortunately, their interest in money comes at our expense. To succeed, companies often focus on making the cheapest products they can (which means skimping on healthy, whole, *real* foods). Then they fortify those products with one or two acceptable components that they can use to promote them (regardless if those acceptable components only make up a miniscule part of them). They then, of course, skip over the *unhealthy* components while marketing the crap out of them. What company is realistically going to say, "Don't forget about the chemical carcinogens you're getting from our products! Those will *really* knock you on your ass"?!

They make their products look like beautiful, heaven-in-your-mouth substances that will send you to your knees from the mind-blowing orgasm you'll have while consuming them. EVERYBODY. MUST. HAVE. SOME. This is how the majority of food companies work, and I want to tell each of them to sit on a fork and spin.

For example, in 2014 a story appeared in the news about Coca-Cola being sued over their "Pomegranate Blueberry 100% Fruit Juice Blend." One could assume this juice was predominately made up of pomegranate and blueberry, right? Especially since the picture on the front of the bottle depicts both, right? Wrong. Here are some numbers: 0.3, 0.2. Those are the percentages of pomegranate and blueberry juice concentrate in the drink, respectively. That means 99.5% of the liquid is something other than what the drink boasts. Hence the false advertising lawsuit.

As for the "100% Fruit Juice Blend" claim, one should also be able to assume the only ingredients in this concoction are different fruit juices, right? Well, here are some ingredients for you, all of which are thrown in there: natural flavors, modified gum acacia, DHA algal oil, ascorbic acid, citric acid, choline bitartrate, alpha-tocopheryl acetate, soy lecithin, vitamin B_{12}.[23]

Regardless if those "other" ingredients are healthy for you or not, how can they claim the juice is "100% fruit juice" if it's clearly not? Answer: because they can do whatever the fuck they want, that's why.

Coke's reasoning? "[Consumers] know when something is a flavored blend of five juices and the non-predominant juices are just a flavor."[24] Oh really? If consumers knew how to see through labels, they wouldn't buy 90% of the shit on the market today. Consumers *don't* know, and assholes like YOU, Coke, need to stop trying to mislead them and fuck with their health purely to get money in your pockets.

Back to the all-mighty cookie I invented above. It sounded amazing, didn't it? Well, what I failed to mention to you is the following:

- I can call my damn cookie whatever I want to call my damn cookie, because it's *my* damn cookie. I'm sure as hell going to pick a name that lures you in and makes you *think* it's natural and good for you, because that sells, and I want to sell the shit out of it.
- It has zero real chocolate. Instead, it has a man-made chocolate substitute that smells and tastes like chocolate, but is cheaper to make, and will wreak havoc on your body. Because, let's face it, all I care about is money.
- By pre-making this cookie, I can shove whatever the hell I want in it (e.g. high fructose corn syrup, MSG, fillers, colors, preservatives), and unbeknownst to you, you get to eat that addictive shit! I don't care. Because, money!
- *Of course* the cookie is low fat — it's a *cookie* and it's fucking 99% sugar! And sugar is cheap . . . which means a larger profit margin for yours truly.
- It's "reduced calorie" because I filled it with artificial sugar. I'm sure hoping you don't notice, because that shit probably causes cancer (and when it comes down to it, I could make a piece of cat shit reduced calorie, but that doesn't make it healthy). I sure do love money.
- The vitamin A that I used is actually a synthetic chemical, and is absolute crap compared to natural vitamin A from *real* food — which you would be getting enough of if you friggin' used your pie-hole as intended. By the way, you don't need 1,000% of anything. But, by the way, I need more money.
- The "30% more" antioxidants actually means 30% more than *another* similar cookie, which barely has any antioxidants. Meaning, my cookie *still* has a miniscule amount of

antioxidants. For example, if my cookie has 30% more than the 0.05mcg of antioxidants found in the other cookie, it still only 0.065mcg of antioxidants. Still JACK SHIT. Ha! I sure fooled you! Now I'm going to go take a money bath.

- The word "natural" on its own means zilch. Sugar is "natural" for fuck's sake. So are maggots. If someone pissed in your cookie they could still call it natural. In addition, unless the product reads "100% Natural," it means only *some* of the ingredients are natural. Anyone can throw the word "natural" onto their product—even if those products are genetically modified and contain toxic pesticides, growth hormones, and antibiotics. Best false advertising EVER, yet consumers flock to "natural" products. Don't be fooled by the words that are thrown on packages. I could throw the word "hydrating" on a bag of poop, and I wouldn't be wrong (poop is about 75% water). But wait, is it "natural" to sleep on a pillow of money? Because I do.
- I know, as a billion dollar marketer, that the more people I promote my cookie to, the more people are going to eat it. I also know that Olympic athletes endorse all sorts of horrible shit, and little kids want to be just like them. So I'm definitely going to get some of them to endorse this masterpiece. Game over. Now show me the money!

All of that trickery is warranted though, because you get 1,000% of your (fake) vitamin A for the day, and a miniscule amount of antioxidants!! Congrats! You're going to be a fake-vitamin-toting cancer patient! Get my point? And please—take a step back for a second. It's a fucking *cookie*. That ought to be the first hint it shouldn't be a regular guest at your table.

What it boils down to, is that the products that are marketed the most (usually deceitfully, as shown above), and are therefore *seen* the most, are eaten the most. This even holds true for supposedly healthy foods. You want calcium; you drink dairy milk, right? You want vitamin C; you drink orange juice, right?

That's because the dairy and orange juice industry have a fuckload of money to pump into advertisements, and we therefore see their ads more than anything else. We also believe them when they say they're the best options for calcium and vitamin C.

There are other options we never hear about that have calcium and vitamin C in much more of an abundance than dairy milk and orange juice. For example, almonds (and almond milk) are busting with calcium—way more than what's found in dairy milk. Red bell peppers are full of vitamin C—double what an orange has. Unfortunately, the pockets of the almond and bell pepper industries are nowhere near as deep as the pockets of dairy and orange juice industries. Thus, we wind up reaching for the most marketed product, when it has absolutely *no* association with its nutritional makeup, how healthy it is, or how much we even need it. We're just supporting the people with the big pockets.

Think about it: what would we be eating if billboards, commercials, and magazines were full of ads for *real*, whole, organically grown foods. Imagine Olympic athletes promoting asparagus and cashews. Imagine pictures of garlic, kale, broccoli, flax seed, quinoa, carrots, and basil sprawled all over consumer advertisements. Better yet, imagine *coupons* for those foods (I'd become one of those extreme couponers in a heartbeat). That's what we'd *know* because that's what would be in our faces 24/7, and therefore that's what we'd buy. On the other hand, something highly processed and packaged in a box with long hard-to-pronounce-ingredients would seem so insanely bizarre to us.

Unfortunately, most people can't see past the attractive, deceitful slogans and packaging. They also fail to look at the ingredient labels of the foods they buy (some people don't even know ingredient labels exist), and if they did, they'd notice that many of the products they're buying hardly contain any real food. You must stop putting your trust in companies that are trying to make money and have zero regard for your health.

Take the highly trusted company, Subway. Their franchisor name is conveniently "Doctor's Associates, Inc.," yet the two founders of Subway were nuclear physicist and a high school graduate. *Neither* of them were in the health or medical fields, yet both probably knew that if they printed the words "Doctor's Associates" on everything they owned and sold, they were going to be taken more seriously and sell more products.[25] You certainly have game, Subway, I'll give you that.

I can hear some other companies now, "Hey now, that's not fair. We *do* care." Well I'm sorry (not really), but if companies gave a shit, they wouldn't be making destructive, harmful, food-like products, and misleading customers to believe they're something else. They'd sell health-promoting, *real* food. Period. Heck, I'd estimate 90% of the "foods" and "beverages" on the shelves of a conventional supermarket would be *goneski* if it were decided only *real* food should be sold as food.

We consumers have been mind-fucked by the very companies that are supposed to be nourishing us. We have essentially been convinced that pre-made, packaged, processed products that are highly marketed, put on the shelves for us, and perhaps have one or two good components (or misleading words on the packaging) are REAL foods and are SAFE to eat. Wrong, and wrong. In reality, they are void of the actual nutrients we need. What a fucking joke.

How did it even get like this—where it's okay to eat something that literally isn't even food? There are people out there who genuinely don't have a clue what actual real food is because of how far our food system has shot down the shitter. Or, sometimes they do, but don't have a clue what to do with it. Perhaps *you're* one of them. The good news is that if you start to steer away from processed, packaged foods, and learn to eat, use, and cook with whole, untainted foods, you can avoid the marketing and mind-fucking completely. Booyah!

Enter the Food and Drug Administration (FDA)
(Or, in my words, "Fraudulent Dumb Asses")

The worst part about all of this deceitful madness is that all "foods" and "beverages" have to actually be approved before they are put on shelves for consumers. This rant, therefore, not only includes the companies that make the products, but also includes organizations like the FDA, who do the approving. I wonder if they realize they're approving foods that aren't 100% food. I'm sure they're either ignorant, in bed with the food companies, or they're getting some hefty bribes. In other words, the FDA is either dumb, or corrupt. And what's their slogan? "Protecting and Promoting *Your* Health." What's that card game I used to love as a child? Oh right—BULLSHIT.

The way I see it, the FDA assumes all products and chemicals are "innocent until proven guilty." They seem to approve food additives faster than I can say "horseshit," and *then* decide to ban them ten years down the road once they've been vigorously studied and it's realized that they cause something like cancer. Get this: in 2014, the deputy commissioner of the FDA said, "we simply do not have the information to vouch for the safety of many of these chemicals."[26] Great, so quick question then: why are you vouching for the safety of these chemicals?

A food or food additive should *not* be approved until long-term studies on its health effects have been done. Period. If they approve it prior to that, then they are, in essence, treating us as guinea pigs. Shit— perhaps we *are* their long-term study?

Cue the Food Guides

Another baffling concept that we were sucked into was the good ol' Food Pyramid that showed up in the early '90s. You know, that "simple" tool that was promoted for *years* and told us how much food we needed to get from different food groups. Well, here's an interesting fact: There was a press release in 2000 that presented results from two different studies on the food pyramid.[27-29] Both studies demonstrated that the food guide had the *opposite* effect on improving nutrition and fighting disease than intended (i.e. it made people sicker). Big fuckin', "oops" there! The woman who led both studies stated that "the food guide pyramid shape conveys the message that all fats are bad and that all carbohydrates are good, despite evidence to the contrary." She also declared that "the studies suggest instead that the dietary guidelines need to be improved or made more specific."[27] Agreed! Why did it take a friggin' *decade* to figure this out though? During that decade, everybody trusted that the food pyramid was "right" and followed it like their life depended on it. More guinea pigs!

The conclusions of the above two studies could have occurred for a variety of reasons. My guess is that not only were people getting sick because the food group amounts on the pyramid were a bit skewed, but it also didn't provide enough information when it came to *choosing* foods from each food group. For instance, if someone is supposed to have "meat," does that mean pasture-raised chicken, or does that mean a chunk-o-salami deli meat? Even if I choose pasture-raised chicken, do I fry it in a gallon of canola oil, or do I bake it with organic spices? Broccoli and french fries were both considered "the same" when it came to a serving of vegetables for fuck's sake. This food guide pyramid—which everyone was told to follow for good health—was a complete sham and waste of time. You cannot put some pictures on a little friggin' pyramid and suddenly have the public become nutritionally literate. Consumers need nutrition *education*, and lots of it.

Side note: there *is* actually a complex guideline "manual" that comes out every five years (published by The US Department of Health and Human Services and the US Department of Agriculture) entitled "Dietary Guidelines for Americans," but it's boring and confusing (and still inaccurate), and, well, how many times have *you* heard about it?[30]

Without education, everyone interpreted that damn pyramid in their own way. It didn't provide any significant nutrition improvement, and therefore I'm thrilled it has been thrown out the window (took way too long though if you ask me). It evolved several times over the years, but always failed to provide all of the necessary information to the consumer so they knew what foods to choose (if it did, nobody would be wandering around so fucking confused). Instead, the diagrams usually focused on *simplicity* so it would be "easy for the consumer to understand" (like a picture of a plate with distinct types of food filling each quadrant).

Unfortunately, with simplicity comes lack of information. Thus, when you couple all of the millions of new "foods" and "beverages" out there with a simple plate that needs filling, it is having the opposite effect. A billion and one food options exist per food group for people to potentially choose, and most of those options provide shitty nutrients. Thus, everyone winds up finding their own clarity in the guides. For example: "Half of my plate is supposed to be veggies? Great! I'm going to eat a pile of fries every day for the rest of my life! Problem solved!" They think it's easy to follow because they make it work for *their* food preferences. "A" for effort, Food Guide gurus, but the problem hasn't come close to being solved.

You're going to love this next tid bit. In the year 2000, *more than half* of the advisors on the Dietary Guidelines Advisory Committee (who are part of the US Department of Agriculture, and are responsible for coming up with food recommendations) "had financial ties to the meat, dairy, or egg industries that may have made it more likely that unhealthy foods would remain in the government's diet plan."[31] The committee kept this secret while making dietary recommendations for all of America—which of course included copious amounts of meat, dairy, and eggs to directly benefit them, and had little to do with actual health recommendations. This happened to be a violation of federal law. The outcome? They wound up knee-deep in Federal Court. Take that, fuckers.

As Dr. Neal Barnard, President of the Physicians Committee for Responsible Medicine, put it, "Having advisors tied to the meat or dairy industries is as inappropriate as letting tobacco companies decide our standards for air quality." Amen, Neal.

You have to realize that many individuals (and the companies they work for) have ulterior motives and hidden agendas, and it's now up to *you* to do the research on what nutrients you actually need—and which ones simply benefit someone else's pocket. If someone throws a pyramid, plate, or guide in front of your face, research the shit out of it before attempting to follow it.

Screw the Food Guides,
We Have Scientific Research Articles!

Bada-bing, bada-boom! Thank goodness for scientific research articles! These little gems hold the TRUTH! Actually, they don't. They merely provide probable cause and effect reasoning (in other words, if you eat *this*, the effect will most likely be *this*). They never provide "proof." However, as a woman of science, I have read approximately ninety-four million scientific research articles in my time (I also make numbers up), and I can tell you a few things from my experience: First off, unless you have a background in science, don't bother reading scientific research articles. It will be like trying to learn Swahili while playing the ukulele during a shark fight—way too much going on. They are not only filled with science and medical jargon, but are also overflowing with numbers and graphs that will make you want to pull your hair out. Instead, you'll want to find a reputable source (like a well-known periodical or professional) that *paraphrases* the study for you. Then, you'll have to hope like hell they've paraphrased it accurately (and don't have ties to that industry), because unfortunately, there are a heck of a lot of people out there that will distort study outcomes in order to generate fame and followers.

Take this 2015 headline found plastered all over social media: "A glass of red wine is the equivalent to an hour at the gym, says new study!" Right. How many people do you think flocked to that post (yay! "Followers!"), and then flocked to their wine rack— without actually hunting down the real study? "Seven glasses of red wine, and I've run a fucking marathon! Give me my medal of honor!" Not quite. The study *actually* showed that if you drink red wine *while* you exercise, a component of it can act like a performance-enhancing supplement.[32] Well, at least it can in rats. See where I'm going with this? People will say anything to get attention—even if it means distorting facts.

Secondly, the authors of the articles may have conflict of interests with the research being done (i.e. they may work for the company for whom they're providing *amazing* study results—like when the meat and dairy industries made meat and dairy recommendations). You will see this with a company called Monsanto, who I will refer to throughout this guide. Due to intellectual property rights, Monsanto is the *only one* that is allowed to do research on their products. They offer zero transparency, and who knows how they're manipulating their study outcomes if no one else can look at them. If that doesn't shout "fishy business," I don't know what does. To be reputable, products, foods, additives, etc. need to be studied by third parties that *don't* have associations with the industry involved.

Thirdly, many studies—specifically nutrition studies—are not relatable to real life. Meaning, a study may isolate one specific food additive and test it to see if it causes cancer. In reality, "isolation" never occurs in nature. Therefore, while a scientist may determine that a simple food additive is safe on its own and doesn't cause cancer, it is completely unrealistic to translate that conclusion to real life. Millions of reactions between the numerous chemicals in our environment are occurring and interacting together at all times, and unless you can replicate that complicated scenario (if your name isn't MacGyver, don't even try), the isolation studies are kind of bullshit. You could take that "non-cancerous" chemical, cuddle it up to other chemicals in your environment, and POOF, suddenly it *does* cause cancer.[33]

Similarly, many studies make claims that are a bit deceiving. For example, a study may tell you that kids who eat carrots are less likely to get ADD. Hold your horses though—maybe kids who eat carrots simply have healthier lifestyles in general, and kids who *don't* eat carrots (or healthy foods in general) sit in front of the TV for eight hours per day and eat a bunch of junk. Perhaps it's the *lifestyle*, and has little to do with the carrots. Therefore, the next time you hear a claim like, "acai berries can improve weight loss," please pause before you go buy stock in acai berry production. That claim *may* have come from a study that looked at people who consumed acai berries, but those people may have also added a workout routine and eliminated a bunch of shitty foods from their diet. The acai berries may be wonderful, but they're not the sole cause of weight loss. Mind-blowing, over-sensationalized claims about *single* foods, nutrients, or products that "cure your whatever" should always raise a flag. There is no single solution for anything.

Lastly, studies can have holes. This means that the scientist or author forgot to control part of the study, which renders it inaccurate or unreliable. For instance, let's say a study provides the suggestion that alcohol consumption causes third nipples. That could kind of be a cool party trick . . . but wait, how *much* alcohol does it take? I don't know, because the study forgot to control how much alcohol their subjects were consuming. They also forgot to control what their subjects were eating. Perhaps alcohol only causes third nipples if ninety bottles of absinthe are consumed alongside a plate of fireworks. Shit like this happens with studies all the time; studies get published and then pulled because they were found to be flawed.[34]

Not all studies are corrupt, unrealistic, or flawed though. There are plenty of great ones out there. So, just for funsies, let's say a reputable study *does* get published and *does* provide excellent insight into a certain mystery or hypothesis. Guess how long, on average, it takes that information to be circulated into clinical practice? You'll never guess, so let me tell you: seventeen *years*.[35] Seventeen-friggin'-years. There are nearly two million scientific articles published annually, which means a practitioner would have to read approximately 5,500 articles *per day* to keep up.[36] Ha! May as well forget about their patients! By the time our doctors even hear about a fantastic study outcome, it may be too late, or there may be new information that negates *that* information. There is so much information out there, that, quite frankly, professionals can't keep up. Hopefully this guide will take you less than seventeen years to read, and we can kill a bajillion birds with one stone.

At Least We Have Our
Doctors and Professionals . . . Right?

Wrong. On top of all of the "false" food advertising, vague food guides, and corrupt government agencies, we have masses of health professionals (e.g. personal trainers, nutritionists, medical doctors), to whom we seek for health and nutrition advice who are often nutritionally illiterate. Even *nutritionists*.

As someone who has worked in the health field — from medical offices to gyms— I can tell you that there are many quacks out there pulling nutrition advice out of their assholes that I fear for the safety of people approaching them for guidance. They come from different walks of life, they all preach different diet fads and recommendations, and they all have different levels of degrees or certifications. Most of them have little-to-no nutrition training, yet still tell their clients or patients how they should be eating. There is no standard. Or, in the case of the nutritionists, they *do* have substantial nutrition training, but it's often based on food guides or heavily influenced by certain food industries. In reality, most nutritionists simply promote information about the food industries with the most money — because those industries are the ones who paid to have their information in the coursework.

Here's a good example of someone preaching from their ass: Eons ago, I worked for a woman who owned a personal training studio, and much of her time was spent helping people lose weight. I would first like to stipulate that this chick was genuinely a wonderful human being. Unfortunately, nutrition was a foreign language to her (but I give her credit because she never claimed to be an expert). First off, her personal nutrition was horrible. She would regularly leave and go get fast food for lunch, and then bring it back and eat it in front of her clients. Secondly, her famous line—which she would spout to all clients—was that "it was okay for her to eat that way because *she* wasn't overweight, and as soon as they reached *their* goal weight, they could eat whatever they wanted as well!" Holy smokes. Is this really the message that professionals are sending? That *size* solely matters, and *health* doesn't? Yes, yes it is.

It gets worse. Even doctors have minimal nutrition education—you know, the information on the fuel that makes our bodies function. In fact, most of the doctors I've spoken with are absolutely clueless about nutrition. Did they not pay attention in med school? Or did the med schools fail to provide nutrition education? The University of North Carolina has a Nutrition in Medicine Project that did some digging and found that between 2004 and 2009, the number of US medical schools that met the *minimum* requirements for nutrition training decreased from 38% to 27%.[37] For you non-math folks, this means that in 2009, 73% of medical schools were not properly educating their future doctors on nutrition. Say WHAT?! How is that even possible? Don't answer that question—I already know the answer—it starts with "b" and ends with "ajillion dollar pharmaceutical industry."

Basically, when we feel like shit, the people who we seek out to make us feel better, simply don't have extensive knowledge about the best way to make us feel better (head straight to chapter 14 if you want to read more about this issue). Even in Nursing School—which I attended in order to receive my Exercise Physiology degree—there was a completely unbalanced emphasis on *pharmacology* (i.e. prescription medications, also known as "the study of poison" if you're into classic Greek) over *nutrition* for health and healing. We *did* have a nutrition course, but if I remember correctly (keeping in mind my brain was fueled with cafeteria food and $2 vodka at the time), it was simply about memorizing the different nutrients and recommended daily allowances (RDAs). *Not* how each nutrient could fix, cure, or heal certain ailments caused by malnutrition. Yet, when it came to my pharmacology course, learning shifted toward "the right way to determine which drugs would fix which problems within the body." We even learned how to write prescriptions.

In 2013, the journal *Medical Care* published a study that showed that today's primary care physicians spend less time than previous generations of doctors talking to patients about what they eat.[38] Probably because the "food" and "beverage" industries are becoming more and more ass backwards and confusing. Probably because doctors don't know enough to feel comfortable discussing nutrition (of course they don't—the medical schools aren't providing the education). Perhaps it's that they've seen the same advertising we have, and therefore believe it. Or, perhaps it's because they have the same shitty nutrition habits that most people do, and therefore feel they can't preach what they don't practice themselves (I have definitely worked with and met my share of unhealthy doctors over the years). Realistically (most definitely), it's because they have drug reps knocking on their door every five seconds with "miracle pills" that will easily solve the problems their patients face on a daily basis. Talk about easier, and far less time-consuming than discussing nutrition changes! Whew! Now they'll have more time to read their 5,500 scientific articles every day!

It has come to this: The majority of doctors are quick to prescribe medications with a long list of side effects that don't usually *solve* the problem simply because they are unaware or uncertain about *real* nutrients.[39] Unfortunately, these prescription meds merely help manage the symptoms of ailments that could easily be fixed with nutrition changes (with zero side effects). Doctors have become programmed, robotic pill-prescribers. Some of them even refuse to believe that nutrition could have anything to do with healing. In 2011, a California bill mandating only *seven* hours of nutrition training (to be completed within *four* years!) was struck down because opposing doctors felt it would get in their way of working, and they didn't need to be micromanaged by the government.[40, 41] I kind of feel like strangling someone . . . I'm just not sure who to jump at first.

I don't want to sound like a complete a-hole though. Obviously doctors are highly intelligent people. I have friends who are doctors. And, just like it's not your fault you don't know how to eat, it's not their fault they haven't been adequately educated. I urge you to always attempt to discuss nutrition options with them though. If they're honest they'll most likely tell you they don't feel confident enough to give nutrition advice, but may point you in the direction of someone who can. Alternatively, some of them may make shit up, hoping you'll be submissive and won't question their "intelligence" (I have a few personal examples of this, which you will hear about later on). Then again, there are plenty of doctors out there who are starting to educate themselves, so you may land on a good one. They're discovering how to cure their malnourished patients with *food*, and are starting to take a stand. You just need to find one of them before you start reaching out to a doctor who doesn't have nutrition knowledge, will scoff at the "nutrition can heal" concept, and will shove a toxic pill down your throat to keep the pharmaceutical industry alive.

Don't Do Drugs, Kids!
Wait . . . Definitely Do Drugs!
And Other Ridiculous Treatments, Too!

Speaking of the pharmaceutical industry, I want to strangle a drug rep every time I see an advertisement for some "miracle" pill. As mentioned previously, the word "pharmaceutical" comes from the classic Greek word "pharmakeia," which means "the art of poisoning." To back that awesome definition up, here's a little fact for you: in 1998, the *Journal of the American Medical Association* reported that pharmaceutical drug reactions were somewhere between the *fourth* and *sixth* leading cause of death in America.[42] That's right: prescription meds are killing a shitload of people, and are ranked right up there between cancer and diabetes. By the way, that ranking only included deaths in *hospitals* under *monitored conditions* and with prescription drugs that were *properly prescribed and administered* (i.e. only included drugs that were used in hospitals as intended). This statistic didn't take into account deaths *outside* of hospitals or deaths from *misusing* medications. If we add in the millions of more reactions and deaths that *weren't* accounted for (accidental overdoses, improper administering, kids getting a hold of their parent's pills, etc.), I'd be willing to bet a kidney that pharmaceuticals are the *leading* cause of death in America. Talk about your all-time backfire.

To put it briefly, it was well known back in the '90s that pharmaceutical, "poison" drugs were killing us. A lot of us. But I guess that's all kosher and shit because the pharmaceutical companies cover their asses by listing "death" as a side effect in their disclaimer. "We put it on the package, so not our problem if someone keels over!" I'm sorry, but "death" should not be considered a side effect. It should be considered murder. Pills sure do make a lot of money though. So, forge on pharmaceutical companies! FORGE THE FUCK ON!

Let's examine one of the most prescribed pills out there: Simvastatin Oral (otherwise known as "Zocor").[43] This magical pill was manufactured to help lower bad cholesterol and help raise good cholesterol—something that is definitely "required" based on the current status of public health. The only issue is that a proper diet *automatically* does this. I have had clients bring their cholesterol levels back to normal within *weeks* of changing their diet, and with no side effects whatsoever (unless "feeling like a kickass superhero" is a side effect).

Unfortunately, Merck (the manufacturer of Zocor), saw an opening for profit, and stole the show. They produced this wonderdrug that allowed people to lower their cholesterol without having to change a thing about their diet. Pass the gravy, that's AMAZING! Hold up though—let's look at the side effects of Zocor, listed on the Mayo Clinic's website.[44] I would have used the information directly from Merck, but they have a *twenty-two* page document that explains how to take Zocor, and the dangers associated with it.[45] Red flag much?

Simvastatin (Zocor) Side Effects

Check with your doctor immediately if any of the following side effects occur:

More Common

1. Dizziness
2. fainting
3. fast or irregular heartbeat

Less Common

1. Bladder pain
2. bloody or cloudy urine
3. blurred vision
4. body aches or pain
5. chills
6. cough
7. dark-colored urine
8. difficult, burning, or painful urination
9. difficulty with breathing
10. difficulty with moving
11. dry mouth
12. ear congestion
13. fever
14. flushed, dry skin
15. frequent urge to urinate
16. fruit-like breath odor
17. headache
18. increased hunger
19. increased thirst
20. increased urination
21. joint pain
22. loss of consciousness
23. lower back or side pain
24. muscle cramps, spasms, or stiffness
25. muscular pain, tenderness, wasting, or weakness
26. nasal congestion
27. nausea
28. runny nose
29. sneezing
30. sore throat
31. stomachache
32. sweating
33. swelling
34. swollen joints
35. troubled breathing
36. unexplained weight loss
37. unusual tiredness or weakness
38. vomiting

Incidence Not Known

1. Blistering, peeling, or loosening of the skin
2. bloating
3. burning, crawling, itching, numbness, prickling, "pins and needles," or tingling feelings
4. constipation
5. diarrhea
6. difficulty with swallowing
7. general tiredness and weakness
8. indigestion
9. large, hive-like swelling on the face, eyelids, lips, tongue, throat, hands, legs, feet, or sex organs
10. light-colored stools
11. loss of appetite

12. pains in the stomach, side, or abdomen, possibly radiating to the back
13. pale skin
14. puffiness or swelling of the eyelids or around the eyes, face, lips, or tongue
15. red skin lesions, often with a purple center
16. red, irritated eyes
17. skin rash, hives, or itching
18. sores, ulcers, or white spots in the mouth or on the lips
19. tightness in the chest
20. troubled breathing with exertion
21. unusual bleeding or bruising
22. upper right abdominal or stomach pain
23. weakness in the arms, hands, legs, or feet
24. yellow eyes or skin

Some side effects may occur that usually do not need medical attention. These side effects may go away during treatment as your body adjusts to the medicine. Also, your health care professional may be able to tell you about ways to prevent or reduce some of these side effects. Check with your health care professional if any of the following side effects continue or are bothersome or if you have any questions about them:

Less Common

1. Acid or sour stomach
2. belching
3. burning feeling in the chest or stomach
4. dizziness or lightheadedness
5. excess air or gas in the stomach or intestines
6. feeling of constant movement of self or surroundings
7. full feeling
8. heartburn
9. lack or loss of strength
10. pain or tenderness around the eyes and cheekbones
11. passing gas
12. sensation of spinning
13. skin rash, encrusted, scaly, and oozing
14. stomach discomfort, upset, or pain
15. tenderness in the stomach area
16. trouble sleeping

Incidence Not Known

1. Being forgetful
2. depression
3. discoloration of the skin
4. hair loss or thinning of hair
5. inability to have or keep an erection
6. loss in sexual ability, desire, drive, or performance

Other side effects not listed may also occur in some patients. If you notice any other effects, check with your healthcare professional.

TOO MANY WORDS. Let me take the liberty of summarizing for you: ingest Zocor and be prepared to reenact Major Toht's death scene in *Raiders of the Lost Ark*. Google that shit if you don't know what I'm talking about.

After seeing how that crap can affect you, if you *still* consider pharmaceuticals to be the answer for solving ailments like high cholesterol, please close this guidebook and violently hit yourself over the head with it. That list is *insane*. Think about all of the people who are on *multiple* prescriptions at once (because they obviously have to manage the side effects of the *original* pill they took). Multiple pills means exponentially *more* side effects due to their interactions with each other. I can't even begin to imagine how shitty those people must feel (whether they know it or not). The worst part? Their cholesterol problems aren't even cured; they're merely being managed by a synthetic chemical coursing through their veins.

Their cholesterol problems could be 100% cured, quickly and painlessly, if their health professional knew to discuss nutrition with them. Real nutrients (from real food!) can be incredibly powerful when it comes to ailment-fighting and prevention (on any level), thus this healing extends far past cholesterol issues. So, why on *Earth* are we not reaching to them for healing? Because there's no profit in having patients eat properly, and you certainly don't get return customers, that's why. Instead, we keep the pharmaceutical business alive by repeatedly reaching for chemical pills to manage our shitty habits.

Pharmaceuticals are *not* our body's preferred method of healing, and more often fix one problem and then create ten more (or three hundred more, if you're taking Zocor). Or, maybe you *think* they're doing a fantastic job managing your disease, when in reality, the problems they're creating show up decades later. One example is group of drugs, called "anticholinergics," that when taken chronically increase your risk of developing dementia and Alzheimer's.[46] They can be used to treat anything from asthma, to incontinence, to depression, to sleep disorders. Congrats! We "fixed" your asthma! What's great is that you won't remember you ever had it once the Alzheimer's sets in!

So hold up—don't you feel that *pharmaceuticals* should be considered the "alternative method?!" For shit's sake—anyone who knowingly wants to chronically chomp down some Zocor (or any other drug), with its long list of side effects and possible adverse drug reactions (which sometimes include murder . . . I mean "death"), over simply eating healthy *after* knowing the facts, is extreme and alternative if you ask me. Fucking hell, you're basically playing Russian roulette and asking to be in pain.

Somehow though, everything has gotten flipped around, and we now **consider** healing through nutrition to be "alternative," when that is, in actuality, the way our bodies are meant to heal. Yet, pills are so *easy*, and *easy* is what everyone wants. No one wants to improve their nutrition then wait for their body to heal itself. "Psshhh. I ain't got time for that!"

Another great example is the fact that lifestyle and nutrition changes can *cure* heart disease—the number one cause of death in the world.[47] Making lifestyle and nutrition changes could easily eliminate 30% of world-wide deaths. Thirty-friggin'-percent. Yet, instead of attempting to prevent or *cure* the disease (even though the World Health Organization clearly states that "heart disease and stroke can be prevented through healthy diet, regular physical activity and avoiding tobacco smoke"[48]), people run to their doctors in a frenzy (or get carted there on a gurney). They start popping dozens of daily pills and putting metal expanders in their heart vessels. They often have their chests ripped open. Sometimes they have healthy blood vessels removed from various parts of their body that are then sewn onto their hearts in order to assist the clogged arteries that have failed. Who the heck doesn't find all of *that* radical and extreme?! Just eat a fucking carrot!

By the way, none of the above mentioned conventional heart disease "treatments" actually fix the problem *or* prolong the patients' lives. They purely make them feel temporarily amazing by allowing blood to be momentarily pumped through their body.

They don't heal, and will most likely have similar treatments for the rest of their lives. To support that statement, you might be interested to know that patients who control their blood pressure with pharmaceuticals have a *higher* risk of death from heart attack and stroke than people who naturally have low blood pressure from a kickass diet.[49]

Speaking of these ridiculous, invasive treatments, Dr. Nortin M. Hadler (professor of medicine at the University of North Carolina at Chapel Hill) stated back in 2005 that bypass surgery "should have been relegated to the archives 15 years ago."[50] Fifteen years prior to that would have been 1990. Ummm . . . yeah. Keep rakin' in that dough, heart-surgery industry (they pull in $100 billion per annum).[50] Chaaa-ching.

It all seems a bit backwards and wacky when you think about it, doesn't it? Dr. Dean Ornish, who runs a program for reversing heart disease (with Former President Bill Clinton being one of his steadfast followers) stated, "I don't understand why asking people to eat a well balanced vegetarian diet is considered drastic, while it is medically conservative to cut people open and put them on cholesterol lowering drugs for the rest of their lives." Great point, Dean. I don't suppose anyone really thinks about it, as that has become the norm.

What a great money-making scheme. Convince millions upon millions in the world who are diseased or fighting ailments, that a little, easy-to-take pill will make their *symptoms* go away . . . but fail to mention that they don't actually fix the problem. That way, these people need to continue to take those drugs for eternity. And maybe some other drugs to manage the side effects. How many times have *you* been convinced by a health professional that a pill is the solution?

Take a step back for a second, and really think about this. Imagine all of the lives that would be saved if people shifted away from prescription pills (bye bye adverse drug reactions—one of the leading causes of death), and toward lifestyle changes (bye bye heart disease, diabetes, stroke, certain cancers, a million other ailments—all of which are leading causes of death in developed nations). Perhaps this is someone's sick way of keeping the world population under control. Well played, whomever-you-are, well played.

Thankfully, there are already instances upon instances of people forgoing pharmaceuticals and other insane procedures, and curing their malnutrition issues simply by implementing lifestyle and nutrition changes. Why don't we hear about them? Those cases are considered "alternative," that's why. Also because you often can't do a scientific, controlled, double-blind research study on different changes to different lifestyle habits. It *is* easy, however, to produce scientific, controlled studies on who takes what specific pill and gets what specific result, and *those* studies are the ones that are funded, peer-reviewed, published, distributed, and advertised to the world as mainstream healing.

Side note: Pharmaceuticals *can* help in some instances (I don't want to sound like a complete fuckwad here and say that drugs are complete crap). However, I would argue that those instances are mainly *acute* instances (e.g. trauma care—like pain management for a bone sticking sideways out of your leg). However, when we're talking about *chronic illness*, they are usually far more damaging, involve many unnecessary side effects, and bring more long-term health issues than benefits. Pharmaceuticals create more customers than cures. Fact.

* * *

What a clusterfuck. With this whole confusion nightmare going on, we have veered far from healthy eating and are making it more and more difficult for ourselves with every passing day. Everyone—including the FDA and food & beverage companies (yeah, that's right bitches, listen up!)—needs to cut the bullshit. We need to start focusing on *health* before we waste billions more on non-effective treatments for preventable diseases like heart disease, certain cancers, and diabetes—and eventually kill ourselves off. Hey, I have an idea! Let's put those billions of dollars towards nutrition awareness (and I'm not just talking about a fucking picture of a multi-colored food plate)! You know, let's spend some quality time educating people in order to steer them away from malnourishment.

Side note: from here on out, every time I refer to someone as "uneducated," please understand that I'm not calling them a moron. I literally mean they haven't been taught something. Don't take it personally. There's a lot about the world that I don't know. I am uneducated about tree frogs and seventeenth century art, just like a lot of people are uneducated about nutrients and food. We are all uneducated about *something*, but thankfully have the ability to learn.

Unfortunately, instead of being educated on proper nutrition, the food industry has evolved into what it is now, where we've been *turned away* from education and sucked into their advertising, their skewed diet recommendations, and their easy-to-eat products. We also take their word that this crap is safe. Well, fool me once, shame on you. Fool me twice, shame on me. With the knowledge I now have, I will certainly *not* be fooled again. And, now that *you* know, you can decide whether or not to be shamed as well.

It's insanely frustrating because we *know* we have the ability to heal ourselves. I mean, we don't go screaming to the doctor every time we get a paper cut or bruised shin, right? We *know* our bodies are capable of fixing those types of injuries. That is a prime example of nutrients healing our bodies as intended. Most of us will have no problem taking care of a little cut or bruise, because those ailments don't require much fuel, and our bodies can scrounge it up easily. Some people may take longer to heal, or may wind up with secondary infections, but that's because their immune systems aren't optimally fueled.

Well guess what? If you can sort your nutrition out, this works on a much larger scale as well. The body is perfectly capable of preventing or healing itself from more serious ailments if it has the proper fuels to do so. I'm not talking the splintered bone sticking sideways out of your leg—that shit would take some serious Jedi mind tricks. I'm talking about chronic *illness* like diabetes, certain cancers, heart disease, and autoimmune disease. Most of them can be 100% *cured* by eradicating malnutrition. Thus, I would argue that, on a grand scale, we don't even have chronic disease problems, we have *malnutrition* problems.

To sum everything up, I'm irritated that shitty "foods" and "beverages" exist and are approved by administrations we should be able to trust, when they clearly have horrible, destructive reactions within our bodies. Hundreds of studies show how dangerous and harmful some food additives are (just wait for chapter 21). I'm irritated at money-hungry weight-loss programs that solely focus on getting people smaller, and not giving a shit about the state of their insides. I'm irritated that doctors are rarely educated on nutrition—the *main* way our bodies prefer to heal. I'm irritated that someone believes millions of people will suddenly know how to eat simply by staring at a fucking plate or pyramid. I'm irritated that the right kind of nutrition education isn't out there for the general public so everyone can at least make educated choices on what they put in their pie-holes. I'm irritated that people reach for pills before anything else—and consider that normal! I'm irritated that we've essentially created this world of "ease," without any concern for health (i.e. it's easier to pop a pill than to change your lifestyle, and it's easier to drive through a fast food joint than to cook your own meal). I'm about as irritated as one can get. Watch out world—you know how women can get when we get irritated (insert potty-mouth nutrition book here).

If we put all of our focus on nutrition awareness to improve the current health crisis, we could turn this depressing situation around. Nah, that would bankrupt too many food and beverage companies, health professionals, and pharmaceutical companies. And THAT certainly can't happen. Wait . . . can it? Answer: of course it can. We just need to get the majority of consumers on the same page.

Moral of the Story:
Our food and healthcare systems are completely fucked up
and have left people more confused than a fart in a fan factory.
It's not your fault you don't know how to eat, but it *is* your
responsibility to figure it out.

Chapter 7

Malnutrition Costs What?!

If everyone were to adopt a whole-food, plant-based diet,
I really believe we could cut health care costs by 70 to 80 percent.
—T. Colin Campbell, PhD

With all of the confusion that surrounds food and nutrition in today's world, what I said in the intro is true: most people haven't got a fucking clue how to eat. They follow misleading advertisements or nutrition instructions from people who aren't fully educated on nutrition, and unfortunately wind up sick. The problem is now escalating to the point of madness. As an example, the US spends more on healthcare than any other country—*two and a half times* more than the average spending. This amounts to nearly *$4 trillion* annually.[51, 52] With the US spending that much on healthcare, everyone should be a friggin' poster child for health. Instead we're the opposite. We have become world leaders in chronic disease and death.

In 2000, the World Health Organization reported that the US ranked number one in per capita health spending. Unfortunately, it also confirmed that somehow—even with all of that money being pumped into healthcare—the US ranked *seventy-second* on *level* of health (i.e. the state of health in America does not line up with the money spent on it).[53, 54] Many developed countries had similar results—we're all blowin' cash faster than a casino junkie.

Yes, that report was from over a decade ago, but trust me, not much has improved. The US is still one of the **most** obese and unhealthy countries in the world, and advancement is lagging behind most other developed nations (i.e. life expectancy is increasing, but not at the rate of other developed nations)[51]. The fact that we expect to magically get healthy without changing course and trying something new, is embarrassing and quite frankly makes us look real fucking stupid.

Something has gone terribly wrong, and it's about time people start owning up to it. It's *us*, it's what *we've* done to our food system, and it's what *we're* putting in our pie-holes. There aren't freaking disease fairies flying around random parts of the world sprinkling cancer and diabetes dust on us. What *we're* consuming (or not consuming) is causing malnourishment. This is why I laugh when people use the argument that a product or food is "okay" because they've been "consuming it for decades." Um, correct me if I'm wrong Sherlock, but if we're sicker than we were decades ago, shouldn't we look at the very foods we've been consuming the *most* as the probable culprit?

An indirect correlation exists between the decline of our food industry, and the rise of disease (meaning, as our food industry started to drown in shitty food products, disease skyrocketed). Completely shocking, I know. I *totally* would have thought we could eat chemically-laden, genetically modified, highly-processed, nutritionally-void foods for decades without any consequence. I also totally would have thought we could then "fix" our ailing bodies with diets, pills, and bypass surgeries! That *has* to work, right?? As Chef Gordon Ramsay would say, "Fuuuuuuuuccccckkk me."

So yeah, over the past few decades, as all of the shit and confusion exploded into our food system, diseases have crept up on us. Actually, some of them aren't creeping. Some of them are forging full-steam ahead, faster than McDonald's can deliver a Big Mac at their drive-thru window. Rather than get to the root of the problem, the "healthcare" industry—sorry, I need to pause for a second, but what a paradox! Not only does the "healthcare" industry clearly not represent *health*, but they sure as shit don't seem to *care*! Anyway, back to my point. The "healthcare" industry decided to treat the *symptoms* of diseases. In other words, they wait for people to get sick and *then* try to help them rather than trying to prevent diseases from taking hold in the first place. I'll let you guess which one profits more. In reality, we don't need new miracle treatments or cures; we need to STOP THE FUCKING DISEASES FROM SHOWING UP IN THE FIRST PLACE (sorry—I tend to shout when I get frustrated).

If you think about it, these chronic diseases are only *symptoms* of malnutrition. They're showing up because people are fucking up their pie-hole usage. If you simply try to cure the diseases, yet continue to live in a malnourished state, that disease will keep coming back to bite you in the ass. It is imperative that we stop focusing on the symptoms. Cure the malnutrition and don't allow your body to be a feeding ground for disease.

Need some facts and figures to back all of this up? Have no fear, the stats are here! I have chosen some (horrific) information for you to mull over that relates to disease and our food system. Try not to shit your pants while reading these (but if you do, save that skid mark for chapter 26, when we talk about what your poop should look like).

Autism Spectrum Disorder (ASD)

ASD describes the range of conditions that effect communication, social skills, and behavior (including autism and Asperger's syndrome). Back in the 1980s autism was estimated to effect 1 in 10,000. In the 1990s it became 1 in 2,500. A decade later that number became 1 in 88. Then, in 2010, 1 in 68 (I wish I were making this up).[55-57] Those numbers are staggering. Do we really believe our genes change this rapidly, and people are suddenly exploding with autism? (The answer is "no," by the way.) Alternatively, do we suppose something we're *exposing* ourselves to could be the cause?

In 2012, a list of the top ten chemicals that were suspect in causing developmental neurotoxicity (in other words, "a fucked up nervous system")—which includes ASD—was released. Guess what?! Many of the chemicals can be found in or on the foods we eat![58] Yum! And guess what happens if a pregnant mother unknowingly ingests a nice dose of these chemicals as the child inside of her is trying to develop? Developmental neurotoxicity, that's what! You're going to want to sit down for this next statistic: mothers who live near certain pesticide-sprayed-crops are 60% more likely to have a child with ASD. SIXTY PERCENT!! From the fucking chemicals being sprayed on our food! That's no joke. How close are *you* to a chemical-happy food farm?

If ASD continues to rise at this alarming rate, the US (and other developed nations) will eventually be run by people with developmental disabilities. I'm not suggesting people with developmental disabilities are incapable of running a country, I'm simply saying **it's** fucking awful that they're being disabled by our food system. Don't worry though, there's a whole chapter dedicated to saving our children later on. First, let's throw out a statistic: in 2011 alone, it was estimated that the US spent over $9 billion on care of children with ASD. [57, 59]

Food Allergies

Food allergies are a funny thing. Not "funny ha-ha," but funny because people assume they happen "just because," and there's nothing they can do to prevent them or get rid of them. *Au contraire*. In 2013, the Centers for Disease Control and Prevention (CDC) released a report on a survey that suggested 1 in 20 kids in America had food allergies.[60, 61] That would be a 50% increase from the late '90s. That's purely *food* allergies. Since I believe certain skin allergies (e.g. eczema) are also caused by food, I'll mention that the survey also stated that 1 in 8 kids had a skin allergy, which would have been a 69% increase since the late '90s. I have no problem saying, in my opinion (and yes, it's my opinion), these sharp increases have everything to do with the shit we've added to our food in the past several decades. It only makes sense. You put toxic shit in your body, your body reacts.

For example, in 2014, a study was published that queried why a ten-year-old girl was having a reaction to a blueberry pie (that didn't have any ingredients in it that she should have been allergic to). It turns out that blueberry pie still had some antibiotics hanging out in it that were causing the reaction (they had been used as a pesticide on the blueberries).[62] Whoops. It's getting hard to escape this shit.

Since we're keeping tabs, you may be interested in knowing that the cost of children's food allergies in the US was estimated at nearly $25 billion per year.[60, 63]

Heart Disease

From the previous chapter we already know heart disease is the number one killer in the world, *and* that it is completely preventable by adapting a "healthy lifestyle." However, since numerous people have no idea how to define a healthy lifestyle, the number of people suffering and dying from the disease continues to plague us. In 2010, about 45% of men and 31% of woman aged fifty-five and over reported being told they had heart disease (that doesn't mean you folks under age fifty-five are safe!). This doesn't include congenital heart *defects*, this only includes preventable heart *disease* that comes from shitty lifestyle choices. As of 2011, heart disease was costing the US a whopping $108.9 billion annually.[64, 65]

Obesity

In the early 1960s, over 50% of the population was actually considered to be at a healthy weight (rock on!), with only 13% considered obese. Between 2007 and 2010 the number of healthy Americans was nearly cut in half, while obese (not simply overweight, but *obese*) Americans skyrocketed to over 35%.[64] There are now more obese Americans than healthy weight Americans. Embarrassing. Obesity goes hand in hand with many diseases, so I'm going to leave it at that and call it the "gateway" ailment to disease. If obesity rises, so do diseases like cancer, heart disease, and diabetes. In 2008 alone, overweight and obese Americans cost the US an extra $147 billion.[66]

Diabetes (Type I and Type II)

In 2010, over twenty-five million people in America were diabetics. TWENTY-FIVE-FRIGGIN'-MILLION. Not including those twenty-five million, an estimated additional *seventy-nine* million were considered pre-diabetic (i.e. on the road to becoming a diabetic). While many people live "comfortably" with diabetes for their entire life, diabetes often leads to complications like kidney failure, heart disease, blindness, stroke, amputations and death (diabetics are twice as likely to die early than non-diabetics). Sounds like a carnival ride—put me on it! Contrary to popular belief, diabetes can be reversed and even cured via improvements in nutrition (definitely Type II, Type I looks promising).[67-72] Lastly (drum roll please), in 2007 it was estimated that diabetes was costing the US around $174 billion per year.[73]

Let's add all of this terrifying information up. Each year the US spends roughly:

- $9 billion on autism spectrum disorder treatments;
- $25 billion on food allergies treatments;
- $109 billion on heart disease treatments;
- $147 billion on obesity treatments; and
- $174 billion on diabetes treatments.

That's a grand total of $464 billion—almost a half a trillion dollars—spent annually on diseases that, in my opinion, are mostly preventable by making improvements in nutrition. I guess that's money well spent if you're only concerned with treating people's *symptoms* (and making money off those treatments), rather than reversing or preventing disease.

Remember that this is merely a *handful* of diseases I chose to discuss. There are plenty more that could be added to this list. As mentioned at the beginning of this chapter, the US spends nearly $4 trillion on healthcare every year. If you read the quote that kicks off this chapter—stated by a renowned nutrition expert with decades of nutrition research under his belt— you'll see that we could possibly save upwards of *$3 trillion annually* if we updated our eating habits. Hey America, want to get out of debt and get healthy?! STOP FUCKING WITH THE FOOD SYSTEM AND TEACH PEOPLE HOW TO USE THEIR MOTHERFUCKING PIE-HOLES. The more I shout, the more people will hear me, right? Here's hoping.

If you think I forgot about cancer, I didn't. There's a whole chapter dedicated to that asshole later on. In a nut-shell, our food system has gone down the shitter, and is bringing us with it. If we don't do something about this disease nonsense, it will win. And by "win," I mean eradicate the human population.

Moral of the Story:
We're spending a buttload of money intervening and treating diseases, rather than focusing on preventing them from ever happening in the first place. That makes sense how?

SECTION II

The *Amount* of Crap People Cram in Their Pie-Holes

Chapter 8

The Nutrition Triad

Enough of the depressing, "we're all dying," "someone-completely-fucked-up-the-system" shit. Let's get on to the fun "fix-my-pie-hole" stuff!

Even though all of the previous information may have seemed quite disheartening, it should have demonstrated how ass-backwards many food and beverage companies and organizations are, and how uneducated the general public is (which unfortunately includes most of our health professionals). We're killing ourselves simply because we've lost touch with what's acceptable to put in our mouths.

The good news is that *you* have control over what goes in your mouth. *You* control what foods and beverages you buy, and *you* control how you prepare and cook them. So really, once you do some good ol' "edumacating," you should be golden! Now, translate this to a larger scale: *we* as consumers could have full control over our food system based on which foods we buy (or refuse to buy) or grow in our own gardens. There are a buttload more of *us* than there are of "them" (you know, the food and beverage companies hell bent on profiting at our expense). *We* have the upper hand. How exciting! Let's all hold hands, sing Kumbaya, and get this shit done!

Enter the Nutrition Triad. What's the Nutrition Triad, you ask? GREAT question! It's my badass approach to nutrition. It's a three-sided concept that, when followed, ensures you avoid malnutrition. It represents what it takes to be a spandex-loving superhero at the *top* of the nutrition spectrum. Unfortunately, most people only focus on one, *possibly* two, parts of the triad, and are thus on a train bound for the bottom half of the spectrum.

In order to use your pie-hole properly, you need to look at how *everything* interacts together; I mean *everything.* Have you seen the size of this guide? What the fuck did you think was filling the rest of the pages?! The three principal focuses however—the three parts of the triad—should be the 1) *amount*, 2) *type*, and 3) *variety* of nutrients you consume. That train, my friends, will whisk you away to a world where disease doesn't exist, energy is abundant, and unicorns frolic in your fairy garden. Hell yes!

Let's break this triad concept down further. The *amount* of fuel your body requires is measured by the calories you consume. The *type* of fuels you consume are based on the foods or beverages you choose. Lastly, *variety* is also extremely important in order to get an adequate range of nutrients. The following diagram will help with this concept. If you only focus on one of the factors, you may find yourself heading straight to the pits. Focusing on *two* of those factors will certainly help you climb a bit higher on the nutrition spectrum, but chances are you'll still be malnourished. However, if you can center yourself between all *three* factors, so your body receives the correct amount, type, and variety of nutrients, every process in your body will run as intended. This includes your immune system, which will turn into Chuck Norris and put a big ass sleeper hold on anything that comes near it! KER-POW!

The Nutrition Triad

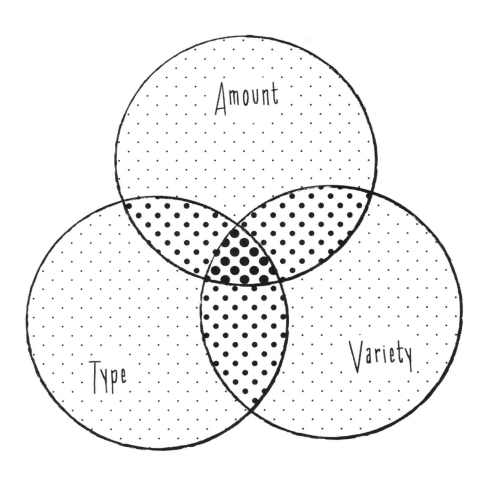

- **Amount**
- **Type**
- **Variety**

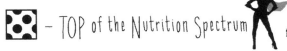

- ▨ – TOP of the Nutrition Spectrum
- ▨ – MIDDLE of the Nutrition Spectrum
- ▨ – BOTTOM of the Nutrition Spectrum

To recap: Nutrients are our fuel, and are used to adequately supply every simple or complex process in your body. Everything we do requires fuel. What you choose to shove down your pie-hole, matters. If something is lacking in your diet, whether it's not enough food in general, or not the right type or variety of food, you become malnourished and shit begins to shut down. When your body begins to shut down, you become a miserable, sick bastard—men usually more than woman. C'mon, you know that's the truth.

The transition to optimal pie-hole usage won't happen overnight. It will take some time to adjust to real food, learn how to grocery shop, discover new recipes you love, and most importantly discover your magical formula of amount, type, and variety of nutrients. However, it is 100% doable, and 100% worth it. The journey begins: we will begin to dig deeper into the three triad factors within the next few sections of this book, and will begin to start piecing together *your* magical nutrition equation. Hot dayum, let's do this!

Moral of the Story:
Nutrition is fucking COM-PLEX. But, you can't let that deter you. The Nutrition Triad concept—which will help factor in the amount, type, and variety of what you're shoving down your pie-hole—will let you discover how to adequately fuel yourself *and* fit into your Captain America suit.

Chapter 9

Amount:
How Much *Should* You Eat?

This is the component of the Nutrition Triad that most people focus on when they diet or attempt to get healthy: how much to eat (or not eat). "Keep those calories down, and you'll shed five pant sizes in just two days!" *Oy vey*. While being aware of calories *does* have some importance, it's worthless on its own, and is far less important than the other two nutrient factors (when it comes to *health* anyway). However, it's the easiest component to tackle, so we're starting here.

Every person on this planet requires a different amount of fuel. Why? Um, because I'm not you, and you're not me. Everyone is running and regulating millions of *different* processes every day, at *different* rates, and for *different* durations than the next person. Even if two people did the exact same thing for a day, they would still require *different* amounts of fuel, because their bodies are *different* and therefore they use energy *differently*. Letting someone put you on a generic calorie-restricted diet because it worked for them, or because they sell weight-loss programs is a wasted effort. Let's get this straight: WE ARE FUCKING DIFFERENT. Therefore, we all need a *different* amount of fuel. Get it? DIFFERENT.

To be clear: this chapter is not how much you *want* to eat, but how much you *should* eat. If you can't differentiate between the two, you obviously slept through chapter 5. The goal is to eat for *health*, not for *hobby*. There are several ways to estimate how much fuel you need for optimal health, but ultimately it is always going to be precisely that—an estimation. It is impossible to know *exactly* how much fuel your body requires, especially when that number is constantly changing (because you never do the same exact thing every day). Keep that notion in mind when you get to the end of this chapter—you may need to eat a little more or a little less fuel than you estimated (due to several factors like your activity level, air temperature, you get pregnant, etc.), and no cookie-cutter formula can tell you that.

This is why certain weight loss programs that offer, for example, two different "programs" (e.g. a 1,200 calorie program and a 1,500 calorie program) to millions of people have an array of results. It's absolutely fucking idiotic to try to funnel millions of people into just two caloric diets when everyone requires different amounts of fuel. However, when those companies start showcasing the select few people for whom it *did* work (who *hasn't* seen a Jenny Craig or Weight Watchers commercial?!), everyone starts panting and drooling and believes it will work for them as well. And still—for those few people who do shed some weight—they've still only focused on *one* of the Nutrition Triad factors ("amount"), and have not given two shits about the others ("type" and "variety"). This means there's a good chance they're still in jeopardy of health issues, regardless of what the scale says.

Thus, it's important for everyone to try to hone in on their own *individual* calorie requirement to avoid disease. Most people overshoot their calorie requirement, but what happens if we *under*-consume? As stated previously, fuel is required to run and regulate all of our bodies' necessary tasks. If our bodies try to complete all of their daily tasks and run out of fuel before doing so, what the fuck do you think is going to happen? You are not an energy wizard who can whip up extra energy with your sorcery-stick. You're *human* (on your way to becoming *super*-human), and your body will begin to slow down, or even worse, break down. Eventually you will become diseased.

Need a clearer picture? Let's pretend you need to drive to Miami for the weekend and your car runs out of gas with fifty miles to go. Unless you want to push that pile of metal, it ain't moving until it gets more fuel. Or, taking it further, let's say you ditch the car and hitchhike to Miami, leaving the car sitting there, unattended, without fuel, while you funnel beer down your throat for a year. It's going to require *a lot more* than just fuel to get that bad boy going (new oil, new battery, who knows what else—I'm not a fucking mechanic).

Similarly, if *your* body doesn't get enough fuel, it will begin to shut down like a car would. It will sit there in protest and declare: "either you roll me like a sack of potatoes, or fuel me up bee-ach!" Let's just hope you fuel it up before *you* need a new battery.

I have had obese clients come to me confused beyond belief as to why they're not losing weight on their 1,200 calorie diet. It's because they're not eating enough! Their bodies have completely shut down and are no longer capable of functioning as intended. Can you see why starving yourself is as much of a dumb fucking idea as over-eating? It's important to get as close as you can to your specific caloric "sweet spot," so you don't run out of fuel or have too much fuel left over. This is important because—drum roll please—a shift in either direction can lead to disease.

How on earth does one ascertain how much to eat? Initially this may seem challenging and will most likely make you want to incinerate every calculator in existence. However, once you learn how to listen to your body and understand what it feels like to have too much or too little fuel, finding your caloric sweet spot will actually become second nature and quite obvious (and you can feed your calculator to the folks down at your local weight-loss center who will forever be counting calories).

"Calories!? Eeeek! I've heard of those horrible motherfuckers—keep them at bay!" Stop. Calories are simply the amount of energy provided by the food we eat. Calories are not bad; they're actually required. They're *energy*.

There are several complicated and confusing equations that will help you determine a ballpark daily calorie amount, but when it comes down to it (like I mentioned earlier) you're never going to get an exact number. In addition, remember that no one else's number should be the same as yours. The energy *your* body needs is entirely based on how much energy *you* use each day—which may also vary daily. Why the hell are we doing this then? Because some people have no clue about calories, and whether or not they're supposed to consume two calories or two million calories. I used to be one of them—I didn't give a shit about calories, and ignored them completely. For you geniuses who believe you already know how much you're supposed to consume, well now you can see just how smart you are! Game on!

Let me start by saying that these estimates don't consider "special populations." Meaning, this won't be as accurate for children who are growing, woman who are pregnant, women who are nursing, body builders, or that guy who sang Gangnam Style. This is for the average Jane or Joe. Therefore, if you are growing, nursing a baby, packing on the muscle, or running around like you're riding a horse, you will have to eat slightly more or less depending on your specific situation. However, regardless of your circumstances, you must remember that these numbers aren't the end-all, be-all anyway. They are a *guideline* to determine if you're eating anywhere close to what you should.

The equations that follow can be used to give you that starting guesstimate, and I've given examples using my personal information to show you how this works. Grab a calculator and get ready to bust out your fifth grade math skills (groan). I'm going to make this as easy as possible for you, so even if you have the math skills of a potato, you should be able to work this shit out. Use a pen, pencil, crayon, eyeliner, whatever to write your information on these pages as we go along. Ready to math-ersize? Buckle up—this is the point of no return.

Step 1

Your weight needs to be converted to kilograms (kgs). Most everyone on the planet has figured out that the metric system is the shiznit and has already uses kgs. Unfortunately, if you're from Myanmar, Liberia, or America, you most likely haven't. Use equation 9.1 to help determine your weight in kgs. Pick the option that pertains to you, and dive right in. If you already know your weight in kgs, you can beam yourself to Step 2!

Equation 9.1: Calculating your weight in kilograms (kgs)

OPTION 1: IF YOU ALREADY KNOW YOUR WEIGHT IN POUNDS (LBS)
WEIGHT IN LBS ÷ 2.2 = WEIGHT IN KGS
MY CALCULATION: 138LBS ÷ 2.2 = 62.7 KGS
YOUR CALCULATION: _____ ÷ 2.2 = _____ KGS

OPTION 2: IF YOU ALREADY KNOW YOUR WEIGHT IN STONES (STS)
WEIGHT IN STS X 6.35 = WEIGHT IN KGS
MY CALCULATION: 9.87 STS X 6.35 = 62.7 KGS
YOUR CALCULATION: _____ X 6.35 = _____ KGS

OPTION 3: IF YOU ALREADY KNOW YOUR WEIGHT IN UNICORN TURDS
I JUST WANTED TO MAKE SURE I STILL HAD YOUR ATTENTION.

Let's generate some excitement over the fact that we just did some math! Hoo-rah! Don't go all hexadecimal on me yet though; we have a few more steps to go.

Step 2

Now that we've discussed unicorn turds (or did you miss that part?), and know your weight in kilograms, we can calculate what's called your basal metabolic rate, or in laymen's terms, "how much energy your body needs to survive." We'll simply call it your "survival number" because that's an easier term to remember, and "basal" reminds me of "basil," and makes me crave pesto.

Basically, if you laid in bed all day doing absolutely nothing (we all have those days, right), you still need energy to do things like beat your heart, expand your lungs, and excrete urine (hopefully you get out of bed if there's a need). This step will take age and gender into consideration since people of different ages and sexes expend various amounts of energy. However, I **could** find two women of the same age and weight that are like polar opposites when it comes to how much energy it would take them to survive. This explains why all of this formulating can be a crock of shit. Keep plugging along though, because we're doing this simply to piss you off . . . I mean to get a *general* idea on calories we need, so onwards and upwards! Who doesn't love reading and doing math at the same time?! Don't answer that.

Use table 9.1 to help with this step. Find your age in the left column (making sure you choose the right gender), and then use the corresponding equation to calculate your survival number:

Table 9.1. Equations to assist in calculating your survival number

If you were born with a *penis*	
age 18-30	15.3 x kgs + 679
age 31-60	11.6 x kgs + 879
age 61+	13.5 x kgs + 487
If you were born with a *vagina*	
age 18-30	14.7 x kgs + 496
age 31-60	8.7 x kgs + 829
age 61+	10.5 x kgs + 596

I was born with a vagina, and I'm in my thirties, so I would use the equation second from the bottom (and so would someone almost twice my age; how accurate does *that* sound?!). I then head to equation 9.2 so I can see how to nerdily throw the weight that I calculated in Step 1 (62.7kgs) into that equation.

Equation 9.2. Calculating your survival number

HERE'S WHAT MY EQUATION LOOKS LIKE:

8.7 X 62.7 + 829 = 1,374.49 SURVIVAL CALORIES

NOW, FOR SHITS AND GIGGLES, YOU CAN CALCULATE YOURS

(WRITE YOUR SPECIFIC EQUATION FROM TABLE 9.1 HERE, AND SUBSTITUTE
YOUR WEIGHT IN KILOGRAMS, WHERE IT SAYS "KGS"):

_____ X _____ + _____ = _____ SURVIVAL CALORIES

My body needs around 1,374 calories purely to *survive*. Thus, how fucking stupid does it sound when weight loss programs dish out 1,200 calorie meal plans to millions of people?! Answer: really fucking stupid. I'd be dead on that plan.

We're obviously not interested in simply surviving for the rest of our lives though—well, I'm not anyway. I mean, there's no point in wearing a superhero suit if you can't put it to good use. I want to know how much energy my body needs to *thrive*. SPOILER ALERT: this math shit is about to get serious! Bear with me as we head to Step 3 to account for our activity levels.

Step 3

This is where we determine how many *extra* calories we need to add to our survival number based on our lifestyle. Refer to table 9.2 and choose whichever option describes you best.

Table 9.2. Activity level multipliers

Category	Description	Multiplier
The beached seal	Let's face it, you're not riding the fitness wave. Your daily activities include things like sitting, standing, driving, sewing, ironing, playing cards, reading, typing, and desk work, and napping. You contemplate peeing in the nearest jar when nature calls.	0.2
The chinchilla	You like to dabble in the art of raising your heart rate, but don't quite like to break a sweat. Your daily activities include things like garage work, carpentry, house cleaning, playing golf, sailing, and light exercise.	0.3
The dingo	People wonder where you get your energy. Your daily activities include things like gardening, cycling, tennis, skiing, dancing, heavy exercise, and little sitting. You probably know more about nutrition than most if you have this much energy.	0.4
The honey badger	You're a fucking firecracker. Your daily activities include things like heavy manual labor, leaping tall buildings in a single bound, or playing high-performance, competitive sports. You're fucking NUTS.	0.5

If you're in the beached seal category, please try not to take one of your naps until this shit is over. If you're *not* in the beached seal category, please be honest with yourself. There's no point in pretending you're a dingo if you're not; it will only make this less accurate for you, and what's the point of doing this if you're not going to be honest with yourself? No one is going to know what you choose except you. (This is when you go back and make sure you chose the right category).

On another note, if you're someone who lives in a location where extreme climates are present (e.g. harsh winters and hot summers), and you feel your activity level may fluctuate throughout the year, you may want to perform a couple different calculations relating to different times of year. Or, pick something in the middle. I don't care how you do it, just *do* it.

Personally, as a competitive athlete who gets my ass kicked daily, I'd fall into the psycho honey badger category. Thus, I need to multiply the survival number I calculated in step two, by 0.5.

Equation 9.3. Amount of extra calories needed for activity level

SURVIVAL NUMBER x ACTIVITY LEVEL FACTOR = CALORIES NEEDED

MY SURVIVAL NUMBER WAS 1,374.
THEREFORE: 1,374 x 0.5 = 687 EXTRA CALORIES NEEDED TO BE A HONEY BADGER

YOUR SURVIVAL NUMBER WAS _____.
THEREFORE: _____ x ____ = _____ EXTRA CALORIES NEEDED

That's how many *extra* calories we need on top of our survival number to withstand our activity levels. Thus, we need to add those extra calories to our survival numbers (see equation 9.4).

Equation 9.4. Adding activity calories

SURVIVAL NUMBER + EXTRA ACTIVITY CALORIES = CALORIES NEEDED

MY SURVIVAL NUMBER WAS 1,374 AND MY EXTRA CALORIES WERE 687.
THEREFORE: 1,374 + 687 = 2,061

NOW YOU'RE GOING TO ADD YOUR EXTRA CALORIES
TO YOUR SURVIVAL NUMBER:

_____ + _____ = _____

Annnnnnd, just when you thought we were done, there's one more step. If you haven't used this guidebook as toilet paper yet, you're doing bloody brilliant.

Step 4

Remember how I said that everything you do requires energy? Well, apart from our physical activity which we just sorted out, eating and metabolizing the shit you put in your pie-hole actually uses a substantial amount of energy—about 10% of your total daily energy in fact. Therefore—you guessed it—we're going to add another 10% of our calories to the number we came up with in step three to cover our eating habits.

Good thing I stayed awake in high school math class and know that "10%" is the same as "0.10." Thus, using the final calorie number from Step 3, we can now determine our final caloric estimation.

Equation 9.5. Calculating pie-hole usage calories

FINAL CALORIE AMOUNT FROM STEP 3 X 0.10 = EXTRA CALORIES NEEDED

MY CALCULATION: 2,061 X 0.10 = 206 EXTRA CALORIES NEEDED

YOUR CALCULATION: _____ X 0.10 = _____ EXTRA CALORIES NEEDED

That's how many *extra* calories we need for digestion and metabolism. Now we head to equation 9.6 to add those bad boys into our running calorie tally.

Equation 9.6. Adding pie-hole usage calories

FINAL CALORIE AMOUNT FROM STEP 3 + EXTRA CALORIES NEEDED TO EAT = ULTIMATE, FINAL, CALORIE ESTIMATION

MY EQUATION: 2,061 + 206 = 2,267 DAILY CALORIES NEEDED

YOUR EQUATION: _____ + _____ = _____ DAILY CALORIES NEEDED

Wahoo! We did it! Get up and bust out your favorite dance move! Even you, beached seal!

In the end, I determined that I need approximately 2,267 calories per day in regards to my age, gender, activity level, and energy it takes to eat and stay alive. However, knowing myself well, I know that some days I don't push as hard during my workout. On the contrary, some days I spend twenty hours nailed to my desk writing this fucking book. Therefore, that number is not—I repeat, NOT—100% accurate (have I repeated that enough yet?). However, it *does* provide a starting point in determining your caloric sweet spot, which will help those of you who initially may have had no concept of calories whatsoever.

I'd estimate my sweet spot to be within around 300 calories of the final calculated number of 2,267, depending on my activity level for the day (so anywhere between 1,967 and 2,567). If I then went and calculated how much I've *actually* been eating (cue the next chapter), and found out it was around 6,000 calories, it would be clear that I've been a gluttonous piggy, and I would need to sort my shit out and train my body to eat less.

Go ahead and add and subtract 300 from your final calorie amount and you'll get a range as well—hopefully representing your daily sweet spot (or, the amount of calories in one Sonic milkshake) .

Moral of the Story:

Your body requires a specific amount of fuel. That amount can change daily, and is impossible to pinpoint. However, for those of you who have absolutely no fucking clue how much food you're supposed to be eating, initially learning about calories can help you understand them and provide you with a range to shoot for.

Chapter 10

Amount:
How Much *Have* You
Been Eating?

Now let's determine how many calories you've *actually* been throwing down the chute, so we can compare *that* number to the one we figured out in the previous chapter. If you have no idea how to do this, you're not in the minority. Before I learned about nutrition I had no idea what a calorie was, much less if an apple had ten calories or ten thousand. Don't sweat it—there are some great tools out there to assist you. For starters, there are hundreds of calorie and nutrient tracking websites, books, and applications. You'll want to find a tool that *you* find user-friendly that clearly depicts how much you chow down on daily (e.g. your total calories). Finding a tool that also provides specific nutrient amounts or percentages (e.g. percentages of fat, carbohydrates, and protein) would also be beneficial, as we'll be discussing percentages in the next section.

My favorite nutrient-tracking website is *www.cronometer.com*. I use Cronometer with clients because it gives a detailed breakdown on all nutrients with easy to read visuals. My suggestion (do it!), is that you track your food for a few days.

Whatever tool you choose, please realize that most of them are weight-loss based and will ask you how much you're trying to lose. If you're not trying to lose weight, just indicate so. Also, don't worry about tracking any exercise—we merely want to find out how much food you've been stomach-smuggling. Before you start, here are a couple of pointers:

1. Try to avoid changing your nutrition habits first. Eat how you've been eating to make this as accurate as possible.
2. It will be in your best interest to log *typical* days; not days where you fly to Vegas to celebrate your sister's bachelorette party and get TAAANKED on 15,000 calories of Mai Thais. The goal is to determine how much, *on average*, you consume. Don't throw that average off by logging a binge-fest.
3. Be as accurate and specific as possible. Every little thing you put in your mouth should be tracked (e.g. meals, snacks, chewing gum, beverages), because I can tell you this: most people underestimate the shit they put in their mouths by upwards of 40%, especially when they eat out.[74] They convince themselves they're eating a lot less than they actually are—sometimes 1,000 calories less. That approach won't get you anywhere. Break *every* meal down and log the shit out of it (i.e. log the *ingredients* of the sandwich—bread, mustard, lettuce, tomato, etc.—not simply the sandwich).

Remember, you're only doing this for a few days, so while it may seem like the end of the world, you'll be done in two shakes of a lamb's tail. If you are eating processed foods that come with labels and bar codes, most calorie tracking apps will allow you to scan them in for easier tracking. However, this doesn't mean you get to be proud of the fact that you're eating processed foods.

Once you track your food for a few days, you can come back and pick this book up again. Enjoy your break!

(Queue obnoxious elevator music.)

If you're reading this paragraph before logging, you're not helping yourself. GO AWAY AND LOG. I mean it—get the fuck out of here.

(Queue hypnotic food-logging music.)

Welcome back! It's time to assess your daily calorie consumptions from your food logs, and ask yourself the following:

1. Is my total calorie consumption close to what I calculated in the previous chapter (within 300ish calories)?
2. Is my total calorie consumption nowhere near my caloric sweet spot?
3. Is my total calorie consumption consistent from day to day? Or, does it fluctuate significantly (e.g. 1,300 calories one day and 3,200 calories the next)?

These results should help you determine whether you're (on average) shoving too much, or too little shit down your pie-hole.

On a side note, if you obsess over calorie counting you're losing sight of the bigger picture: *learning* how to use your pie-hole. Calorie counting on its own means jack diddly (tell that to the fifty-four billion people currently counting calories like a boss), and is much less meaningful than the type and variety of your fuel. Knowing how much fuel your body needs will eventually become second nature, so don't let it consume you. I don't count calories, I never *want* to count calories, and you shouldn't have to either. *But*, if you need to at first, to get a good understanding of what a calorie is, approximately how much it may take to fuel your body, and how much you've actually been fueling your body, then it's a good idea (and if you're reading this, then you should have already done it).

The good news is that your body will actually tell you when it needs more fuel (or has received too much fuel), and you will learn to recognize these signals. I'll assume we all know what eating too much feels like: having a heavy, aching tummy, feeling bloated and lethargic, and feeling like you're about to slip into a food coma. On the other hand, eating *too little* brings on other symptoms like lightheadedness, dizziness, confusion, and fatigue. Thus, if you calculate your estimated calories and find you're lightheaded on a daily basis, you probably need more food. Listen to your body and trust your judgment. But be patient—don't make an adjustment, feel like shit for a day, and then give up because you're fucking staahhhhvin'.

It's important to wait a week or so after adjusting your intake to make sure your body has actually become accustomed to your new habits. Initially, you may experience what I like to call some "adjustment" symptoms (i.e. if you're used to eating 3,000 calories and you drop down to 2,000, you're going to be pretty fucking miserable). Take baby steps and wait it out. If you still feel those symptoms after a week or so, adjust your food intake up or down slightly and see what happens. If you feel better, *great*! If you don't, keep adding or subtracting until you do. Remember, we're breaking habits here—that shit can take time and can feel like hell. Regardless, always try to give your body time to adjust to your new routine first.

Furthermore, check this shit out: calories become even *less* important if your diet consists mainly of plant foods (e.g. fruits, vegetables, grains, legumes, nuts, herbs). That's right, it has been well documented that people who eat a plant-based diet can consume more calories, and maintain a slimmer weight and healthier body than their animal-food-hoarding counterparts.[75-77] This is due, in part, to the fact that people who eat more plant-based, whole foods have an increased metabolism, allowing them to burn more fuel.[78] A plant-based diet simply means that the *majority* (not necessarily all) of your calories come from plants.

Hey, I *love* to eat, so this was reason enough for me to adapt a plant-based diet! The more food, the merrier! It's extremely difficult to over-eat on a plant-based diet simply because of the fiber in plant foods (try, I dare you). Therefore, if you are someone who consumes more plant foods than animal foods, this whole calorie-counting ordeal becomes even less valuable. Your instructions basically become, "shovel it in!" We'll learn more about plant and animal foods in the next section. Until then, go eat some carrots.

Moral of the Story:

Finding the right amount of fuel is important, and will eventually become second nature. If you hate calorie counting and want to enjoy larger portions, focus on whole, plant foods.

Chapter 11

Hydration

Aside from *calorie* amounts, we also need to discuss the amount of non-caloric fluids we ingest. Being hydrated is the key to your body functioning efficiently and effectively, thus it is extremely important to understand how to stay hydrated. For the sake of this section, we're purely going to discuss water. Once we get to the "type" section, we'll discuss other types of fluids.

It's strange to think that our bodies are actually 60%–80% water. Thank goodness for cell membranes or we'd be in a puddle on the floor! But wait, why the heck are we so full of water? Well, you see, water is our internal, high-speed transportation train that delivers the oxygen we inhale, and the nutrients we consume, to our trillions of waiting cells. It also helps flush waste out of our bodies (hurray for easy pooping). All hail the mighty water!

Basically, water is pretty friggin' essential. Without it we cannot digest, transport, or absorb food, and pooping becomes a nightmare. Before you know it, you'll start sportin' sunken eyes, raging headaches, and begin to stumble around like a dizzy, drunk fool. We can last for a few weeks without food, but without water we will curl up and die within days. Dehydration is serious shit. Perhaps now is a good time to go get a glass of water?

What many people don't realize is that water is in most foods. Therefore, the amount of water you need to ingest on its own relies heavily on how much water you're already getting from the foods you're consuming. Guess which foods have the most water? It sure as shit won't be the highly-processed, stripped-down crap that you find in a box! Nope, it's the whole, fresh foods like fruits and vegetables that pack a punch. Take a second and skim through Appendix C to see what I'm talking about. The more real, whole foods you eat, the more hydrated you'll be. If you eat a lot of processed shit, well, have fun pooping.

After reading all of the previous information thus far, you can probably guess where I'm about to head when I mention the recommendation that "everyone should drink eight glasses of water per day." Holy shit, here we go again. The reason this statement was made (and usually refers to eight, 8-ounce glasses by the way) is because it was figured that people would find it "easy" to remember eight, 8oz glasses. Fucking hell. Health should never be about "ease," it should be about what's *right* for our bodies. The greatest part about this recommendation, is that there isn't even research to back it up![79] The "right" amount of water consumption depends largely on an individual's diet, the environment they live in, their activity levels, and how much they sweat. Yet, most people I know who are trying to improve their hydration strive like hell to hit that generic, mythical 8-glasses-per-day mark. Therefore, I'm going to remind you that, as with caloric intake, no one can tell you *exactly* how much water you need. However, like before, there *are* ways to estimate how much water you need.

Let me first say this: most people live in a dehydrated state (probably because all of the shitty, highly-processed foods they're consuming are void of water, and also because they choose beverages like energy drinks over plain water). Therefore, one of the first recommendations I can make is to increase your water intake. Lube that body up and let 'er roll! My clients who start hydrating are amazed at the instant results. They immediately sleep better, their skin clears up, they don't have headaches, they have more energy, and they're not miserable, whiny bitches (they're words, not mine!). If you didn't already, go get that glass of water and enjoy it while you continue to read.

Seriously, go get some water. I'm not going anywhere. I'm a fucking book for fuck's sake.

On a side note, for those of you looking to lose weight and have heard the ol' "water helps you lose weight" myth, I would actually argue that it's somewhat true. Being hydrated will make your body function better and run more efficiently at all times—including while you're on the weight loss wagon. Thus, while water itself doesn't *directly* make you lose weight, I would say that staying hydrated certainly does.

A good way to determine if you're hydrated is to do a piss check. Don't splash around in it; *observe* it. If it stinks like desert-toasted coyote carcass, and is a dark yellow or amber color, you're most likely dehydrated. If it's free of odor and light yellow, you're most likely hydrated. If it's somewhere in the middle, you're somewhere between dehydrated and hydrated (duh). Some factors may alter this test, though. Taking certain vitamins and eating certain foods can sometimes disguise the smell or color of your urine. This is when you can turn to your poop (yay, poop!). Is your poop dry, hard, or hibernating? If it is, and you also have dark, aromatic urine, you're dehydrated. Tackle that faucet like you mean it.

Now, to make things more complicated (because that seems to be the theme here), I want to mention that not all water is created equal. Therefore, it's my recommendation to drink *filtered* water to avoid certain chemicals that naturally occur, or may be placed, in your water supply. Like fluoride.

If you're one of the lucky folks who live in an area where some genius decided that drinking fluoride would help with tooth decay, this especially pertains to you. Let's discuss this for a second. Think about it—you're *drinking* fluoride (which is linked to a myriad of mental and behavior disorders, including a lowered IQ, autism spectrum disorders, ADHD, and dyslexia).[80, 81] *Drinking* something means it goes past your mouth, through your digestive system, and gets absorbed into your bloodstream . . . to then mingle with every cell in your body. Little Mr. Fluoride molecule is *not* smart enough to realize that it needs to jump onto your teeth and hold on like hell in order to reduce your tooth decay when the rest of the water molecules around it head straight down your throat. Instead, as always, we're robotically following the advice of the people that profit from the sale of it.

Dr. Dean Burk, a former senior chemist for the National Cancer Institute, once stepped forward and said:

> Fluoride causes more human cancer deaths than any other chemical . . . it is one of the most conclusive bits of scientific, and biological evidence that I have come across in my fifty years in the field of cancer research . . . fluoride amounts to public murder on a grand scale.[82]

Well that's awesome. They must have some pretty convincing salespeople out there for this shit to still be pumped into public water systems.

So who's regulating how much fluoride people are consuming? Answer: no one. I don't know what the strategy is these days, but when I was younger we were forced to swish the shit around in our mouths in primary school—because we lived in a community that hadn't filled our water supply with fluoride yet. The school nurse would walk around with trays of fluoride shots like a resort bartender, making sure that everyone got a good swish in . . . and I have stained, pitted teeth to thank for that. Say "hell no" to fluoride (or to your school nurse). Why? Past not wanting to die from cancer, how about the fact that the US puts fluoride in most of its water supply and *still* has a higher rate of tooth decay than countries that don't.[83] Thankfully, in 2015, the US got their shit together and recommended—for the first time in over fifty years—*lowering* the level of fluoride dumped in public water.[84] Regardless of the amount of fluoride in your water, it won't fix a shitty diet. And *that* is the problem—not lack of fluoride. If you don't eat an abundance of toxic, nutrient-depleted foods, your teeth won't rot out of your head. End of story.

Thus, I recommend doing some research on water filters and buying one for your home. Then, buy a glass or stainless water bottle and drink out of it throughout the day until your urine runs clear. One of the silliest things you can do is try to be fantastic with hydrating and filtering your water, and then drink out of a plastic water bottle that may leach chemicals right back into your water. Put your smart hat on and get a water bottle that won't poison you, and use it over and over. I always (always!) have my stainless steel water bottle with me. And, I actually *use* it too, because while simply carrying it around may look trendy, it actually doesn't do a fuckin' thing for your health unless you drink out it.

* * *

Before we move on to the next section, I'd like to point out that in order for your body to consistently run properly, it needs a steady supply of both calories *and* water. This means you don't eat all of your calories, or drink all of your water, in one big binge at some random hour of the day. It means you have meals, snacks, and water spread throughout the day. It means you try not to go more than a few hours without shoving something healthy down your pie-hole. Personally, I get headaches and get light-headed if I go more than three hours without food or water. That's me though, and you'll figure out your optimal fuel frequency by trial and error.

Most folks who preach the "it's better to go long periods without eating" (i.e. fasting) concept, are solely concerned with weight loss, and not whole-body health. If you're going to be using your body constantly, it needs fuel and water constantly. Simple. We're not here to try to trick our bodies into thinking we're starving, and we're not here to "reset" our system. We're simply staying fucking fueled and hydrated. Period. You don't run your car around on empty because it will magically run better once you *do* fuel 'er up again, do you?

Moral of the Story:
Drink more water, dammit.

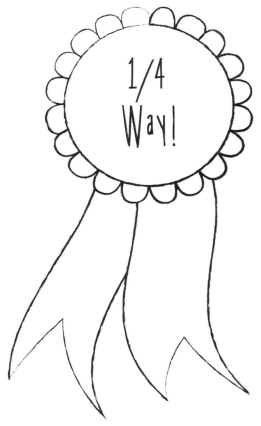

Congrats! You're 1/4 of the way done. That probably sounds pretty shitty, but hey, here's a ribbon!

SECTION III

The *Types* of Shit People Throw Down Their Pie-Holes

Chapter 12

Type Trumps Amount

Spoiler alert: this section is going to be fun. Fun with a capital "F," if you catch my drift. Please feel free to give the food industry a big ol' high-five (or kick to the crotch) for providing me with ample crap to bitch about. Buckle up—things are about to get fucking wacky.

Before we dive in, let's take a second to celebrate. We tackled the first nutrient factor (amount), and survived! Fuck yeah! I have to be honest though . . . doing all of those calorie calculations may have been a big, fuckin' waste of time. Mainly because if you figure this nutrition shit out, the amount you eat becomes a bit irrelevant. We'll discuss this more in depth later on, but just realize that if you choose the right *types* of foods, you can pretty much eat all you want. You're not going to get fat eating carrots and beans; the fiber in those foods will make you explode well before that ever happens. So why'd we do all the calculations then? Because this is about *learning.* Understanding what a calorie is and how it relates to what you're putting in your pie hole is still an important part of the puzzle—especially if you're not yet ready to give the types of foods you eat an overhaul. Being knowledgeable about calories will give you a better understanding of the big picture, and that's the point of all of this. If you hate me a little for making you dust off your calculators, I'm okay with that. Shake it off.

Let's move on and explore the second nutrient factor: type. The *types* of food you eat are undeniably more important than the *amount* of food you eat (said no weight loss program ever). This is why simply counting calories is of little value on its own (which is, unfortunately, the path most people take). You could get your allotted 2,000 calories from hot dogs. And, while that may be the right *amount* of fuel for your body, that shit won't provide the nutrients you need to function at Captain America capacity.

Remember, we're talking about pie-hole usage for whole-body *health* here, not simply for weight loss or muscle gain. So, please repeat after me: My goal is to be *healthy*, not simply skinny or buff. My goal is to be *healthy*, not simply skinny or buff. My goal is to be *healthy*, not simply skinny or buff . . . feel free to keep repeating. You will not get healthy by counting calories, but you *will* improve your health by eating the right *types* of foods (which will also result in you becoming slim and buff—it's a win-win).

As stated above, weight loss programs typically only focus on *amount* and not *type.* They do this simply by limiting your fuel intake (i.e. a restricted calorie program that involves keeping you focused by counting points or something). Sometimes, they even provide you with shitty, packaged, highly-processed "foods" that are full of salt, sugar, and chemical additives (yet are a set number of calories). Yum! They rarely teach you about the *types* of fuel you should be eating to stay healthy (providing you with a pyramid-like-tool doesn't count). They merely show you that if you eat less food you can lose weight. "Wait—I can be on the program and eat all the bacon and ice cream I want and *still* stay within my points!? Count me in!"

Here's where I high-five you in the face. Stop trying to "beat the system" by following ridiculous point systems, or by choosing well-advertised shitty types of food. You know damn well that copious amounts of bacon and ice cream won't provide your body with kick-ass nutrients. You should also know that Coke Zero and Diet Coke are no better than Coke. Sugar-free gum is no better than regular gum. They are *still* just soda and gum no matter how you look at them; they're all just processed shit. Thus, the focus is all wrong. Rather than searching for the "better" of the shitty options, we need to search for the *best* options—which would be actual whole, untainted foods.

Speaking of options, one of my biggest pet peeves is when people label themselves based on the types of foods they eat (e.g. vegetarian), and assume that simply bearing that title equates to them being healthy. Any nutrition label (e.g. vegetarian, vegan, raw foodie, carnivore), can be broadly defined. For instance, a "vegetarian" could consume nothing but Doritos and Red Bull, and also chain-smoke all day. However, a "vegetarian" could also eat a wide variety of organically grown fruits, vegetables, beans, lentils, whole grains, nuts and seeds. One would clearly be a malnourished health nightmare, while the other would be fighting crime in their superhero suit. Yet, since neither of them eat meat, by definition they're both "vegetarians." Put the fucking diet labels away and focus on eating healthy.

When people ask me about my eating preferences, they wind up utterly confused: "Are you a vegetarian?" No. "Are you a vegan?" No. "Then what the hell are you?" I'm a human, and I eat real foods (mainly plant foods) that make me healthy. Simple as that. My diet doesn't need a label, and labels don't equate to health. Heck, I know vegetarians who outright refuse to eat vegetables.

So, where do we start? Well, if your body needs, for example, 2,000 calories for the day, than it's up to you to start focusing on getting those 2,000 calories from as many fantastic, health-promoting foods as you can. In a perfect world (humor me for a sec), all 2,000 of those calories should be from healthy, nutrient-dense foods. Anything else is a waste of calories that will pull you away from optimal health and push you towards the bottom end of the Nutrition Spectrum. You'll suddenly go to jump into your Captain America suit and rip a bigass hole up the crotch ("but I don't get it, I stayed within my points?!"). Unfortunately, Captain America and crotchless pants do not go hand-in-hand (when it comes to **crime** fighting, at least—I'm not saying I wouldn't want to see him in crotchless pants). Until your calories come from nutrient-dense foods, stay away from the suit.

Keep in mind, what your body "needs" and what you "want" are most likely vastly different right now. However, as you learn about nutrition and begin to eat *real* foods and drink *real* beverages, you may find that you actually start craving *real* food and *real* beverages. Yes, your taste buds will "change," and the gap between what you "need" and "want" will diminish. You will start to actually crave the nutrients your body needs. In the beginning, finding the types of foods that make your body thrive *and* that you enjoy, will seem like a challenge, but everyone loves a good challenge, right? RIGHT! WHO'S WITH ME?! (Stands in superhero pose, adjusts cape, and jumps out the window.)

Moral of the Story:

The *types* of nutrients you consume are far more significant than the *amount* you consume, or any diet label you feel like giving yourself. Choose the *healthiest* nutrients, and you'll prevent a ginormous crotch-hole from forming in your pants.

Chapter 13

Put the Whole in the Hole

Every time you eat is an opportunity to nourish or neglect your body. Some options will catapult you towards Captain America status, and others will send you plummeting to the depths of Diseaseland. Thus, it is crucial that you start making conscious decisions about what gets near your mouth, and whether or not it's going to harm you or help you. Ideally, if you want to live a disease-free life packed full of rainbows and fairy dust, you'll want to steer away from all of the harmful shit, and aim for as many health-promoting, immune-boosting, kick-ass nutrients as possible. If that sounds brilliant to you, your goals should be to:

1. stop shoving useless shit down your throat;
2. stop considering "better" options of shitty foods to be okay (e.g. the amazing calorie-free Coke Zero)—because in reality, they're all still just shitty, processed foods; and
3. stop focusing on what to *eliminate* from your diet (e.g. calories, carbs, Frappuccinos, grains, gluten), and instead, focus on powerful foods to *add* to your diet.

Side note: If you make a decision to put something shitty down your pie-hole, you need to own it. *Know* that you've made a conscious decision to exchange something harmful for something nurturing. And then don't come crawling to me when you feel like shit.

Ideally though, every time you eat you should asking yourself, "which kick-ass nutrients do I need that will give me enough energy to fight a bear?!" If you can refocus and do this, and start *adding* kick-ass superfoods to your diet, those foods will begin to replace the shitty foods. Before you know it, your diet will be full of awesomeness, and you *will* be fighting bears. Let grandma patch up the crotch-hole on the Captain America suit because shit's about to get wild again!

What are these mysterious kick-ass foods that everyone should focus on? None other than real foods. As in, *whole* foods. When I say "whole," I mean "hasn't been fucked with." As in, the difference between a carrot and carrot cake. Whole foods, to me, are mainly untainted by humans (okay, someone planted the damn seed, but you get my point). They grow on their own in a field, on a tree, or in the ground. They don't come in a box, and they don't have an ingredient label. They are organically grown and free of toxic chemicals. Heck, if anything they might have bugs or bird shit on them, and THAT'S A GOOD THING! It means they're actually *fresh* and weren't sprayed, highly processed, stripped, wrapped, and put on a shelf for three years!

To help herd you in the right direction, I have supplied a list of whole foods that I regularly plow into. From them, I can create some of the most delicious, mouth-watering meals—meals that will literally make me want to hump my plate for days. I have cooked these meals for people of all walks of life—even steadfast meat-and-potato consumers—and they have licked their plates clean. Once *you* start learning and experimenting with real, whole foods, you'll be able to make endless options of easy, gourmet-like cuisines in the comfort of your own kitchen. Exciting, I know.

apples	lentils	sunflower seeds
blueberries	beans	coconuts
mangoes	quinoa	basil
avocadoes	barley	cilantro
tomatoes	oats	mint
dates	wild rice	parsley
carrots	cashews	cinnamon
spinach	almonds	ginger
broccoli	walnuts	garlic
cauliflower	chia seeds	cumin
beets	flax seeds	turmeric
pumpkin	pumpkin seeds	vanilla beans
peas	sesame seeds	cacao beans

Looking at that list, I *know* with simple common sense you're aware it's filled with healthy foods. Remember though, I'm talking about buying them in *whole, unprocessed* form (i.e. roasted, salted, tamari almonds are *not* the same as plain, organic almonds). If they have been highly processed, put in a box with sugar, salt and other additives thrown in, they are no longer the nutrient-packed food they used to be . . . because the damn humans got a hold of them!

Does this mean you have to eat the foods on that list? NO. Not only is that list incomplete, but it represents a small portion of the whole foods *I* enjoy eating and that make *me* thrive (head to Appendix B for a longer list). When I eat those whole foods, I get all of the nutrients my body needs. I have no clue if they'll make you thrive, if you're allergic to them, or if you even like them. It will be up to *you* to come up with your own list of whole foods that you enjoy—foods that make you feel heroic, that you can concoct into any recipe your wannabe-superhero ass desires.

When I get to this part of the transition process, the panic usually sets in and I hear the following: "I don't know where to find healthy foods," "healthy foods cost too much," or "I don't have time to prepare healthy foods." Let's address these concerns, because either I'm defying the odds, or this shit is actually doable.

"I Don't Know Where to Find Healthy Foods"

I have lived in several different climates around the world, and I always find healthy food. You know why? Because healthy food is real food, and real food exists everywhere.

There are challenges, however. For instance, in climates that have extreme winters it becomes slightly harder to get fresh foods. In that case, you do the best you can. Perhaps you freeze your fresh foods from the summer months. Perhaps you buy frozen foods that are shipped in from somewhere else that *can* still grow those foods. Sure, they may not have the same amount of wonderful nutrients by the time you consume them, but reduced wonderful nutrients are better than a bunch of shitty nutrients.

In the warmer months or climates, a local farmers market or a Community Supported Agriculture program are *excellent* places to find some fresh, seasonal, whole foods. "Natural" or "Organic" grocers are starting to pop up everywhere as well, so search your area—there may be one near you! And, here's the kicker: you don't need Birkenstocks, patchouli, and a joint to shop there. *Everyone* is allowed to buy healthy foods! You simply need to have enough motivation to get your ass in there and ask someone to help you navigate the new territory.

Even better, why not scrap the buying altogether and grow food? You know, start your own garden. You city dwellers can even make gardens *inside* your house (say whaaaa?! YES!). Find a local garden nursery (hopefully with organic options) and ask for help. Depending on the climate you live in, there are a wide variety of foods that you may be able to grow on your own (which can save a butt-load of money). Get that thumb GREEN!

"Healthy Foods Cost Too Much"

I spend less money on food than most people for a few reasons. For starters, I don't pay for the packaging of the processed stuff. Most of what I buy is whole and package-free, which is great since most of the healthy foods that people consider to be overly-expensive are *processed* "healthy" foods (i.e. they come in a box or package with some healthy-sounding word slapped on it). Secondly, some of the most expensive foods are absent from my diet (e.g. meats and cheeses). Lastly, I buy foods that are *in season.* "In season" means cheaper. If a food is *out of season*, it means it has been shipped in from somewhere else. This requires jet fuel and packaging—neither of which are cheap.

For you "I-need-numbers" people, check this out: according to a 2013 study, healthy eating only costs *slightly* more than shitty eating—$1.48/day more to be exact.[85] The study also indicated that "it is possible to choose more nutritious foods . . . without spending more money and . . . improvements in dietary choices does not invariably cost more."[86] Whether or not it *does* cost more depends largely on the *types* of foods you choose to buy. For example, if I choose to have beans rather than beef, I'm going to save some dough. Beans, on average cost $1.07 per pound, while beef costs $5.28 per pound (and one will provide me with healthy fiber, iron, and a plethora of other nutrients, and the other will give me cholesterol and saturated fat).[87] While I'm at it, I may as well go and start a college fund for my kid!

If you truly want to keep costs low, it simply means cutting down on some of the more expensive foods. If you choose to eat expensive foods, you can't bitch and moan about costs. Also, let me remind you that if you can find a way to pay for shampoo, movie tickets, chewing gum, beer, lotion, nail polish, music, your car, TV, and internet (all of which you don't *need*— but please let me remind you that you *need* nutrients), you will find a way to buy the less expensive, healthy food.

To summarize, you're not allowed to get your panties in a bunch over the price of healthy foods anymore—you simply need to educate yourself on how to find the ones that fit in your budget. How much does a carrot cost? Are you buying any beverages? Why? You only need water, right? If you buy expensive foods, that's your *choice.* Stop crying over your own choices.

"I Don't have Time to Prepare Healthy Foods"

Guess what? There are an *infinite* number of recipes out there. So, c'mon folks, if time is an issue for you, THEN YOU FIND THE RECIPES THAT TAKE THE LEAST TIME TO PREPARE. Do I really need to say that?! I'm a perfect example: I have no more than thirty minutes to get dinner on the table when I get home. Thus, every whole-food, power-packed, mouth-watering meal I make is made in less than 30 minutes. I have a few meals that take longer, and my strategy is to prep those meals earlier in the day so I can hit them hard when my thirty-minute countdown begins. So yeah, sorry to rain on your parade, but "lack of time" is also a bad excuse to not eat whole, healthy foods. Don't worry, there's a whole chapter on preparing healthy foods later on—we just need to do a little more learning first.

* * *

Those excuses aside, many people actually *do* have good intentions when it comes to eating whole foods, but unfortunately wind up with a completely skewed ratio of whole foods to shitty processed foods. Like eating "an apple a day" when everything else they're consuming is highly processed crap.

As an example, let's revisit the 2,000-calorie-per-day scenario: You leave the house in the morning after throwing your apple-a-day down your throat (100 calories gone), and head to the gym. After you toss around some weights, you decide to stop off at Starbucks (because you broke a fucking sweat you bloody hero). Without hesitation, you grab a healthy-looking blueberry scone which rings in at 420 calories. Then you snatch a 560-calorie Tazo green tea frappa-shit-accino. Before you know it, *half* of your calories are gone for the day, and the only beneficial thing you ate was an apple! A scone and drink from Starbucks—regardless of how healthy they appear—are *not* going to nourish you; both are packed with shit your body is definitely not holding out for.

Since you technically need 2,000 calories of *healthy* foods, but have already wasted 1,000 calories on shitty foods, you're either going to come up short on beneficial nutrients for the day, or you're going to have to *over*-consume to get all of the good nutrients you need. Neither method works, by the way. If you really give a shit about the one and only body you will ever have, you will pack it full—not half-full—of the best nutrients possible.

On a side note, excuses like: "It's okay that I eat this scone, because I courageously went to the gym this morning," can be filed under "dumbass justifications." But hey—congrats for getting your ass to the gym! Now get your head out of that ass. Going to the gym is *never* an excuse to put destructive things in your body. Furthermore, working out hours earlier is *not* going to burn off the nutrient-deprived scone you attack an hour later. Are you crying yet? Stop crying. And wipe that scone off your face.

Before we move on, I want to discuss meat and dairy. Both are often staple foods, but don't technically fall into the "whole food" category—unless you are ripping into a live chicken, or suckling directly from a cow's teat. I generally hear doors slamming in my face when I begin to discuss meat and dairy. Remember folks, I grew up in friggin' rural *Vermont* surrounded by dairy farms and chicken coops. My back yard was littered with cow shit, "manure" was a common scent in the air, and I once had a calf named after me. I'm surprised I didn't drop to all fours and start mooing when I hit puberty. Even though I hardly ever consume meat or dairy, I'm not demanding everyone follow my lead. What I want to point out is that meat and dairy are usually the "whole" food groups everyone *assumes* they need, but don't (fuck you, food pyramid).

Here's an important life lesson I will repeat an obnoxious amount of times throughout this guide: you don't need specific "foods," you need specific "nutrients" (e.g. fats, carbohydrates, protein, vitamins, minerals). Where you *get* those nutrients is your choice (i.e. you get to pick the foods you eat). You don't *need* meat and dairy like you don't *need* apples and broccoli. Nutrients are everywhere, and part of learning about how to use your pie-hole, is learning about your choices (check out Appendix B). I'll say it again: there are a million and one whole food options out there.

It's going to be up to *you* to choose whatever the fuck ones you want!

I'm "well-learned" about this topic because I turned a blind eye on the foods that were advertised most, did my own research on what whole foods contained which nutrients, and discovered the foods that made me feel like a rock star. For example, red meat is high in iron—but so are cashews. I have never been a steak lover, but LOVE ME SOME CASHEWS. Dairy milk has calcium, but broccoli and almond milk have *more*, and they don't make me feel bloated and backed-up like dairy does. So naturally, I choose to get my calcium from sources other than dairy. Drum roll please . . . holy *shit* I'm still alive!

I don't give a rat's ass about product advertising, how healthy something is marketed to be, or which foods have been eaten daily for the past however-many years. It's all about learning about which (real) foods contain the best nutrients for you, and more importantly, how they make you feel. It's funny (not really) how much research people do before they buy cars, electronics, engagement rings, etc., yet don't seem to give a flying fuck when it comes to researching the stuff they're putting *inside* themselves. If you start researching where to get the best nutrients, you will wind up landing on whole foods time and time again.

In the following chapter, you will be guided through a medical shit storm by a distinguished cardiologist who knows all-to-well what happens when whole foods are avoided. Pay attention, take notes, and I'll see you on the flipside.

Moral of the Story:

Whole foods are the key to health. Find the ones that turn **you** into a plate-humper, and then shove them into the depths of your pie-hole as often as you're able.

Chapter 14

Frankenstein Medicine and the Metabolic Syndrome

Doctors are men who prescribe medicines of which they know little, to cure diseases of which they know less, in human beings of whom they know nothing.
—Francois Marie Arouet Voltaire

Contrary to public belief, the biggest threat to our country isn't terrorism or our dependence on foreign oil. It is rather the ever-increasing "unwellness" of our population.

We have discovered the truth about the absurd amount of money being pumped into the healthcare system, and how our state of health doesn't line up. As a doctor who has worked with numerous service members, I can also, unfortunately, confirm that this scenario extends to our military force—which becomes a terrifying thought. If the men and women of the military are sick, what does that mean for our safety?

In 2012 the Washington Post published an article on the increasing incidence of service members failing fitness tests. The author reported that *obesity* was the leading cause of ineligibility for people wanting to join the Army. It wasn't that they weren't strong enough or mentally tough enough; it was because they were too *unwell*. Consequently, military officials now see "the expanding waistlines in the warrior corps as a national security threat."[88] Meaning, if we do not optimize our nutrition habits and start turning this health epidemic around, we will become the unhealthiest population in our nation's history, supported by a military too unfit to defend us.

What is the cause of this debilitating "unwellness"? It is an epidemic known as "the metabolic syndrome," is caused by poor lifestyle choices, and can be linked to most modern diseases. Truth be told, metabolic syndrome is, perhaps, the greatest threat to our society. It leaves us in a vulnerable state and inhibits us from performing at all levels. As a precursor to most western diseases, it is undeniable that preventing the metabolic syndrome should be a focus of healthcare providers. Yet, that is rarely the case.

As an example, in a 2006 review of the causes, patterns, and effects of heart failure (a common condition caused by the metabolic syndrome, where the heart can no longer pump enough blood to meet the body's needs), the author recognizes *primary prevention* as a necessary step in the approach to eliminate heart failure, but then never develops the theme further. Instead, she rather focuses on the role of medical interventions and testing.[89] This has become the trend—to treat disease rather than prevent it.

To defend this notion further, I was recently struck with a sobering realization while attending a medical conference on a similar condition called "heart failure with preserved ejection fraction," or simply "HFpEF." You see, no modern day medical development has yielded a demonstrable impact on the arresting, reversal, or cure for this prevalent disorder. Yet the conference revolved around the various tests, and multitude of drug trials to treat it. And, although a brief mention was made that the metabolic syndrome was a major contributor to the development of HFpEF, I was most disturbed that not *one* word was mentioned about the only proven method to reverse, arrest, or cure this metabolic syndrome (which would then prevent the development of HFpEF). I'm, of course, talking about optimal nutrition.

What needed to be acknowledged was that HFpEF, as well as diabetes, hypertension, coronary artery disease, stroke, sleep apnea, Alzheimer's disease, and cancer—just about everything that keeps modern day doctors, nurses, hospitals and nursing homes in business—are all merely *symptoms* or *complications* of the metabolic syndrome. And therefore, if we refocused our attention on *preventing* the metabolic syndrome (via proper nutrition), we would eliminate a heck of a lot of debilitating disease.

Moreover, in this conference room packed full of some of the smartest and most educated people in this country (some of whom were innocently drinking their diet sodas—more to come on this), not *once* was there mention of another widespread condition called "hyperinsulinemia." This condition has a central role in the cause of the metabolic syndrome, and the two together could be considered the gateway to most western diseases. They should have been the focus of the discussion. Yet, no mention.

Thus, without discussing the roles of the metabolic syndrome or hyperinsulinemia, the only points left to discuss were *interventions* and *treatments* for HFpEF, and not how to *prevent* it from ever occurring. These professionals simply failed to acknowledge that *nutrition* is the only effective way to prevent, reverse, or eliminate this threat. "Coincidentally," the healthcare industry profits from treatments and interventions, and not from preventions.

With recognition that hyperinsulinemia and the metabolic syndrome are the gateway to most western diseases (and are preventable), the focus for the remainder of this chapter will be prevention of western diseases from a medical standpoint—specifically via proper nutrition. However, it must be noted that everything in this book before you is, in fact, all about how the food you choose to consume will either facilitate or eliminate hyperinsulinemia and the development of the metabolic syndrome. Eliminate those two conditions, and you will eliminate substantial amounts of ailments, disease, medical bills, treatments, and medications. Unfortunately for my profession, it would also eliminate the need for most conventional medical professionals. With this in mind, perhaps doctors of the future can return to their aspirations of becoming actual health care providers rather than disease managers.

* * *

Over the course of the past several thousand years, we have shifted our diet to the consumption of highly processed, nutritionally deficient "foods" and "beverages." Specifically, the consumption of processed carbohydrates and sugars has skyrocketed (e.g. breads, pastas, cereals, flours, pizza, confectionaries, sodas), wreaking havoc on the organ systems' ability to maintain a healthy state.

What most people don't realize, is that a carbohydrate is simply a bunch of sugar molecules connected by chemical bonds. This doesn't mean that all carbohydrates are the enemy, it means the more *processed* and *modified* a carbohydrate becomes (as in the examples given above), the more that food is viewed simply as "sugar" by your pancreas (which has a hand in regulating sugar levels in the body). That's right—as you consume a pizza, pasta, and breadstick meal, your body essentially thinks you're eating sugar. Your pancreas then produces a hormone called insulin to keep the escalating sugar levels under control. In turn, the more processed foods you eat, the more your pancreas is stimulated to pump out insulin to help regulate the ever-increasing sugar load.

What is insulin? You may have heard of it before, but may be unfamiliar with the many roles this hormone plays in the body. Let's take a look.

- Insulin lowers elevated blood sugar.
- Insulin increases appetite.
- Insulin shifts metabolism into storage mode.
- Insulin converts glucose and protein to fat.
- Insulin converts dietary fat to stored fat.
- Insulin removes fat from blood and transports it into fat cells.
- Insulin increases the body's production of cholesterol.
- Insulin stimulates the growth of arterial smooth muscle cells, causing high blood pressure, kidney failure, and arterial plaque build-up.

Note the association of insulin with fat production and storage. Yes, insulin and fat are good buddies. *Fat* doesn't make you fat—too much *insulin* makes you fat. Essentially, an *over*-production of insulin (due to increased ingestion of processed foods—which contain an abundance of processed carbohydrates) will most likely cause someone to gain weight and become diseased. But, like I said above, not all carbohydrates are the enemy. *Complex* (or what I refer to as "slow") carbohydrates—the ones nature provides to us—meaning whole foods such as broccoli, tomatoes, spinach, and barley, do not cause this intense insulin release.

This is where the glycemic index fits in (which you have most likely heard of, and will soon learn more about in chapter 17). This index determines how closely a carbohydrate-rich food resembles a simple sugar, and thus how severely insulin will be released when it's consumed. Remember, more insulin means increased appetite, more fat storage, and more disease. On the following diagram, you can see that—even among the same class of food— there is a large difference in the body's reaction to processed foods versus whole foods (flour made from wheat, versus a grain of whole wheat). Thus, for someone who regularly reaches for processed foods (and is in a constant state of hyperinsulinemia), you may see why, over time, they may be at major risk of developing disease. In fact, current research has demonstrated that hyperinsulinemia leads to a state of ongoing systemic inflammation and cell damage, which is felt to be the first indication or warning sign of most disease.[90-92]

The Effect of Wheat Variations on Insulin Levels

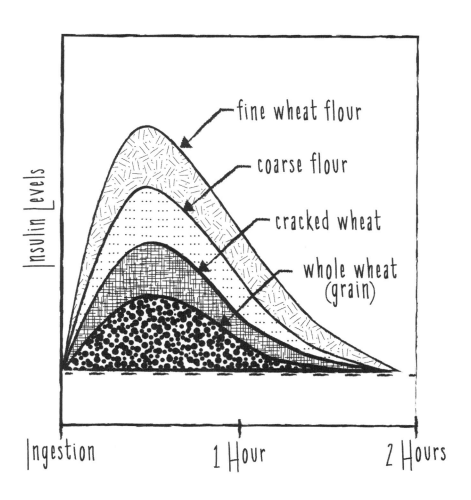

Insulin Levels

fine wheat flour

coarse flour

cracked wheat

whole wheat (grain)

Ingestion — 1 Hour — 2 Hours

This constant state of increased insulin production (termed "hyperinsulinemia") from eating processed foods causes a variety of pathological conditions, now well documented in scientific literature. In order to characterize these conditions as one disorder, we have created a new "disease," and have labeled it "the metabolic syndrome." This syndrome encompasses several ailments, including but not limited to, obesity, sleep apnea, high blood pressure, elevated blood sugar, diabetes, increased clotting, stroke, kidney failure, plaque build-up, heart attacks, congestive heart failure, failure to thrive, depression, and premature death—many of the main causes of modern sickness and death. Hence, why the metabolic syndrome should be considered the greatest threat to our existence.

Over time, as someone continues to eat processed foods, their pancreas will start spewing out so much insulin that matters get worse. This brings us to another syndrome called "insulin resistance"(or "pre-diabetic"), created to define this defective state. Take a guess on how doctors are trained to deal with this. That's correct: prescribe a drug that forces your body to synthesize *more* insulin (which was the problem to begin with), and eventually a second medication to push out even *more* insulin, and then another medication to make your cells more *sensitive* to whatever insulin is floating around. The ludicrous part about all of this is that NONE OF THESE MEDICATIONS TAKE CARE OF THE HYPERINSULINEMIA OR REVERSE OR CURE THE METABOLIC SYNDROME. In fact, most of these medications are simply managing your symptoms, while at the same time causing serious side effects like GI distress, kidney failure, liver failure, acidosis, anemia, congestive heart failure, allergic reaction, and possibly death.

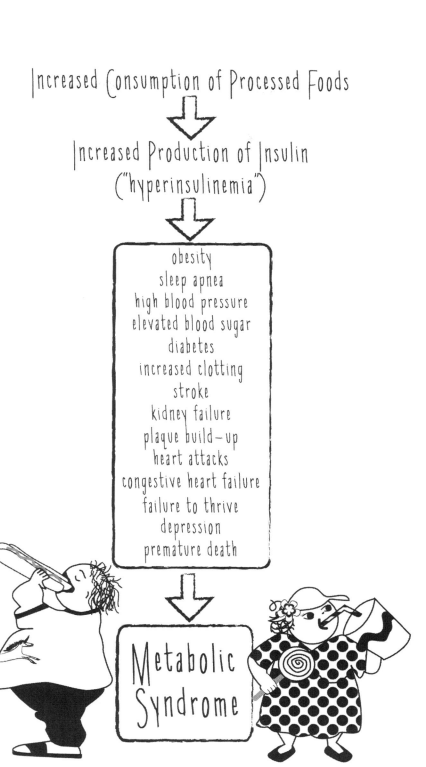

Down the road, once these prescribed medications have completely burned your pancreas out and it can't make any more insulin (hello, diabetes), what do we doctors do? We prescribe insulin! Heck, if your pancreas can't make it, you can buy it—even if it won't solve your problems!

And this vicious, unavailing cycle will continue unless there is great change from all sides of the health industry. You see, even when people become sick enough to be admitted to the hospital for more aggressive assistance, they're probably worse off. When I do rounds on my hospital patients who are suffering from all of these disorders, instead of helping them get better by serving them whole, fresh foods, they are actually being further poisoned by being served highly processed foods such as canned vegetables, sweetened juices, sodas, artificial flavors, white flour, sugary deserts, and burgers. Instead of recovery to health, it's a perpetuation of the killing fields—all from eating the highly-processed foods that have been presented to them by the people who are supposed to be helping them.

At the end of the day, we have a society of people reliant on treatments and medications for their metabolic syndrome symptoms (obesity, hypertension, diabetes, high cholesterol, etc.), which sounds like a win-win for the pharmaceutical companies, if you ask me. All the while, these patients still feel awful, and are not cured. I have come to call this Frankenstein Medicine: where we health care providers—excuse me, *disease managers*—"fix" all the numbers, but the patient feels like a walking zombie and will never get better.

To validate this concept, table 14.1 depicts a list of medications and associated costs on a patient I recently saw who suffers from a variety of illnesses caused by the metabolic syndrome. Don't ask me to list the hundreds of associated (horrific) side effects.

Table 14.1. List of medications presented to a patient being treated for complications of the metabolic syndrome

	Prescription	Cost
1	Lyrica 75mg, 1 by mouth, twice daily	$428.10
2	Oxycodone 5mg as needed	$19.47
3	Meclizine 25mg every 8hrs as needed	$47.66
4	aspirin 325mg 1 by mouth daily	$4.00
5	Humulin R 100unit/mL solution insulin pump	$143.27
6	Amlodipine 10mg 1 by mouth, in morning	$2.00
7	Betamethasone Diproprionate 0.05% cream, apply twice daily	$101.29
8	Fenofibrate 54 mg 1 by mouth, in morning	$28.51
9	Glucosamine-Chondroitin Complx, 1 by mouth in morning	$18.93
10	Pantoprazole DR 40mg, 1 by mouth in evening	$52.55
11	Lamsulosin ER 0.4mg, 1 by mouth after meal	$78.96
12	Triamcinolone acetonide 0.5% cream, apply twice daily	$20.96
13	Oxycontin ER 10mg, 1 by mouth, twice daily	$228.08
14	Insulin NPH 100 unit/mL (70-30) via insulin pump	$283.56
15	Metoprolol Tartrate 100mg, 1 by mouth, twice daily	$4.00
16	Tizanidine 4mg, 1 by mouth, three times daily	$235.91
17	Diazepam 5mg, 1-1/2 by mouth in evening	$14.76
18	Cymbalta DR 60mg, 1 by mouth, twice daily	$238.37
19	Acetaminophen 325mg, 2 by mouth, twice daily	$10.99
20	Lovaza 1g, 2 by mouth, twice daily	$285.82
21	ProAir HFA 90 mcg/actuation HFA aerosol inhaler, as directed	$111.04
22	Nitrostat 0.4mg, as needed for chest pain	$27.52
23	Plavix 75mg, 1 by mouth daily	$4.00
24	Isosorbide mononitrate ER 30mg, 1 by mouth daily	$31.15
25	Lisinopril 40mg, 2 by mouth in morning	$8.00
26	Lipitor 40mg, 1 by mouth daily	$4.00
27	Mirtazapine 45mg, 1 by mouth at bedtime	$96.28
28	Glyburide 5mg	$27.34
29	Victoza 1.8mg subcutaneous daily	$192.25
30	Invokana 100mg, 1 by mouth daily	$602.99

30 medications costing a total of $3,351.76

This is classic Frankenstein Medicine, at a cost of over $3,000 *per month* in prescriptions. You would at least hope that this investment is helping him . . . yet, I can assure this person still feels poorly, is gaining weight, has no energy, and is getting progressively *more* unhealthy by the minute. Let's not forget he has now succumbed to spending his days mapping out his drug routine. Multiply that by the millions of patients in this country with a similar fate, and you can see where this is going. This is not atypical and could someday be you or your children if we don't implement a serious change in our view of nutrition. Here's a late breaking news flash:

EVERY COMPLICATION, AND IN FACT THE DEVELOPMENT
OF THE METABOLIC SYNDROME, CAN BE COMPLETELY PREVENTED BY
A WHOLE FOOD, PLANT-BASED DIET.

Furthermore, if you already suffer from any of these previously mentioned disorders, you can reverse and possibly cure them by switching to such a lifestyle. This is bad news for the medical industry, but I challenge you to ask any health professional if this is not the case. They will likely agree, but will respond by saying something like, "yeah, but who the hell is gonna do that?"

You see, my colleagues may be aware of such a lifestyle, but are generally unfamiliar with how to prescribe such a diet, or follow it themselves. These are often the same health professionals you'll see slurping down diet soda—the same ones that sat next to me at the HFpEF conference. They clearly had no clue that diet soda contains an artificial sweetener which raises insulin levels in a similar manner to sugar—both of which have the same short and long-term deleterious health effects. These doctors were none-the-wiser, drinking the very problem they were discussing.

Frankenstein Medicine

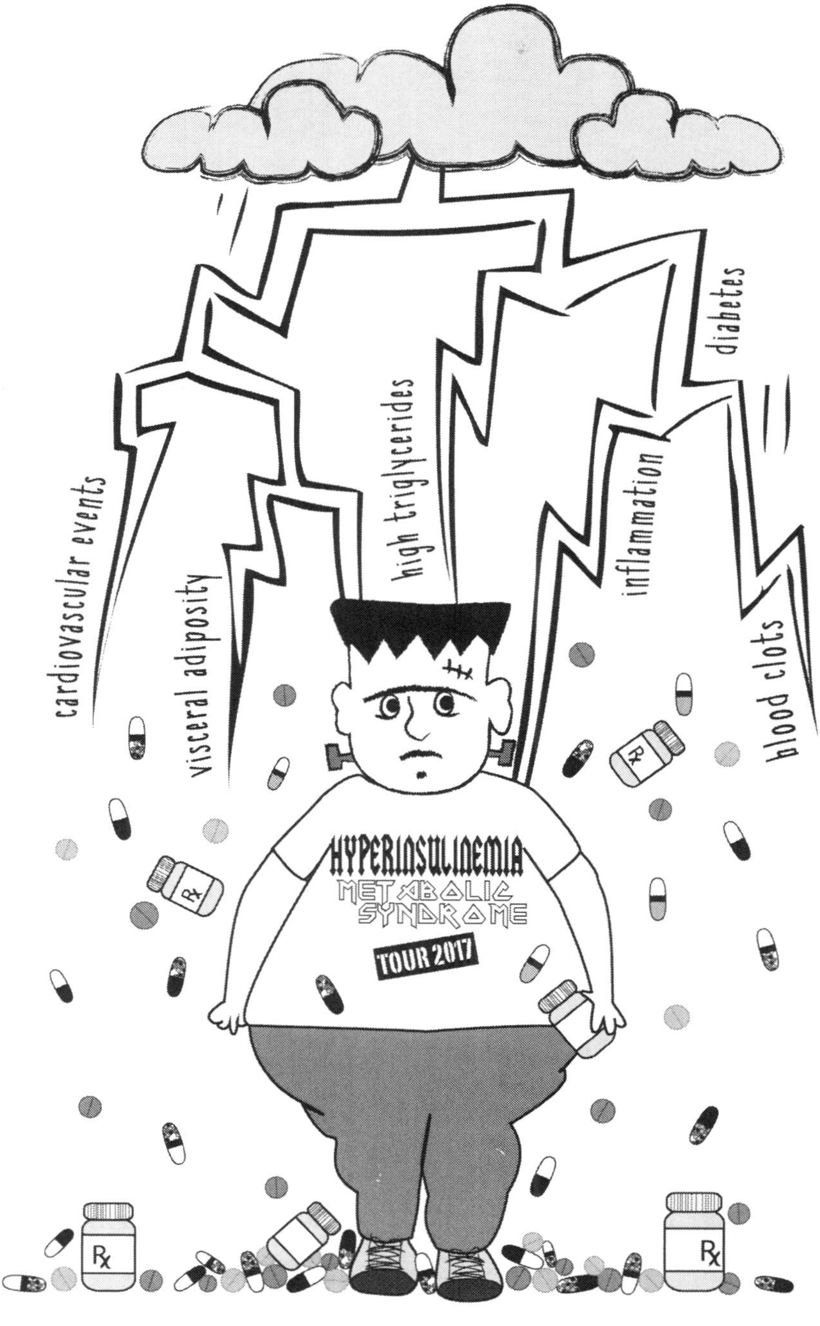

In summary, the professionals out there, with the most extensive medical training in the world, who are supposed to be talking care of you, have for the most part completely given up on you. They are resigned to the fact that they will have plenty of job security for the rest of their careers if they keep playing the pharmaceutical game.

In other words, the general medical field and pharmaceutical industry are enabling you down a one-way street to "unwellness," and are flourishing by your choices as you ease on down that road. This is further compounded by a medical reimbursement system that scores, judges, and reimburses doctors and hospitals by meeting certain benchmarks—which includes the dispensing, administration and monitoring of drugs, and performance of tests and procedures. Conversely, there is NO widespread recommendation for the evaluation, or financial reimbursement for good nutrition.

Please read on and prove the medical establishment wrong. Learn about whole foods and plant foods, and discover how your body thrives off them. Learn how to maintain a healthy, nutritious lifestyle and prevent the development of the metabolic syndrome (and the multitude of other diseases that may come with it). Do not get sucked in to the vortex of processed foods, poor health, expensive polypharmacy, and dependence on a medical system not equipped to pull you out and help get you better.

—Jeffrey A. Rosenblatt, M.D., F.A.C.C.

Chapter 15

What the Fuck is So Special about Whole Foods?!

*We pay the doctor to make us better, when we should
really be paying the farmer to keep us healthy.*
—Robyn O'Brien

What's so special about whole foods? Why should we be
putting the whole in the hole? Did you read the previous
chapters?! Whole foods are made up of the wonderful, untainted,
health-promoting nutrients that rock our bodies' socks off. These
game-changing nutrients are the same gems that get kicked to the
curb once foods are processed, stripped down, packaged up, and
shipped across the world to sit on a shelf for three years. By
having these nutrients be the focus of your diet, you can eliminate
or improve your aches, pains, and disease, and at the same time
steer clear of the doctors who want to pump you full of pills to
manage your shitty diet symptoms. What are *nutrients*?! Calm the
eff down—we're about to find out.

Nutrients are the little parts, or building blocks, of food. Food
is comprised of a shitload of these parts, many of which we're not
even going to discuss. Some are even yet to be classified (in case

you get bored and decide you want to go for a Nobel Prize). In the next few chapters we're going to examine the *largest* nutrients, as well as discover some of the "good" versions and the "not-so-good" versions. We're also going to discuss some trendy terms that people seem to naively use, yet couldn't define if their life depended on it.

The large nutrients we'll be discussing are fats, carbohydrates, and protein, which together are called "macronutrients" (or, in other words, "big-ass nutrients"). If you're still picturing nutrients being the "building blocks" of food, these big-ass nutrients are the blocks that take up the most space in your food. They are also probably the nutrients you have heard about most. We require each big-ass nutrient in a specific amount, and each has a specific function within the body.

Fats

Fats aren't simply the good ol' mounds of "fun" hanging onto your hips. They actually have a purpose, and are used for insulation, protection, and regulation of body temperature. They are also our main source of energy while we're resting. Yes, that's right—you burn more fat at *rest* than you do when you exercise. Take *that* to your next trivia night. Past that, fats also help us keep our skin smooth, hair shiny, and cells functioning properly. Sounds kind of important, right? You might want to mention that to someone next time they tell you they're "cutting out fats."

Carbohydrates

Carbohydrates are the body's main source of energy—specifically for the central nervous system (this includes your *brain*). They're also "protein-sparing," which means they give our bodies energy, so we don't break down our precious protein for energy instead. Fad dieters will most likely tell you to do the opposite: use protein for energy and stay the fuck away from carbs. Please don't (we'll address this topic shortly). People on true low-carb diets are legitimately starving their brains and putting themselves at risk of permanent organ damage. Want to drop your IQ and feel like shit? Cut out carbs.

Proteins

Proteins are used for structure, and provide the framework for hormones and enzymes that help deliver and start chemical reactions within our bodies. They also play an important role in our immune function and fluid balance. Contrary to public belief, they are *not* a main source of energy, nor are they the "best" nutrient. Therefore, next time someone is low on energy and says, "I need to get some protein," punch that person in the protein (e.g. muscle), and then feed them a banana (e.g. carbohydrate).

There you have it: the big-ass nutrients we'll be focusing on. We'll learn about each of their specific roles when it comes to nutrition, and how much of each **we** need. Most importantly, it's important to note that we need all three of the big-ass nutrients to work in unison, and none should ever be considered better than the other. DO YOU HEAR ME? Wrap that concept around your head right now, because it's going to piss me the fuck off if I hear one more person talking about cutting out fats or carbs. You need *all* macronutrients working together at *all* times. That is, if you don't want to look and feel like the Grim Reaper.

Fats, carbohydrates, and protein all have "good" and "not-so-good" options though, and this is where "cutting out" actually becomes important (i.e. you want to cut out the bad options of all three, and aim to consume the beneficial, nourishing options). For instance, a banana is mainly carbohydrates, but so is caramel . . . Pop quiz time! (You must score 100% to continue reading.) Which food—a banana or a piece of caramel—is the *whole* food that contains the health-promoting nutrients?

(Cue Jeopardy theme song.)

I'm not even going to answer that. Can you see why choosing the right *type* of foods becomes so important?!

We also need to understood that most foods contain a combination of fats, carbohydrates, *and* proteins. For example, even though grains are mainly carbohydrates, they also contain fats and proteins. For fuck's sake, spinach is nearly equal parts protein and carbohydrate—who knew? I did! It is nearly impossible to find foods that are *all* fat, *all* carbohydrate, or *all* protein, which has become a huge misconception. Most whole foods contain all *three* macronutrients in various percentages (along with water, fiber, and many other smaller nutrients). Table 15.1 breaks some common foods down for you so you can have a better understanding of this concept.[93]

Table 15.1. Macronutrient percentages in common foods

Food	% Fat	% Carbs	% Protein	% Water
Foods that have more *fats* than carbs or protein				
almonds	50%	22%	21%	4%
pumpkin seeds	50%	11%	30%	5%
cashews	44%	30%	18%	5%
avocado	15%	9%	2%	73%
olives	11%	6%	1%	80%
Foods that have more *carbs* than fats or protein				
black beans*	<1%	24%	9%	66%
wild rice*	<1%	21%	4%	74%
apple	<1%	14%	<1%	86%
raspberries	1%	12%	1%	86%
broccoli	<1%	7%	3%	89%
Foods that have more *protein* than fats or carbs				
spirulina (dried)	8%	24%	57%	5%
chicken breast*	4%	0%	31%	65%
wild salmon*	8%	0%	25%	60%
mussels*	4%	7%	24%	61%
eggs*	11%	2%	12%	75%

*cooked versions

OHMYGOD! Almonds are full of protein?! Pumpkin seeds have the same protein percentage as chicken?! Mind blowing, I know. Foods aren't purely made up of one nutrient—if you want more evidence, head to Appendix C. If you're a super sleuth who realized that none of those percentages add up to 100%, that's because I didn't list all of the smaller nutrients (e.g. vitamins, minerals, phytonutrients), which we will discuss in upcoming chapters. You probably also realized I included water content. Remember when we discussed hydration and how, if you ate plenty of un-fucked-with foods, you'd be closer to being hydrated? I wasn't lying! Check out the amount of water in those bad boys! If you can't stand *drinking* water, eat it.

Before we move on, I want to categorize foods for you. We already discussed this a bit in the last section, and we will discuss it many more times throughout this guide. Pay attention because *where* a nutrient originates makes a huge difference in how it will affect the body. In other words, a protein molecule from a duck will have a different effect than a protein molecule from a carrot, and both will have a different effect than a protein molecule from a processed, piece-o-shit, made-in-a-factory product.

Animal Foods

Animal foods come from an animal—bet you didn't see that one coming. If you're confused about whether or not something came from an animal, ask yourself if it once had a face, or came from something with a face (e.g. a chicken has a face, and an egg came from something that has a face). If you carve a face into a pumpkin, it doesn't count. Examples of animal foods are meats, eggs, and seafood.

Plant Foods

Plant foods come from plants. Catching on yet? If you eat something that never had a face and grew on something attached to or in the ground, it's a plant food. Examples of plant foods are fruits, vegetables, whole grains, herbs, nuts, seeds, and legumes.

Processed Foods

Processed foods are man-made and generally come in a package with an ingredient label. They usually contain a mix of animal foods and plant foods, as well as a bunch of other additives that will hold the newly concocted food together, or to make it look or taste better. Examples of processed foods are yogurts, cheeses, cookies, crackers, pastas, breads, cereals, pastries, sauces, condiments, dressings, microwave dinners, fast foods, and restaurant foods. If someone else has already fucked with it, it's processed.

To summarize, animal foods usually have to be minimally processed or cooked to be consumed, while plant foods can generally be consumed whole or raw. However, most all animal and plant foods will contain a mix of fats, carbohydrates, and proteins. Who knows what processed foods will contain, and frankly who gives a shit, because we're going to start avoiding them anyway.

Here's a fact that will blow your mind: healthier and tastier versions of all processed or packaged foods can actually be made with whole foods, in your own kitchen, with your own two hands. That's no lie. While they would technically then be included in the "processed" category, and would no longer be "whole," at least *you* did the processing, and know exactly what went into it.

Moral of the Story:

Food is made up of numerous types of nutrients, and can also be categorized into animal foods, plant foods, and processed foods. If you give two shits about your long-term health, you'll learn which types of foods to avoid, you'll head straight for the whole foods, and you'll chow down on the best, most untainted nutrients.

Chapter 16

The Facts on Fats

Remember what the doc said: you don't get fat by eating fat. You get fat by having a fucked-up diet, which leads to an over-production of insulin, which leads to the metabolic syndrome . . . which leads to saddlebags, muffin tops, and caskets.

As we have already discussed, fats are available in most foods and are a vital part of our energy needs. Thus, it's imperative we pie-hole them. We just need to be sure we're make wise choices, as there are foods that offer "good" fats, and foods that offer "not-so good" fats.

"Good" fats are generally liquid when isolated (think oils), and are found in abundance in foods like avocados, nuts, and seeds (i.e. plant foods). Notice how I said they're found *in* those foods. I'm talking about eating those foods *whole*—not slurping up the oil. Less optimal fats are generally solid at room temperature (think white chunky stuff), and are generally found in, or attached to, foods like beef, chicken, and pork (i.e. animal foods). Last but not least, the *really* shitty, destructive, damaging fats are—drum roll please—made by humans!

Side note: please stop buying low-fat or non-fat foods. Why? Let me ask you this: when was the last time you saw a low-fat avocado or a non-fat almond? None of the "good" fatty foods have low-fat options—they're simply whole foods. If something *does* have a low-fat option, it automatically means it's been highly

145

processed in order to have the fat removed (and most likely had a lot of sugar or other shit added). The less a food is fucked with, the better. Put the whole in the hole, remember?

Ideally, the average individual needs around 20%–35% of their calories from "good" fats.[94] For those of you who haven't jumped on the math wagon yet, that's around a *third* of your calories from fat (so you better be damn sure you're getting the right kinds). To help you understand where the "right kinds" come from, here are some fat-related terms for you to familiarize yourself with:

Trans Fats

You've probably heard of these jerks, but may not know quite how to define them. These would be the man-made fats that are highly destructive to the body and should be avoided at all costs. I'm not joking. If you regularly consume trans fats, you will most definitely wind up with a pretty shitty disease. Why are they being made by man if they're so destructive, you ask? GOOD FUCKING QUESTION. Apparently, they are "needed" in processed foods to make them more stable and less likely to spoil—because shelf life is obviously more important than health. Avoid processed foods, avoid trans fats.

Trans fats naturally exist in some animal products as well though, and the verdict seems to still be out on whether or not they're on the good list. They appear to be "less destructive" than the man-made versions, but the studies also seem to have been funded by the same industries being investigated. Sirens! Red flag! More sirens![95-97]

In my opinion, if something has trans fats in it (specifically the man-made ones), it should have an alarm that flashes bright red lights and blares the following warning at you if you get near it: "Hello Consumer! If you pie-hole me regularly, you will most likely get heart disease. You may also wind up with Alzheimer's, cancer, diabetes, liver dysfunction, infertility, and depression!! PUT ME THE FUCK DOWN IF YOU WANT TO LIVE!!"

Many countries have completely banned the use of trans fats in foods because of how shitty they are— some for over a decade![98] In the US . . . not so much. The scary thing is, in the US not only are trans fats allowed, but if a product contains less than half a gram, the manufacturer can pretend they're not there and officially claim "zero trans fats" on their label.[99] *Any* amount of trans fats are bad though, so the fact that some foods might have them, yet claim "zero trans fats," is terrifying and infuriatingly wrong—because who is keeping track of how many of those "zero trans fats" foods someone is packing away? That shit adds up! Do you feel that? That's the feeling of you being screwed by companies that are supposed to be trustworthy and provide us with healthy food. If you're not angry, check your pulse.

Since trans fats are packed into processed foods, it means they should have a nutrition label, and should be listed (unless the amount is less than 0.5g, then hey, let's pretend they're not there). To fool you even more, trans fats may also be listed as "partially hydrogenated oil" in the ingredient list. So, if something claims "zero trans fats," yet has partially hydrogenated oil listed, it *does* have trans fats, and you should throw it in the incinerator. Here's where the little bitches can commonly be found:

- baked goods (e.g. cookies, crackers, cakes, pie crusts, pizza dough, hamburger buns);
- fried foods (e.g. donuts, french fries, fried chicken, chicken nuggets, taco shells);
- snack foods (e.g. potato chips, corn chips, tortilla chips, candy, microwave popcorn);
- solid fats or spreads (e.g. margarine, vegetable shortening); and
- pre-mix products (e.g. cake mix, pancake mix, drink mixes).

Now, at this point, I shouldn't have to say it, but none of those items listed above should be of concern to you if you're focusing on whole, healthy foods. However, because I feel the need to expose the bullshit that food companies are pulling—even if it's irrelevant to the foods you *should* be eating—I will continue to try to burn down their integrity and character. Because, I can.

Check this out: It was back in *1999* when the FDA first proposed that trans fats may not be safe and should be labeled. Seven (seven!) years later, that proposal was put into effect, and all processed foods had to label their trans fat content. Seven fucking years. Fast forward another seven years, and in 2013 the FDA finally recognized that trans fats *were,* in fact, the devil. They requested scientific information from researchers so they could potentially ban them from consumer products . . . yet no ban in the US as of yet.[100] This trans fat danger debate has now been going on for fifteen years and has not been resolved. Case in point: don't fucking trust the additives the FDA approves, because you might be dead before they get their shit together and ban them. Still not angry? I hereby officially declare you a robot.

Ketone Bodies

These little guys are produced from fat molecules, and are used as energy during "times of starvation" (i.e. going without eating for an extended period of time). For instance, if you don't provide your body with the right amount of carbohydrates—which we have learned are our main fuel source—then it will have to compensate by producing ketone bodies from fat instead. This sounds ridiculously awesome to most people, because they merely want to "burn that belly fat!" Unfortunately, it doesn't work like that—and we're not here to trick our bodies into doing anything other than what's naturally supposed to happen—so keep reading.

Most people have ketone bodies running around their system, and most people's bodies can keep up with either using them for energy or peeing them out. However, if the level of ketone bodies rises past "normal," the body is considered to be in a state of "ketosis." Ketosis won't kill ya, it simply means you may get some bad gas or your breath might stink a bit (but both should still be considered red flags that you're headed in the wrong direction on that Nutrition Spectrum).

The situation could get worse if the level of ketone bodies *continues* to rise though, and your body isn't capable of clearing them fast enough. This happens, for example, if you continuously follow a low-carb diet, and your body has to continuously produce ketones to try to get energy. What happens next is your enters a state called "ketoacidosis" (another long-ass word you need not worry about pronouncing correctly) . . . and this is where shit really begins to hit the fan. Ketoacidosis *is* dangerous and can cause liver and kidney damage, and in rare instances, death. How do you avoid ketoacidosis? Avoid excess ketones, which are produced if you cut the carbs. In other words, you need to make sure you eat adequate amounts of your (good) carbs, so you have plenty of energy and your body won't go batshit crazy producing ketone bodies for energy instead. It is still entirely possible to "burn fat" and return to a healthy weight by doing this—I promise.

The Omegas

You have most likely heard of at least one of the omegas (omega-3, omega-6, or omega-9), but it's rare for people understand what they *do*. Furthermore, it seems that people want to rapidly and forcefully get omega-3s in their pie-hole (usually via supplement), without knowing if they're getting enough in their diet as it is.

Each omega works its magic in its own, unique way. Omega-3s and omega-6s work together to balance inflammation and clotting within our bodies. One *suppresses* inflammation and break up clots (omega-3s), and one *promotes* inflammation and creates clots (omega-6s). It's a balance system, and as you can probably conclude, if you eat too few omega-3s, and a shit load of omega 6s, your body will be headed straight down inflammation, blood clot lane towards Diseaseland (a common finding in western diets). All disease starts with inflammation, so this is an important topic to master.

The omega-9s can actually be made in our bodies, thus are rarely an issue when it comes to deficiency (since our bodies are kick-ass and know exactly how much we need). Similar to the omega-6s, they also have a healthy inflammation response within the body, and provide benefits like lowering cholesterol.

Overall, the omegas have a lot to do with controlling inflammation and clotting, but need to be consumed in the right ratios in order to be effective. Specifically, your omega-3s consumption should be similar to that of your omega-6 consumption. Unfortunately, most western diets see *omega-6* consumption up to *twenty-five* times that of their omega-3 consumption.[101, 102] You didn't misread that (hence all of the disease floating around in our world). Check out table 16.1 to see which foods contain which omegas.

Table 16.1. Foods with high levels of omega-3s, -6s, and -9s

Omega-3s	Omega-6s	Omega-9s
wild salmon	safflower oil	olives/olive oil
mackerel	grapeseed oil	avocados
anchovies	wheat germ oil	almonds
walnuts	soybean oil	peanuts
flaxseed	sunflower oil	sesame oil
chia seeds	canola oil	pistachio nuts
green leafy veggies	corn oil	cashews

After processing that information, you may be able to see why people wind up with an omega imbalance: the standard western diet offers too many omega 6s (oils), and too few omega 3s (whole foods). Furthermore, this standard diet is generally also full of the shitty trans fats we just read about—which completely interfere with our body's ability to utilize omega 3s. This way of eating obviously allows everyone's omega-6 levels to skyrocket (because there's minimal omega 3s to balance them out), which then starts the process of promoting inflammation and blood clots—both of which open the door to a long list of diseases. Most people are aware of the issues that blood clots can cause (e.g. heart attack, stroke, deep vein thrombosis), but what about inflammation? She's a bitch too. All of the following diseases stem from chronic inflammation:[103]

allergies	celiac disease	GERD
Alzheimer's	Crohn's disease	lupus
anemia	congestive heart	migraines
asthma	failure	multiple sclerosis
autism	diabetes	neuropathy
arthritis	eczema	pancreatitis
carpal tunnel	fibromyalgia	psoriasis
syndrome	fibrosis	rheumatoid arthritis

If you want to avoid that long list of ailments, as well as battle depression, fatigue, ADHD, bipolar disorder, memory loss, dementia, heart disease, stroke, and cancer—all of which omega 3s can improve—you'll balance out your omegas.[104] It's as simple as that.

Most people on typical western diets need to consume more omega-3s, and less oily, greasy foods that are full of omega-6s. Ooooh goody! Omega-3s! I have been doing a good thing by supplementing them in copious amounts on a daily basis! No. While getting more omega-3s in your diet can help you battle all of those above mentioned ailments, you'll want to get them from untainted, whole foods. Once they're in a capsule, or away from the food from which they originated, they become less effective, or not at all effective.[105-109] Stay away from the pills—you are not a pill-popper. You are a food-eater.

On a similar note, since most people are lacking omega-3s (or need to offset their high level of omega-6s), many processed foods are now being fortified with omega-3s. Unfortunately, this is purely another stinky marketing tool, as these products don't provide anywhere *near* a significant amount—or an effective version—of them. They just draw the naive customer in. Eating real, whole foods with real omegas-3s is the only way to truly solve the problem. Now go wipe that oil off your chin and eat some walnuts!

Triglycerides

Triglycerides are the end product of the dietary fat you eat and digest . . . but the story doesn't end there. After you fill your pie-hole, and after digestion, if there are any nutrients *left over* that aren't needed, your body will convert them to triglycerides. These little dudes swim around in your blood and are then stored away in your fat cells, to hopefully later be released and used as energy. Therefore, triglycerides aren't necessarily "bad." However, if you continuously shove too much food down your pie-hole, and continuously have leftover nutrients that your body doesn't need, you will have increasingly higher levels of triglycerides hanging out in your system. An increase in triglycerides means an increase in the risk of heart disease. For the LOVE OF GOD, stop over-packing that pie-hole.

Cholesterol

Cholesterol is similar to triglycerides in that it's a type of fat molecule that circulates in your blood. However, cholesterol has a different purpose than triglycerides, and can also be categorized into a couple different types. Let me first start off by saying that, like triglycerides, cholesterol is not "bad" per se. Your body needs cholesterol, and in fact, makes it all by itself. Wow! What the heck *doesn't* our body do?! Shit we're amazing.

On top of making your own cholesterol, you can also ingest cholesterol (mainly **from** the consumption of animal products). However, like triglycerides, if you have *too much* cholesterol circulating in your system, that's when things become a clusterfuck and you wind up jumping on the disease-wagon.

If you find yourself amid this clusterfuck, you'll want to know about the two types of cholesterol and how they work. HDL (which stands for "high-density lipoprotein," in case you were wondering . . . but you probably weren't) is the "good cholesterol" and can protect against heart disease and stroke. You want to be sure your HDL is topped up at all times.

LDL (or "low-density lipoprotein") is the "not-so good" cholesterol, and you'll want to keep this level low. These little bitches create plaque buildup in your arteries, and will lead to heart attack and stroke. Little party poopers, I say!

Here's the confusing part: it's unclear whether or not eating foods containing cholesterol actually increases your cholesterol levels. Once upon a time, this was deemed the surefire way to get heart disease—eat lots of cholesterol-laden, fatty foods, get heart disease. It doesn't work like that though. Instead, the *types* of fats you consume will have the greatest impact on your cholesterol levels. Therefore, rather than running from cholesterol, run from the processed foods and "not-so good" fats.

* * *

Here are some examples of foods abundant in fats (more are listed in Appendix C). For fuck's sake, please choose whole, organically grown, fresh, unprocessed versions when possible. And run like there's a lion chasing you if you see anything containing trans fats (a.k.a. partially hydrogenated oils).

Foods with Healthier Fats

- avocados
- olives
- nuts (e.g. almonds, walnuts, pistachios)
- nut butters (e.g. cashew butter, almond butter)
- wild fish (e.g. salmon, mackerel)
- seeds (e.g. sunflower, sesame, flax, chia, pumpkin)
- organically grown soy

Foods with Less-Healthy Fats

- deli meats
- high-fat cuts of meat, or meat with skin on
- creams (e.g. sour, heavy, ice)
- spreads (e.g. butter, margarine)
- vegetable shortening
- packaged snack foods (e.g. crackers, chips, microwave popcorn)
- fried foods

Moral of the Story:

A third of your calories should come from fats, so stop trying to hide from them. Instead, rip into the non-processed, whole foods that have healthy fats.

Chapter 17

Cut the Cutting Carbs Crap

If you haven't heard the terms "good carbs" and "bad carbs," you've been living under a fucking rock. Perhaps you're one of those cavemen dieters and you're really trying to play the role. Who am I to judge? Either way, get out from under the rock.

People seem to blab about carbs more than any other nutrition topic. Unfortunately, they usually wind up sounding pretty uneducated—mainly because they consider all carbs to be "bad carbs," or believe that carbs only come from foods like bread and pasta. Alternatively, they simply use the term "carbs" too generically: "Ugghh, I need to stay away from the carbs!" . . . then they go eat a banana, which has around twenty times more carbs than protein. Don't be that guy. Saying you're going to "cut all carbs" is like saying that no one should have a cat as a pet because lions are dangerous. There are, in fact, good versions and not-so good versions. It's time to educate yourself on what "carbs" actually means, and to stop misusing the term—because that's the number one way to shout, "I don't know a fucking thing about nutrition!"

So here we go, it's time to bust into the world of carbohydrates. The amusing part about this is that the more carbs you eat, the more you'll actually be able to learn. You see, carbohydrates power our brains (and therefore the rest of our bodies). Thus, if you want to boost your IQ, eat some carbs. Even if you're a caveman, that tiny-ass brain still needs to be fueled with carbs (how else are you going to discover fire?).

As always though, the *type* of carbs you choose is extremely important. "Good" carbs are found in whole foods like fruits, vegetables, whole grains, herbs, and legumes (beans, lentils, peas). Some of the most nutritious foods on this planet are mainly made up mainly of carbs. Starting to feel like an ass yet? Don't worry, you're not alone. "Not-so good" carbs are usually found in highly refined, processed foods that have ingredients like white sugar and high fructose corn syrup (e.g. cookies, candy bars, ice cream). They also include refined bread, pasta, and rice. If you need a refresher about our society's addiction to processed carbs, head back to chapter 14 and re-read. It's the processed carbs that are fucking us up.

There are studies that have shown that kids who eat more sugary junk food (i.e. "not-so good carbs"), and less veggies, beans, and grains (i.e. "good carbs"), will have a reduced IQ and attention span.[110] Makes sense. Thus, if you choose to regularly give your child "bad carbs" (i.e. highly processed, shitty food-like-substances), you are undeniably dumbing them down. If you didn't know, it's not your fault. Now that you *do* know, please go purge your fridge and pantry of all things sugary and processed so your brain (and everyone else's brain) can breathe. I'm serious—I'll wait.

For those of you who believe that completely "cutting out carbs" is the answer, please remember that carbohydrates are hiding out in most all whole foods. If you truly want to eat carb-free (please don't), then be prepared to live off of the following:

butter	oils
non-processed or cured fish	organs
non-processed or cured meats	shellfish & mollusks

Bon appétit! Can't wait to see the variety of gourmet meals you can dream up from that list of edibles! Fruits, vegetables, beans and whole grains would be goners. If you think for a second you can survive (much less be healthy) on those no-carb foods, then you need to head straight back to page one and start this guide over (I'll wait right here if you need to—no hard feelings). It would be *impossible* for you to get all of the wonderful disease-fighting nutrients that are only found in "good" carbohydrate-rich foods. You would definitely wind up sick, and most likely have the IQ of a fork.

Ideally, the average individual needs about 45%–65% of their calories from "good" carbohydrates. Yes, you read that right. If you're hyperventilating and need to head to a meeting for carbophobics, now's your chance). *Half* of your nutrients should come from carbohydrates.[94] Again, I'm talking about *whole* foods with untainted, health-promoting nutrients. Processed carbs should be kicked to the curb; especially the ones boasting "low carb" levels. Let's take some time and boost your brain power by discussing some carb-related terms.

Fiber

Fiber, or more specifically, "dietary fiber" (not to be confused with optical fibers, clearly) is only found in plant foods, and is crucial for optimal health. It has shown to significantly reduce one's risk of certain ailments like colon and breast cancer.[111-113] Another point to the plant foods! Here's how fiber can specifically help you:

- Fiber provides a feeling of "fullness" by increasing food *volume* without increasing calories. It is nearly impossible to over-eat if you consume high-fiber foods.[114, 115] Thus, if you're struggling with over-eating, try consuming a ton of plant-derived, whole foods, and you'll zap that problem in no time. Whoop!
- Fiber helps regulate blood sugar levels by controlling the absorption of sugar in the stomach (therefore reducing the risk of diabetes).[114, 115] Whoop whoop!

- Fiber helps lower overall cholesterol as well as the "not-so good" (LDL) cholesterol (therefore reducing the risk of cardiovascular disease).[114, 115] Triple whoop!
- Fiber helps reduce your risk of certain cancers.
- Fiber helps regulate your bowel movements by moving foods through your pipes and by making your poop more tolerable (fiber binds water to poop, which makes it softer, reduces constipation, and therefore likely reduces the risk of colorectal cancer).[114-116] No more razorblade poops! So many WHOOPS!

Fiber is extremely important and only comes from plants. Therefore, eat your damn plants if you want to decrease your risk of disease and encourage the sandpaper poop that's been stuck in your bowel for a week. But first, here are some facts that will be handy to know before you start shoveling high-fiber foods down your pie-hole:

- If you don't eat much fiber now, and suddenly pack your system full of fiber, you're going to experience some pretty awesome gas and bloating. Fiber is something you want to increase *gradually* over several weeks.
- If you don't increase your water intake at the same time (if you're not super hydrated already), then you're going to wind up feeling like you're pooping glass. Do yourself a favor and gradually increase your fiber *at the same time* you increase your water intake.
- Since fiber has a "filling" effect, it's important to note whether or not you're actually getting all of the nutrients you need before you feel full. I have people tell me they're "not hungry," after they've barely eaten anything. This is because the food they've eaten is so high in fiber that they feel like they can't eat anything else. They then wind up malnourished because they're not actually eating enough food. This is where balance and variety come into play, which we will discuss later **on**.

Glycemic Index (GI)

If you're still panicking about the fact that all carbohydrates are made up of sugar molecules—even good carbohydrates—please take a time out. Remember, it's the *rate* at which carbs are broken down that becomes important—not simply the fact that carbs are made up of sugars. Foods that are broken down *faster* create higher spikes in blood sugar, and can have a more damaging effect on your body if consumed chronically. When I say, "damaging," I'm talking about ailments like type II diabetes, heart disease, infertility, colon cancer, and macular degeneration, to name a few.[117-123] We're talking *chronic* consumption here. People who continuously shove processed foods down their pie-hole will most likely become a permanent patient of a disease manager, and *will* wind up buying a forever-home in Diseaseland.

This is where the glycemic index comes into play, which was touched upon back in chapter 14. This rating system shows which carbohydrate-rich foods will fuck with your blood sugar levels the most. The foods with the higher scores will affect your blood sugar more (stimulating more insulin to be released), and the lower numbers, less. The confusing part is that one food could have multiple numbers depending on how it is cooked or prepared (which is why you may see foods with conflicting numbers on different indexes). Either way, familiarize yourself with it. I know a lot of people who don't eat, for example, oranges because they think they're high in sugar. Then they go on to devour potatoes like they're going extinct, unaware that the potatoes will have a much higher impact on their sugar levels.

This list represents a sample glycemic index and is nowhere near complete.[124] If you're curious about a food that isn't listed here, Google it.

Sample Glycemic Index

103—dates
100—glucose
97—parsnip
92—scone
90—potato chip
90—mashed potato
85—white hamburger bun
85—baked potato
80—pizza
78—rice cake
78—Gatorade
76—waffle
76—donut
75—pumpkin
75—french fries
72—watermelon
72—popcorn
71—white bread
71—millet
70—Weetabix
70—sweet potato
68—cranberry juice
65—white sugar
65—raw sugar
65—couscous
65—cantaloupe
64—white rice
64—raisin
64—beetroot
63—corn chips
63—Coca Cola
61—ice cream

59—pineapple
58—porridge
57—apricots
55—honey
55—brown rice
55—blackstrap molasses
54—maple syrup
54—buckwheat
53—wheat bread
53—sweet corn
53—quinoa
53—kiwi fruit
52—orange juice
52—banana
51—mango
50—canned peas
50—boiled potato
49—muesli
48—bulgur
46—grapes
42—white pasta
42—peach
42—orange
42—All-Bran cereal
40—whole wheat cereal
40—whole grain pasta
40—unsweetened apple juice
40—strawberry
40—fresh peas

39—plum
38—pear
38—apple
35—wild rice
35—Indian corn
35—fig
35—coconut sugar
35—carrot
29—lentils
28—kidney beans
28—chickpeas
25—grapefruit
25—barley
22—cherries
22—cashews
20—black bean
18—soy bean
15—lettuce
15—cucumber
15—bell pepper
15—asparagus
15—artichoke
15—apricot
10—agave nectar
<15—tomato, garlic, eggplant, spinach, zucchini, broccoli, peanuts, cabbage, cauliflower, celery, coconut water, mushrooms

Now does this mean that you should never eat dates again? Of course not. It means that the carbohydrate-rich foods that you *regularly* consume should be low GI foods, thus having less of an effect on your blood sugar and insulin levels, and lowering your risk of disease. Foods that you enjoy consuming that score *high* on the index should not be staples in your diet . . . unless you're on the "scone diet," which I'm sure (at the rate we're going) will be a "thing" some day.

Going further, there are foods you should eat even *less* frequently than infrequently (i.e. never), and most of these foods didn't make it onto my glycemic index. Let's use Mountain Dew as an example. That fluorescent monkey piss is full of refined sugar (thus would wind up high on the glycemic index). It's also full of chemicals and enough caffeine to pogo-stick your way to the moon. Therefore, you still need to use your noggin and eliminate foods that will really screw you up—they're not worth it even *infrequently*.

Something such as dates though—which are obviously a whole food, and are listed with a rating of 103—are interesting. Even though they can spike your blood sugar, sometimes that's needed (and when it *is* needed, reaching for an organically grown, whole food is a much better option than reaching for a lab-concocted product). This mainly comes into play with endurance athletes. After they've burned off all of their stored energy, they need a quick option to get more immediate fuel to sustain the activity they're involved in. They could basically eat anything and burn it right off. The higher on the glycemic index, the quicker that fuel will be available to them. However, even though they're going to burn it right off, they still need to consider their health. Dates are a much healthier choice than the crap-filled bars and gels that are marketed towards athletes these days.

The same concept applies to people who are experiencing dangerously low blood sugar levels. They want to consume the healthiest food option that won't leave chemical residue in their system. In other words, if a diabetic is having a low-sugar issue, and the options are either dates or donuts, feed them dates.

Sweeteners

Everyone has seen some sort of sweetener in their lifetime — whether it be the little packets of artificial granulated chemicals that are so conveniently placed on every restaurant table on the planet, or something like natural, raw, certified organic honey straight from your local beekeeper. Regardless of what type you're getting high on, all sweeteners are comprised mostly of sugar (or artificial sugar). Like everything else, we're going to learn about the healthier sweeteners, and the array of chemical shit-storm sweeteners that are manufactured and advertised to the unknowing consumer as being the "best low-calorie sweetener around!"

Let's not be complete jackasses though; it's always best to eat your food and beverages *without* sweeteners. I don't use any sort of sweetener regularly, and I haven't croaked from over-eating "bland" food yet. I put "bland" in quotation marks because real food isn't actually bland. However, if you're used to dousing everything in a blanket of sweetness, then of course it will taste bland to you and your sugar-craving taste buds. I, on the other hand, can actually taste my food! The actual *food* — not the sugar disguising it. However, I frequently get asked about sweeteners, so I'm going to discuss the current popular and trendy ones. Your goal should be to either learn how to *not* need them, or to use them sparingly enough that you can actually discover what real food tastes like.

Agave Syrup

Sometimes called agave "nectar," agave is a runny, snot-like liquid that is produced from the agave plant (a big, blue-green, spiky thing). It is often compared to honey, but is actually sweeter and has a thinner consistency. Many vegans use agave as a substitute for honey, and many diabetics use it because of its low glycemic number. A lot of people don't use it at all, because there's no need to use it! There is also some controversy surrounding it, as when it boomed onto the market and had to keep up with sales, it suddenly became a mass-produced, nutrient-void, high-fructose syrup. As a result, if you're going to use agave and want to avoid the mass-produced fake crap, your best bet is to go get an agave plant and squeeze the shit out of it.

Coconut Sugar

This sweetener is produced from the sap of a *flower* that grows on a coconut palm tree; it's not extracted from an actual coconut. Since it doesn't come from a coconut, it doesn't taste like coconut (big misconception there); it actually has a slight caramel flavor. It also differs from "palm sugar" which is produced from other palm trees.

Coconut sugar is produced in the same way maple sugar is produced (by "tapping"), can come in different consistencies (e.g. crystals, block, liquid), and is rich in many healthy minerals. It is also considered "safer" for diabetics due to being lower on the glycemic index.

Honey

Commercial honey is produced by the honeybee, and you may want to cover your ears (close your eyes?) for this one, but bees produce honey by consuming and then regurgitating flower nectar. Say what?! Mmmmmm . . . regurgitated nectar (this is why it's a no-go for vegans). Honey tastes fantastic though (I wonder what it tasted like before it came back up . . .), and there are many different varieties, grades, flavors and colors, depending on which flower the nectar came from, or how much it has been filtered or pasteurized (i.e. heated).

Not only is honey loaded with wonderful enzymes, vitamins, and minerals, but it also has a shitload of wonderful antioxidants as well as antibacterial and anti-fungal properties (go ahead—slap it on that jock itch). The coolest thing about honey, though, is that it doesn't go bad when stored properly (so that honey you just put on your crotch should be good until you're six feet under). Archeologists have actually found pots of honey that are thousands of years old and are *still* good enough to throw in your tea.[125] Or, on your crotch. Ah-mazing. If I need a sweetener for something, I choose honey. Preferably a local, unpasteurized, raw honey, because once honey is pasteurized, it loses most of its beneficial nutrients (so search out the more solid, murky honey). I also make a kick-ass throat and cough syrup out of honey, ginger, and lemon. It has been sitting in my fridge for seven hundred years and—to this day—is still soothing throats.

Maple Syrup

I am a maple syrup snob. I'm from Vermont for fuck's sake—my blood is like 30% maple syrup. I refuse to eat maple syrup from anywhere else (especially the fake-ass Aunt Jemima or Golden Syrup imitations).

The delicious golden goop is produced similarly to coconut sugar by tapping and collecting the sap from the sugar maple tree. WARNING: You cannot simply suck the sap out of the tree (I discovered this the hard way around age seven—friggin' GROSS). After processing the sap, the final product is high in antioxidants. But, like any sweetener, that doesn't mean you go drink a bucket of it on its own. Save your 100% pure *Vermont* maple syrup for a special occasion, and then savor the gooey goodness in all its glory.

Molasses

Ahhh molasses, my archenemy. I can't stand the shit, but don't let me deter you. I used to think it was collected from greasy car engines. I was wrong. In actuality, when plain sugar is processed, a dark, sticky, thick liquid is produced, and this becomes molasses. It has some great properties, like being high in potassium, iron, and calcium, but unfortunately smells and tastes like a hockey player's groin after the third period. Okay, that's my opinion, but it does have an extremely pungent aroma and taste, and therefore should be used in recipes that can support it.

"Blackstrap molasses" is a version of molasses that, in all seriousness, resembles tar. Or, meconium (a baby's first poop, for you non-parents out there). It simply comes from older sugarcane and has more health benefits than the molasses produced from the younger sugarcane (including a significantly less amount of sugar). Therefore, if you must consume molasses (don't do it!), choose the blackstrap version.

Raw Sugar

Don't be fooled. Raw sugar is simply a less-refined version of white table sugar, produced from sugarcane (and sometimes the sugar beet). Since it is "less-refined," it still has a bit of the molasses component in it, giving it its brown appearance and slightly different flavor. What is boils down to, is that you're merely consuming a fancier-looking, more expensive version of white sugar. Suckah!

Stevia

I liken tasting pure stevia to being tasered while taking a triple shot of moonshine. It'll knock you on your arse. The extract is something like three hundred times sweeter than sugar. The only problem is that it is extremely rare to find 100% pure stevia these days (which is extracted from a green leafy plant). Most companies (e.g. Truvia) put "other" ingredients in their stevia to dilute it and take it down a notch. This makes them a stevia *blend*, and no longer pure or natural. Pure stevia should be measured in "smidges" or "pinches," never in teaspoons or tablespoons (unless you really *are* looking to knock yourself on your ass). If you buy "stevia" and it says a serving is equal to one teaspoon (or similar), you've purchased a stevia blend that has had other shit added to it (which should be indicated on the label).

If you must buy stevia, stay away from the blends and buy the real thing. The package should only have one ingredient: "stevia," and will most likely be found at a natural grocer. Most people use stevia because it doesn't have any calories. Fuck yeah! Most people also unknowingly purchase the stevia *blends* and are therefore consuming other shit besides stevia. Fuck no! So hey, if you want to get healthy, how about not consuming stevia (or any sweetener), period?

Table Sugar

This is the stuff we blindly scoop by the cup and dump into recipes. It's also the stuff that's deceivingly thrown into most processed food products on the market so they taste halfway decent (even something seemingly good like organic almond milk). Unfortunately, looking on a label won't help the untrained eye, as most food companies try to disguise the fact that sugar is in their product by labeling it something other than "sugar" (e.g. sucrose, maltose, dextrose, fructose, glucose, galactose, lactose, high fructose corn syrup, glucose solids, cane juice, dehydrated can juice, dextrin, maltodextrin, fruit juice, fruit juice concentrate, dehydrated fruit juice). Don't be fooled. It's all sugar, and it's all the devil.

Basic table sugar comes from the sugarcane or sugar beet, and simply by *looking* at it you should know it's highly processed (that bright, white, perfectly crystallized sugar was *not* born that way). There are too many health risks to discuss when it comes to sugar consumption without risking this book becoming several volumes long. Head back to chapter 14 if you want a glimpse into the world of what-happens-when-you-chronically-consume-sugar. If you don't want your teeth to rot, and don't want to wind up with some shitty disease, learn to eat foods without hidden sugars, and steer clear of recipes that call for *cups* of sugar. You may as well just go eat a bag of sugar, because you sure as shit aren't going to taste any of the other ingredients that may be accompanying it. Time to start rockin' that sugar detox, people.

Artificial Sweeteners

These fuckers are in a league of their own. They go by names such as aspartame, neotame, saccharin, sucralose, and acesulfame, and you will find them branded with names such as NutraSweet, Equal, Sweet'N Low, Splenda, and Sweet One. They are found in almost all processed "foods" and "beverages" that boast they're low or no calorie. Basically, if you're eating something that *contains* artificial sweeteners, you're eating something highly processed that's most likely nutrient-void to begin with. If you're *adding* it to something, then you don't get the point of eating for health. "But, they don't have any calories!" Of course they don't; when shit is made in a lab, it won't have calories! Calories-schmalories. This isn't about weight loss, this is about health. This shit will fuck you up and spit you out. If you want to be healthy, you'll eat *real* food, not a chemical powder made in a lab. We'll specifically touch on the evil of all evils—aspartame—later on. That doesn't give you permission to drink your diet soda until then; tip the shit out, I mean it.

Let's pause for a moment and pretend we're not craving something sweet. In the big scheme of things, if you're focusing on filling up your daily calorie allowance on kick-ass health-promoting nutrients from whole foods, sweeteners shouldn't even be a thought in your mind. *Maaaaybe* you soothe your sore throat with honey a few times a year. *Maaaaybe* you use coconut sugar to bake a cake on your birthday. Or, *maaaaybe* you discover that adding something like applesauce, raisins, or dates to a recipe can be a great alternative to a sweetener.

* * *

Whew. We made it through the carb section without getting fat! Here are some examples of foods abundant in carbs (more are listed in Appendix C). Please choose whole, organically grown, fresh, unprocessed versions when possible. Try your darndest to avoid processed foods and beverages, as these are the foods that will, over time, drag you to Diseaseland. And for shit's sake—stop fucking dumping sugar on everything.

Foods with Healthier Carbohydrates
- vegetables (e.g. carrots, asparagus, broccoli, spinach)
- fruits (e.g. apricots, raspberries, cherries, grapefruit, apples)
- whole grains (e.g. brown rice, oats, buckwheat, rye, barley)
- legumes (e.g. green/brown/yellow lentils, garbanzo beans, split peas, kidney beans, black beans)
- nuts (e.g. pistachios, pecans, almonds, cashews, walnuts)
- minimally-processed, home-made foods (e.g. whole grain bread, whole grain pasta)

Foods with Less-Healthy Carbohydrates
- refined grains (e.g. pizza crust, white pastas, breads, rice)
- highly-processed foods (e.g. cake, candy, chips, cookies)
- beverages (e.g. soda, chocolate and mocha drinks, energy drinks)
- sweeteners (artificial and natural)

Moral of the Story:
Fear not the whole, high-carb foods. After all, half of your diet should come from them. Instead, fear the artificial and highly processed, nutrient-void, full-of-additives carbs that have been produced by none other than our very own food system.

Chapter 18

The Protein Pedestal

They say that vegetable food is not sufficiently nutritious.
But chemistry proves the contrary. So does physiology. So does experience.
And again: the largest and strongest animals in the world are those which eat
no flesh-food of any kind—the elephant and the rhinoceros.
—Russell Trall, MD

Proteins are the most worshiped, misunderstood, over-emphasized, and over-marketed nutrient—which means they are generally considered the "go-to" nutrient for people who are uneducated about nutrition. It has been this way for a long time, mainly because people keep putting pride before health. Heck, the word itself comes from the Greek word "proteos," meaning: "of prime importance." The protein pedestal bullshit needs to end.

The protein saga began back in the 1800s with a German chap by the name of Carl Voit. He was one of the first scientists to set protein recommendations for the highly-respected nutrient. This came after he discovered the average person needed about 48.5 grams of protein per day.[126] Yet, when it came time to make recommendations, he suggested *118 grams* instead—more than *double* his findings. Silly Carl (what the fuck, Carl?!). He clearly didn't want to be the one to break the bad news to everyone.

Then—if *that* wasn't bad enough—one of Carl's students went on to organize the first nutrition laboratory at the United States

Department of Agriculture. He set the recommendation at *125* grams per day, because he felt that "a large protein allowance [was] the right of civilized man."[126] What a fucking joke. What's *more* of a joke is that this is exactly what is happening today! Everyone seems to be following suit, putting protein on a pedestal, and consuming far too much of it. For this reason, this chapter is dedicated to busting some myths.

Don't get me wrong, protein is awesome; we couldn't survive without it. However, protein is awesome in the same sense that fats and carbohydrates are awesome: they are all required nutrients. This means your body needs all *three* macronutrients; they all bear the same importance. Therefore, while we definitely need protein, it shouldn't be looked at as the most "vital" nutrient, or a primary energy source. I will repeat that until monkeys fly out of my ass.

The truth is, average Jane's and Joe's don't need a lot of protein. Furthermore, when protein is over-consumed (as is the case in most developed nations), it becomes detrimental to our bodies. Adding to that, if you *are* over-consuming protein, it means you're most likely *under*-consuming something else (because the excess protein is taking the place of that other nutrient). Therefore, not only does the *over*-consumption hurt your body, but the subsequent *under*-consumption of the other nutrient also impairs your health. Protein should not be the focus. Instead, the focus should be the correct amount and balance of *all three* macronutrients, which includes fats and carbohydrates.

What most people don't understand is that protein comes from plant foods *and* animal foods. Therefore—for fuck's sake—protein does not equate to "meat." Remember, the three macronutrients are generally *all* present in whole foods. This means that protein can be found in foods like fruits, vegetables, grains, and nuts. Furthermore, protein from plants, and protein from animals, have *extremely* different effects on the body. Let's discuss, shall we?

Animal Protein

To start, there are a bunch of uneducated (or possibly greedy) farmers who have been pumping hormones, steroids, and antibiotics into their livestock for years. These "enhancers" result in larger livestock that produce more commodities faster than they normally would. Grow animal, grow!! Make the MONEY!! Unfortunately, all of that crap can end up in *our* system if we consume products from that super-juiced animal. We'll learn about how destructive those chemicals are to our system in a few chapters, so keep your eyes peeled. Do all farmers have this fucked up habit? Of course not, but it should keep you on high alert. If you decide to get your protein from animal products, you should be extremely wary of where that animal comes from, and what dangers it may bring with it.

Past that issue though, there seems to be another major predicament, and here's where I usually start to lose people. Even if we consume 100% pasture-raised, organic animal products that are void of added chemicals, it seems we may still be facing a serious problem. Over the past several decades, high animal protein consumption (anything over 10% of our total calories, according to science) has repeatedly been correlated with an increased incidence of disease.[126, 127] This includes diabetes, certain cancers, osteoporosis, kidney disease, autoimmune diseases (e.g. rheumatoid arthritis, multiple sclerosis, type 1 diabetes)—the list goes on and on.[126, 128] This issue will be discussed more in depth throughout this guide.

Despite the proven increased risk of disease with high animal protein intake, the Food and Nutrition Board (the folks who oversee dietary recommendations) *still* recommend a protein intake of up to 35% of total calories—triple (fucking *triple!*) the amount proven to be safe.[115, 129] Want to know why? Yeah, me too. If you need a moment to go get angry and break something, please take it. The Food and Nutrition Board are clearly on the same "Protein is God" train that our forefathers rode. Furthermore, from what I have read, it seems they made the protein recommendation because of money. In other words, the people funding the Food and Nutrition Board's work seemed to be companies that would benefit from higher protein recommendations (e.g. livestock industries). Someone is clearly buttering someone's muffin, if you know what I'm sayin'.

Chronic over-consumption of animal protein *will* make you sick—which is a huge contributing factor to the numerous chronic diseases running rampant these days. Yet, most people in developed nations are still flocking to protein (mainly animal protein) as if it's the miraculous wonder-drug that will give them wings and rid them of their excess fat deposits. Wrong, wrong, wrong. Sofa king wrong.

Plant Protein

Plant protein has the opposite effect of animal protein. Plant protein *promotes* health and has been shown to reverse, heal, or retard all of the diseases triggered by high animal protein consumption.[126] The best part about choosing plant-based protein sources is that over-consumption of protein becomes extremely difficult (not that it would hurt you anyway). This is due to the make-up of plant foods. They have lower protein levels in general and are usually full of fiber, making them extremely difficult to binge on.

Unfortunately, telling most people about this "little" protein issue is like telling them that they may as well fuck off and die. Most people I talk to equate protein with meat, and "can't survive without it." They won't even toy with educating themselves on the subject. Again, I'm not telling you never to eat meat again. I'm telling you there's a big fucking problem with the *amount* of protein that people *think* they need to be consuming, as well as *where* they think they need to get it from. Go read the quote at the beginning of the chapter again. The largest and strongest animals on this planet don't eat meat. Ermahgerd! How the heck are they surviving?!

Now, try not to faint. The average person only needs about 8%–10% of their calories from protein (you probably just had a heart attack reading that, or think I have no fucking clue what I'm talking about).[130] Go take your heart pills and then let's regroup. For many years—even while being an athlete—I have gotten about 10%–12% of my calories from protein, and I'm doing pretty awesome. This is mainly because I don't see protein as the best nutrient, and I don't try to use protein as energy like every dumbass diet tells you to.

In addition, I choose to get nearly all of my protein from plant sources. Not only would I rather choose disease-fighting versus disease-promoting foods, but it also becomes a no-brainer when it comes to one's protein "quota," if you will. If you eat an animal-based diet (i.e. most of your diet is made up of meats, cheeses, dairy, organs, and seafood with rare appearances from fruits, veggies, legumes, grains, nuts, seeds), you *will* be consuming a disease-promoting, high-protein diet; there's no way around it. If you eat a plant-based diet (i.e. most of your diet is made up of fruits, veggies, legumes, grains, nuts and seeds, with rare appearances from meats, cheeses, dairy, organs, and seafood), you will consume a more accurate nutrient ratio, and a health-promoting diet.

Lastly, I can't help but mention that meat consumption plays a *huge* role in the destruction of our planet. I am not here to preach about anything other than nutrition, but I kind of feel like if we don't have a planet to live on, it will be super difficult to eat. Thus, hear me preach for a second: Livestock production contributes *hugely* to pollution, water waste, grain waste, and to be quite frank, the obliteration of our planet. Why? Mainly because the livestock "business" makes up 14.5% of all greenhouse gas emissions.[131] If you don't know what this means, it basically means that the livestock industry (mainly beef and dairy cattle) are emitting a shitload of damaging gasses into our atmosphere— more than *all* of the vehicles in the world combined (yet there seems to be more focus on curbing vehicle emissions these days). I was shocked to discover that fact. More specifically, meat eaters are responsible for two to three times the global warming than are vegetarians and vegans.[132] On the contrary, protein-rich *plant* foods contribute a considerable amount less to greenhouse gasses (i.e. they're healthier for the future of our planet).[133, 134]

Here's something the livestock industry won't mention: meat (especially beef) is ridiculously inefficient to produce. An absurd amount of food is pumped into the livestock industry (i.e. the foods given to the animals) in order to then pump food out to the people. If we cut out the middleman, and instead of pumping so much food into animals, we pumped that food out to the people on the planet, we'd wind up feeding an extra *four billion* people.[135] I'm not saying we should starve our animals. I'm saying that there's a more efficient way to distribute and eat food, and we're far from it.

On top of that, you may have heard of the ongoing water shortages many places around the globe are facing. Well guess what? It's estimated that it takes around 1,600 gallons of water to produce *one* pound of meat. Fucking ONE. On the other hand, it takes only 100 gallons of water to produce one pound of wheat (another good source of protein).[136] The US uses 80% of their fresh water for food production for fuck's sake![137] I'm not finished. If we want to compare that consumption to other countries, there's something called a "water footprint," which estimates the water consumption of a country. The global average is 1,240 m³/cap/yr (don't worry about those letters, simply focus on the number). China comes in at around 700 m³/cap/yr. Go China! Guess what America's water footprint is? A whopping 2,480 m³/cap/yr—*double* the global average![136] What a fucking waste and disgrace! We're living and consuming like we have a spare planet to hop over to once we're done with this one.

If we're trying to be smart and sustainable with our food production, and are also trying to improve our health, it's a no-brainer: we eat more plant protein, and less animal protein.[132] Funny enough, most of the world does! In fact, only about two billion people choose an animal-based diet, whereas around four billion choose a plant-based diet.[137] If you live on animal products, you're in the minority! However, even though there are less animal eaters out there, they seem to eat so much fucking meat, that it causes an enormous issue. Even a *slight* reduction in our meat consumption can help—not only by improving the damage to our bodies, but the damage to the planet as well (man, I really *am* a friggin' hippie). You know that "Meatless Mondays" idea? Yeah, not a bad one.

Unfortunately, if you choose to *completely* cut out meat, there's a stigma attached to it (usually in the form of ridicule—which is bullfunky and shows how little that tormenter knows about nutrition). Therefore, I wanted to take a second to list some names of people who have made it through life (or who are making it through life) without consuming meat or animal products for an extended period of time. They have all changed, or are changing, this world for the better. Athletes, actors, philosophers, you name it—it's entirely possible to be smart, strong, and sexy without eating meat. It is not abnormal; it is simply a choice. Seriously, take note. Some of these people have, in essence, helped shape the world as we know it.

Albert Einstein (physicist)
Albert Schweitzer (musician)
Austin Aires (professional wrestler)
Betty White (actress)
Billie Jean King (tennis star)
Carl Lewis ("Olympic Athlete of the Century")
Charles Darwin (naturalist)
Chris Carter (NFL defensive tackle)
Christie Brinkley (model, actress)
Christina Applegate (actress)
Confucius (teacher, philosopher)
Dave Scott (six-time Ironman World Champion)
David Carter (NFL defensive lineman)
Eddie Vedder (musician)
Edwin Moses (track and field athlete)
Ethan Zohn (MLS player)
Forrest Whitaker (actor, producer)
George Bernard Shaw (playwright)
George Harrison (musician)
Jim Morris (bodybuilder, former Mr. America and Mr. Universe)
Joan Jett (musician)
Joe Namath (hall of fame NFL player)
John Coltrane (musician, composer)
Joss Stone (singer, songwriter)
Kesha (singer, songwriter)
Kevin Nealon (actor, comedian)
Kristen Bell (actress)
Lea Michele (actress, singer)
Leo Tolstoy (novelist, playwright)
Leonardo da Vinci (painter, sculptor, architect, musician, scientist, mathematician, engineer, inventor, geologist)

Lord Byron (poet)
Mahatma Gandhi (political leader)
Martina Navratilova (professional tennis player)
Method Man (hip hop artist)
Michelle Pfeiffer (actress)
Mike Tyson (boxer)
Natalie Portman (actress)
Pat Neshek (MLB pitcher)
Patrik Baboumian (Germany's "Strongest Man," 2011)
Paul McCartney (musician)
Plato (philosopher, mathematician)
Prince Fielder (MLB first baseman)
Pythagoras of Samos (philosopher, mathematician)
Redman (rapper)
Rich Roll (ultraman, considered one of the world's fittest men)
Rob Zombie (musician, songwriter)
Robert Parish (Hall-of-Fame NBA center)
Samuel L. Jackson (actor, producer)
Sarah Silverman (actress, comedian, writer)
Scott Jurek (ultra marathon runner)
Shania Twain (singer-songwriter)
Sir Isaac Newton (scientist)
Socrates (philosopher)
Surya Bonaly (Olympic and professional figure skater)
Tobey Maguire (actor, producer)
Tony La Russa (MLB infielder, manager, and executive)
Venus Williams (professional tennis player)
William Shakespeare (playwright)
Woody Harrelson (actor)

That, my friends, is a list of some powerful people. Some of the smartest brains in history. Some of the strongest athletes of all time. Some of the sexiest minxes to walk the face of this earth. All because they probably found their magical nutrition equation. It just so happened to be without meat—or, for some, without any animal products whatsoever. And there are millions more.

If you do your research and decide that you want to eat animal parts because they make you sparkle like a unicorn making love during sunset under a rainbow, then *great*. All I'm trying to do is bust the myth that you "need" meat (or dairy, or eggs) to be smart, successful, or strong. This is one of the most important topics on which to educate yourself. You have *options* where you get your protein from, and certain options are much healthier than others. One of the most educational books on this topic is *The China Study*, by T. Colin Campbell (who has over fifty years of nutrition research under his belt). Read it. But wait, not yet. Finish this book first.

If you decide that animal protein is, in fact, the best protein source for you to consume (I'd love to hear your reasoning), then buy from the most natural farms that don't involve hormones, specially formulated "feed," or a constant antibiotic drip. Better yet, raise your own animals. If you choose to *not* eat meat (or other animal products), please make sure you find other organically grown, non-chemical-laden protein from whole food plant sources.

Past choosing a protein source or *type*, it's even more important to ensure you consume the correct *amount.* This way you can decrease your chances of ending up with some shitty disease— and at the same time help cut down on pollution, water waste, and gas emissions.

This next bit of info might help you come to terms with low protein requirements: In our first year in life we double in size. What do we consume to do that? Breast milk (hopefully human breast milk—but we'll get to that later). Breast milk is what percent protein? 80%? 70%? 60%? Nope. A mere 5%. That's right; our specially-formulated milk, that makes us *double* in size in our first year, is only 5% protein.[138] Suck it, protein-lovers.

Let's keep going. I have compiled some protein related terms for you to chew on.

Complete Proteins

"Oooh, oooh, I know this one! Complete proteins are the *best* proteins, right?!" Wrong. People certainly assume they're the best though. It's probably because the protein industry tells you they are, and most products that contain them have glorified (misleading) labels slapped on them like "high quality protein"—all of which sounds fabulous and 100% necessary.

A "complete protein" is simply a term given to a protein molecule that contains all of the "parts" our bodies need. On the other hand, if a protein *doesn't* have all of the essential parts, it has been horribly deemed "incomplete," or "low quality." Not only is this concept complete horse shit, but the other (incorrect) assumption is that animal products are the only foods that contain "complete," "high quality" proteins, and plant products contain the "shitty," "incomplete," "low quality" proteins. This is why a lot of people gorge on meat and eggs—because they feel it has the "best" protein. However, many plants do actually contain "complete" proteins (quinoa, buckwheat, and soy, to name a few), as well as a shitload of other kickass nutrients not available in animal foods. Surpriiiiise!

But wait—do we even *need* "complete" proteins? Nope. Even though we need all of the specific "parts" of proteins (called amino acids, if anyone cares), the whole concept of a "complete protein" becomes irrelevant when we factor in digestion. Here's why: As discussed earlier, our bodies break down the foods we eat. Throughout digestion, all of the broken-down nutrients wind up mixing together in the depths of your churning gut. Nothing stays "complete" when it makes it past your pie-hole—including complete proteins.

There's a "string of pearls" example that works well to explain this further. Let's say a string of pearls represents a strand of protein, and a "complete" strand of pearls would have pearls of all colors of the rainbow (red, orange, yellow, green, blue, and indigo). Let's say you eat that complete strand of pearls (if anyone tries to sue me for choking on a pearl necklace, I will sue you back for being a complete jackass). Once that string of pearls enters your pie-hole the digestion process begins, and that strand sure as shit isn't going to stay in its complete form. It's going to be broken down into *separate* pearls, and those separate pearls will swirl around in your belly to be used however and wherever they're needed. You will have little pretty pearls being sent all over your body to the areas that are requesting those specific colors. Neat.

Now let's say you're *not* eating complete strands of pearls, but instead you're eating a wide variety of *"incomplete"* strands. Some are completely red, some are completely orange, some are yellow and indigo, and some may be blue and green. All of those "incomplete" strands of pearls are going to be broken down during digestion into single pearls—and *holy shit*—mix those bad boys together and suddenly you have all of the same pieces a complete protein would have! FUCKING MAGIC!

Basically, if you're eating a variety of healthy proteins, your body will get all the pieces it needs—regardless if they start as a "complete" protein or not. You don't need "complete" proteins. You simply need to eat a bitchin' diet that contains all of the protein parts our bodies need—from as many foods as it takes.

The exciting part is that your body doesn't even need all of the protein parts at the exact same *time*. In other words, different "incomplete" protein sources don't need to be wolfed down together with the hope that they scamper together in the depths of your gut to make one complete magical protein again. They can be eaten at different times, and your body will piece them together when it needs to—because your body is insanely awesome, if you haven't noticed.

For that reason, be wary of sales tactics. Just because something promotes itself as being a "complete," "high quality" protein, does not mean it's the best, most bad-ass protein source out there. In fact, it generally means it's the opposite: a highly-processed, chemical-filled product. Those words are simply marketing ploys to be used on the uneducated public, and generally huge red flags for something *not* to buy.

Protein Powders, Bars, and Supplements

"Eat me! I have fifty million grams of *complete* protein," said every protein-packed product in the universe. Guess what? Foods that boast their protein content are doing so as a sales ploy (and obviously don't know about the ongoing health issues that come with high-protein diets). Protein should never be sought out like it's the "golden nutrient" that will help you blossom into a fearless gladiator. Thus, to all of the supplement hoarders out there (yes, I'm talking to you—the dude or chick with tubs piled upon tubs of powders and pills that promise to give you six packs and burn "8x more fat" or whatever), please know that it is completely asinine to try to get your protein from a tub of powder or a pill that was made in a lab. Well, if you have any concern about health at least. I have successfully trained a wide-variety of clients—from children, to people with chronic illnesses, to high-performance athletes. None of them—not ONE SINGLE CLIENT—has ever been told to take a protein-packed powder, bar, or supplement. Guess what? They all survived *and* thrived.

Unfortunately, since protein is considered the "go-to," "safe" nutrient, people become leeches to highly processed, synthetic foods boasting their enhanced protein content, because they believe they're pumping their bodies full of harmless, protein-y goodness. Instead, they're merely pumping themselves full of processed garbage that had a kick-ass marketing team behind it—garbage that is less effective than real food. They then often wind up with what's called "osmotic diarrhea," which means there's an excess of poorly-absorbed nutrients floating around their gut.

Those excess nutrients then cause water to be drawn out of their blood and towards their bum hole. Their body is basically saying, "get this shit out of me!"

Oh, and do you want to know what else is usually in those highly processed bars, pills, and powders? Trust me, you don't (and the companies want to keep it secret as well). "Protein" is not the only ingredient in those tubs of yours. Most of them are laden with artificial additives that will sucker punch your insides. Fuckin' eat real protein people—real, organically grown, healthy protein from real, organically grown, healthy food.

Side note: There are some—what I could consider—"non-dangerous" supplements on the market. They are certified organic, and are free of all harmful chemicals, genetically modified organisms, heavy metals, and rodent feces (oops, secrets out). If you *truly* feel the need to supplement, please find a certified organic product, made from whole foods, that doesn't contain harmful additives. Then, understand *why* you're using it, so you can use it correctly.

* * *

Whew. I'm sick of talking about protein; we need to move on. Here are some examples of foods abundant in protein (more are listed in Appendix C). Who gives a shit if they're "complete" sources or not. The most important thing is to choose whole, organically grown, fresh, unprocessed versions when possible. Try to avoid anything highly processed, products from factory farms, and nasty-ass deli meat.

Foods with Healthier Proteins

- legumes (e.g. beans, peas)
- sprouted nuts and seeds
- whole grains
- quinoa
- organically grown soy
- spirulina
- pasture-raised meat and eggs
- wild fish

Foods with Less-Healthy Proteins

- protein bars, powders, shakes
- factory-farmed/caged meat, eggs, and fish
- egg substitute
- processed grains
- genetically modified soy
- anything boasting "high protein" percentage

Moral of the Story:

Don't be a protein pirate. Pull protein off its high horse, and put it on the same horse as fats and carbohydrates.

Chapter 19

Liquid Fare

In the last section we discussed the *amount* of water one should consume to stay hydrated and fully functional. I hope you've tapped into a water supply since then. If not, FOR THE LOVE OF GOD, please go drink some water (or eat some whole foods) before I entice you with other shit you shouldn't be drinking. Because, now that we're in the "Type" section, I'd like to discuss some of the common types of beverages one may reach for, and how they fit in with the "health or hobby" concept discussed earlier.

Water

Ding ding ding! Best every-day choice of beverage (I can hear the echo of "booooor-ing" bouncing off these pages as I write that). Quit your temper tantrum. The base of your fluid intake should be plain water, period. Hit it hard and hit it often (but remember, if you're eating whole plant foods that are full of water, you can back off a bit, as they'll help with hydration). I'm talking *plain* water, not "flavored" water. Any idea what that "flavor" is? Don't worry, you'll find out soon enough. Also, please keep in mind that we're focusing on what's *right* for our bodies, not simply what we crave. If it were all about cravings, I'd be hydrating myself with hot chocolate and gin and tonics.

Sports Drinks

Fluorescent-colored sports drinks were specifically formulated to make you grunt harder, sprint faster, and look like Serena Williams. What they usually fail to mention is that they are totally unnecessary unless you have been exercising for longer than around sixty to ninety minutes. You see, this is when the body starts to run out of little things called electrolytes (e.g. sodium, potassium), which sports drinks have been artificially pumped full of, and which plain water doesn't contain. If you run out of electrolytes, it will be hard to sustain prolonged activity.

Unfortunately, these designed-in-a-lab drinks are nowhere close to natural and come bearing some harsh ingredients. They are also high on the Glycemic Index, meaning you're going to get a spike in your blood sugar (which, over time—especially if you're downing these outside of physical activity—they can be detrimental do your health). There's also no evidence they are needed, or even beneficial, despite what the manufacturers claim. Lies! They're all LIES! Sports drinks are one big pile of marketing nonsense.[139, 140] Please see "Coconut Water" for a *natural* electrolyte-replacement choice when you do get off your ass to exercise for long durations. Or, if you're not an endurance athlete (or not exercising), please go see "Water," because YOU DON'T NEED ANYTHING ELSE.

Coconut Water

Coconut water has become the latest and greatest, see-every-celebrity-holding-one-on-a-beautiful-beach fad. This is a good thing and a bad thing. It's a good thing because there's finally a wholesome, natural product in the public eye. Coconut water is nature's perfect electrolyte sports drink and will trump luminous sports drinks any day (Coconut water has a Glycemic Index rating of 3, where Gatorade has a rating of 78). This shit *will* make you resemble Serena Williams. The bad news however, is that because it *is* now in the public eye there are companies (like Coca-Cola) who are pumping out coconut water faster than shit comes out a baby. How do they make their product "the best"? Why, they chuck some other crap in there to enhance taste and increase shelf life! Jeepers creepers, stop the madness!

If you decide to consume coconut water, please remember the following: you do not need an electrolyte drink unless you are continuously exercising longer than around sixty to ninety minutes . . . or, if you need to stay hydrated because you're sick and vomiting (or have the runs) . . . or, if you're a celebrity on a beach. But, if you *do* happen to be an endurance athlete, a celebrity on a beach, or are leaking from either end, you need to act wisely. Either find a whole coconut and crack that sucker open, or find a packaged coconut water that has the following ingredients, and nothing else: coconut water. If there are other flavors, preservatives, colors or stabilizers you don't recognize, or cannot say with 100% certainty are safe, DON'T CONSUME IT. Learn to love the natural thing, because it actually *does* do a body good.

Tea

Tea is awesome, has a million-and-one health benefits (like improving digestion and metabolism), and has little-to-no calories. There are so many different kinds of tea, and they all have wonderful benefits. I usually have at least one a day: I enjoy peppermint when I need to feel "lifted or energized," I enjoy a chai for comfort at the end of a long day, and I enjoy a lemon and ginger if I'm feeling run down—there isn't a tea I don't like. However, tea is also a good example of how something can become a chemical shit storm. Tea comes from plants. If those *plants* are sprayed with pesticides and herbicides, *you're* going to wind up eating those chemicals as you turn your pinky into an antenna and ever-so-poshly sip your tea. Companies also chuck additives into their tea to boost appeal these days. Furthermore, since tea usually comes in a tea bag (and that tea bag usually gets soaked right in your drink), you might want to know what that tea bag is made of (often harmful chemicals). This is why it's imperative you find loose *organic* tea, which will not be covered in chemicals and surrounded by a harmful bag.

In addition, please, please, please don't go ruining your tea with a cup of sugar. Try to enjoy the actual tea. Here's a hint: the longer you let the tea sit in the water (or "steep"), the more potent it will be. Dip that tea bag or infuser only for a second if you're a tea pussy. But try not to be a pussy, because the longer you leave it in there, the more health benefits you'll get from it. Pinkies up!

Coffee

Coffee is a funny thing for me to talk about, mainly because I've never had a cup. SAY WHAT?! Am I fo' real, yo? Yo—I am fo' real. I can't stand the taste of coffee. It tastes like a hippo pissed in my mouth. I friggin' *love* the smell of it though, and every now and again I ask someone if I can try a sip of their steamy, delicious-smelling, fresh-ground goodness. And every time I want to spit it back in their face for trying to poison me. As a result, I've tried a few sips in my lifetime, but have never made it a ritual. Enough about my bizarre non-coffee habits though; let's proceed.

One of the first questions people ask me when we begin nutrition counseling is whether or not they'll have to give up coffee. Of course not. The coffee bean is a natural thing and has some great benefits. What you *should* consider giving up is the following:

- twelve cups per day, ten cups per day, six cups per day, etc. (once you get this nutrition shit down, you won't need to electrify yourself with caffeine anyway);
- white sugar, artificial sweeteners, and artificial creamers;
- non-organic coffee; and
- decaffeinated coffee.

The best coffee consumption strategy is to trek to Columbia, harvest organically grown coffee beans, and grind them yourself. Second to that, buy the organically grown beans or certified organic, pre-ground coffee from your local grocer. Then try to avoid coffee makers with filters (unless you can tell me for certain what those filters are made of— because they are most definitely leeching shit into your hot steamy drink). Instead, use a stainless steel and glass coffee press. Then drink it black, and enjoy a cup every now and again.

"Oh no, I could never drink my coffee black." Shut up; of course you *can*, you just don't *want* to. Some of you aren't even drinking coffee; you're drinking sugar-filled, chemical-cream water with a *splash* of something that resembles coffee. If you truly want coffee—actual coffee—you should train your taste buds to taste the coffee and *not* the sugar and creamer (start the weaning!). If you don't like the taste of coffee, don't attempt to disguise it. Instead, don't drink it.

The reason you should steer clear of *decaffeinated* coffee is because it's like a hooker who only wants to cuddle—it's not natural. How do you think a coffee bean winds up decaffeinated? Decaffeinated coffee has been processed (and even then still isn't caffeine-free). Coffee naturally has caffeine in it, so LET IT BE THERE. If you don't want caffeine, fuckin' drink something that doesn't have caffeine in it.

Side note: coffee is naturally "drug-like" in nature. Therefore, be vigilant with coffee. It *is* addictive, and has been known to cause both physical and mental changes such as increased blood pressure, insomnia, heart palpitations, feelings of nervousness, and panic.[141] As always, listen to your body. If you're having friggin' heart palpitations after you down some coffee, do the logical thing: surrender and STOP DRINKING IT.

Energy Drinks

Would you believe it if I told you I've never had an energy drink? I don't need a can to tell me I'm a "rockstar," and I'm certainly not looking to have wings. Even after working at multiple gyms and "health clubs" where Red Bull, Rockstar, and Monster drinks were sold in order to superboost gym-goers through their otherwise impossible workouts, they just never appealed to me. Because, here's the kicker: if your body is at the high end of the Nutrition Spectrum, it will have all of the energy it needs! You won't need wings—you'll have a fucking cape! What a concept!

I have climbed mountains without energy drinks. I have played in weekend-long athletic tournaments without energy drinks. I have a two year old who resembles the Tasmanian Devil and have never needed energy drinks to keep pace. Undeniably, there is no need for energy drinks. They are one big poop-pile of marketing ploy crap and should be banned, if you ask me.

Banned? "That seems harsh!" You wouldn't think so if you knew the links between energy drinks and disease (and even death). Tens of *thousands* of people wind up at the ER every year for reasons directly related to energy drinks: rapid heart rate, heart attack, fainting, palpitations, increased anxiety and depression, dizziness, development of uncontrollable phobias and fears, high blood pressure, seizures, and sudden death.[142, 143] Well, the folks who experience the sudden death probably don't wind up at the ER—they probably head straight to the morgue. You get my point though.

With the known dangers lurking behind energy drinks, please take a guess on whether or not there's some wizard out there regulating how many of these energy drinks people consume. If you guessed, "fat chance in hell there's a wizard regulating energy drink consumption," then you're right. Find that magical nutrition equation and the energy will find you.

Flavored Water

How could something with a name like "Revive," or "Focus," or "Essential" be bad for you?! I'm referring to Glaceau's Vitamin Water line (owned by Coca-Cola, of course)—and what a great job they've done with their marketing! Well, guess what? They got into a law suit regarding the fact that they were misleading the public to believe their Vitamin Water drinks were "healthy," while, on the contrary, were far from it.[144] They're not the only ones. Several other "flavored" water brands are lurking out there as well, including the little packets of powder that you can conveniently dump and swirl around in your water (e.g. SoBe Life water, Crystal Light, Propel). They are all merely sugar water and chemicals (vitamins?). Don't believe me? Look on the backs of the bottles or packets and you'll see for yourself. Ingredients like crystalline fructose, phosphates, and natural flavors (perhaps from my mailman's ball sweat—that's natural!) will all be listed.

The dumb part about this? Most gyms and health clubs carry this shit, because the products look like healthy alternatives to "boring" water. Listen up: unless you're doing over an hour of intense exercise (pacing back in forth in front of a gym mirror and flexing and grunting like a fierce warrior does *not* count), then you don't need anything more than water. And you *certainly* don't need shit like flavored water while you're sitting in your cubicle looking to be "revived" after a late night of drunken karaoke. If you're looking for revival, try flavoring your water naturally. Drop a real fucking lime wedge or berry in there (crush them a bit first to release the flavor), and learn what *real* flavors taste like.

Carbonated Water

Mineral water, seltzer water, club soda, sparkling water, and tonic water are all just different versions of water infused with carbon dioxide gas bubbles . . . and possibly some other stuff.

Let's start with "mineral water" (which can actually be carbonated or non-carbonated). If it's carbonated, it's usually *naturally* carbonated. It is generally sourced and bottled directly from an underground waterhole that sits next to a natural gas pocket. This would include brands like Perrier and San Pellegrino (both owned by Nestlé, by the way). If you have a desire for bubbly water, reach for carbonated *mineral* water, as it's probably the most natural. Just realize that if you buy the brands mentioned above, you're now supporting Nestlé for all of the other fake-ass garbage they pump out into the world. There are plenty of other lesser-known mineral water companies who aren't owned by large corporations only concerned about revenue (e.g. OnePure, from New Zealand). Find one near you.

Besides natural mineral water, the rest of the above mentioned carbonated waters usually have gas *artificially* added to them (i.e. they're more "processed" and less "natural"). They also usually have other additives chucked in (e.g. flavor enhancers, artificial sweeteners, minerals). This includes tonic water (one half of my good ol' gin and tonic duo—suuuuuck!), which actually takes the "additives" a bit further by adding something called quinine. Quinine was originally used to treat malaria, and then later used to treat leg cramps. It can have an extremely toxic effect if over-consumed. However, if you're consuming it with your gin and tonics, you'll die from alcohol poisoning *way* before you die from quinine poisoning. WHEW. Want to know if your water has quinine in it? Put it under a black light (or any UV light) and it will glow bright blue![145, 146] Neat-o.

Juice

If juice were purely "juice," it wouldn't be an issue. The only problem is rarely does juice simply contain juice (even if it boasts "100% juice"). Suckers! It usually contains additives like sugar, synthetic vitamins, and artificial colors and flavors. If you are a juice drinker, you most definitely want to look for certified organic, cold-pressed juice. This means that nothing has been added, it wasn't pasteurized (which kills nutrients), and the juice was produced merely by squeezing the shit out of the fruit or vegetable. Or, squeeze the shit out of your own produce and make some homemade juice.

Furthermore, juice is one of those drinks that people tend to over-consume because it comes from a fruit or vegetable, so "it must be healthy!" Juice isn't necessarily "bad," per se, especially if it's certified organic, cold pressed juice. However, if you regularly consume a lot of juice, it will send your blood sugar levels into orbit (hello hyperinsulinemia and the metabolic syndrome). Why? Because drinking *one* glass of, let's say, orange juice, is the equivalent of eating about eight oranges. You would never eat eight oranges at once, so don't fucking drink them either.

Beer

Like coffee, beer originates from natural food sources (like barley and wheat), so you should probably drink a few a day. I'm joking. If you think for a second that companies aren't hiding funky shit in their beers, then you're still driving the naive wagon. Many beers contain added stabilizers, preservatives, colors, sugars, aaannnddd—drum roll please— fish bladders!

We have hit an all time low. Fish bladders are used to help make beer "less murky."[147] Some of your favorite beers may boast those ingredients. I'm not going to mention any names (Corona, Guinness, Fosters, Budweiser, Newcastle, Michelob, Coors . . .) but many common beers are contaminated with this crap.[148]

If you're a beer drinker, your best bet is to find a certified organic, local microbrew or craft beer and ask them about their ingredients *before* the beer pong game. Find clean beer. Or, hunt down some German beer. I'm not joking. Germans have had their shit together for quite some time. They established a law back in 1516 called "Reinheitsgebot" (say *that* ten times fast while tipping one back), that requires all German beer manufacturers to restrict their ingredients to water, yeast, hops, and either barley or wheat. They cannot use additives like sugar, colors, and stabilizers.[149] Those Germans are genius (I'm one quarter German, by the way).

At this point I shouldn't have to say it (but I'm going to): if you think your daily caloric allowance should be filled with beer calories, I wish you the best. Please pass this guide onto someone else. In all seriousness, if you love beer, then enjoy one periodically (hopefully a "clean" one). Just keep in mind that the point of putting matter in your mouth is to fuel up. While beer may fuel you to strip down and strap on some rollerblades so you can skate through your town in your birthday suit while belting out "Pour Some Sugar on Me" (I definitely haven't done that), it's certainly *not* going to propel you towards optimal health.

Wine

I know you want to skip over this section (what you don't know, won't hurt you, right?). I can feel the panic attack setting in. "Do. Not. Take. Away. My. Wine." Again, I'm not going to take anything away from you, I'm simply going to give you some info, and you can make your own damn decision. If you're old enough to read this guidebook, you're old enough to do that.

Here's the scoop on wine: It originates from grapes, right? So all is glittery and good in the world, right? Wrong. Like beer, wine companies have been sneaking shit into their fermented beverages for ages.[150] They, of course, want their wine to look, taste, smell, and feel the best, so it sells the most. Thus, once again, you need to do your research. Contact your favorite wine vendors and ask them what additives they use (if they won't tell you, the sirens in your head should go off). Drink the "cleanest" wine possible. I'm going to take a stab in the dark and say it probably won't be the cheap, mass-produced crap you see on the shelf of every store.

One more thing: Some of you may have heard about the resveratrol in wine being a life savor when it comes to inflammation, heart disease, and cancer (which seemed to give everyone the green light to gulp as much as possible). Not so much.[151] Unfortunately, as much as you'd like it to, a wine habit will not cure shitty nutrition.

General Alcohol Consumption

People have been getting tanked for decades. I can guarantee (not really) that much of history was built upon drunken escapades that turned into genius inventions and discoveries. Christopher Columbus *had* to have been totally shit-faced when he ran ashore in the Bahamas instead of Japan. Thank goodness for the crunk juice or America wouldn't be what it is today (although perhaps that's not a good thing . . .). Unfortunately, drinking can come with some serious downfalls.

First off, as mentioned above, you may land in the Bahamas instead of Japan. Secondly, drinking in excess will most definitely cause some internal issues. For instance, woman who have just two drinks per day (wine, beer, spirits, you name it) have about a 40% increased chance of developing breast cancer.[152, 153] Did you friggin' read that? You will have a *forty* percent increase of being diagnosed with breast cancer if you're a woman and you regularly consume merely two drinks per day (and no, men you're not off the hook simply because the above mentioned study focused on people with vaginas). That's pretty effin' significant, folks. In fact, *anyone* who consumes more than just *one* serving of alcohol per day will have an increased risk of colorectal, mouth, larynx, pharynx, esophagus, breast, and liver cancers.[154-156] If you're a smoker, your risks go up even more! Weeeeee! Take my word for it (and all of the scientific studies supporting these statistics): if you are regularly consuming alcohol at a rate greater than one drink per night—especially if you are a smoker—you may as well throw in the towel and kiss good health goodbye.

With that knowledge, if you still decide to use some of your daily calorie allowance on booze-fuel, do so responsibly. Find natural alcohols that don't have added shit in them (electric blue liqueur did not fall off a fucking electric blue liqueur tree). Then, once you find a "clean" drink, have one *occasionally*. Not one bottle, but one *drink* (which means one glass of wine, one bottle of beer, or one shot of spirits—not all of the above).

I understand there may be times when you head out with your posse and want to impress the pants off someone by doing a half-naked interpretive dance while writing your name in the snow with your own piss. As long as those times are few and far between, you shouldn't encounter the issues that stem from "too much alcohol." That is, as long as you are smart, safe, and stay away from things like heavy machinery and bull fights. If you're not-so-smart, then perhaps you should limit your drinking to a padded room.

Moral of the Story:

Have I mentioned that you should drink a bunch of water?

Chapter 20

Amount + Type

We've now covered the major *types* of nutrients. Hopefully, you can now see that choosing the best options of fats, carbohydrates, protein, and fluids is crucial, and that they're *all* important, and *all* play an integral role in maintaining our health. They are also *all* usually found in combination together in most foods (well, *whole* foods anyway).

Let's take what we've learned thus far and piece it all together. If we were to combine the *amount* of food we should be devouring, with the *types* of nutrients that should make up that amount, it would go a little something like this:

- My estimated daily calorie amount calculated eons ago was 2,267. I'm going to round that number to 2,300, because I'm all about making this easier. I also don't care if I eat more because I mainly eat whole plant foods, which won't make me fat or unhealthy.
- I'm then going to throw my math skills into high gear, and separate those calories into the ideal fat, carbohydrate, and protein percentages. For this example, I used the following percentages: 35% fats, 55% carbs, and 10% protein (similar to what I normally consume).
- Beep-bop-boop-beep . . . I determine that I need 805 of my calories from fat, 1,265 from carbs, and 230 from protein.

Ahhh fuck it, this will be much more fun if we go ahead and make a pretty pie chart (mmmm . . . pie). Here's a snapshot of what my daily macronutrient amounts and percentages usually look like, including some of the foods I regularly devour:

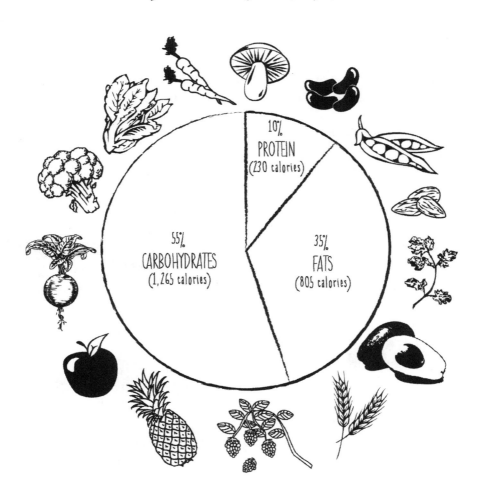

Daily Macronutrient Intake
Based on 2,300 Calories per Day

10%
PROTEIN
(230 calories)

55%
CARBOHYDRATES
(1,265 calories)

35%
FATS
(805 calories)

Side note: that pie chart does *not* represent a plate; it represents my total intake of food for the day. Over the course of a day, if I eat the right types of foods, I will wind up somewhere around those percentages and calorie amounts for each macronutrient. And I'll know that I've hit the nail on the head when abundant energy pours out of my veins.

But wait, how the heck does one figure out how to hit the right percentages (or calories) while you eat?! Frickin' *laser* beams. Wait, what? That doesn't even make sense. How about by *logging your food*, as you did (or should have done) in the "Amount" section? When you logged, the website should have provided you with the total amount of fat, carbohydrate, and protein calories you consumed. Without even touching a calculator, you should be able to see if you're anywhere close to the recommendations (especially if the website provided the percentages for you). Do carbohydrate calories take up half of your total calories? Do the fat calories take up the second most? Do the protein calories take up the least? If the website you used calculated the percentages for you, go ahead and write them in the appropriate spaces at the bottom of equation 20.1.

If the website you used *didn't* provide percentages for you (sucks to be you), and you really want to get accurate, you can calculate them yourself (you bloody over-achiever). This is not something that *needs* to be done; this is the nitty-gritty. I'm only including this step because I know there a lot of over-achievers out there. If you'd rather simply look at your total calories and guesitmate as to where you're at, go for it. If not, equation 20.1 will take you through the calculation gauntlet.

Equation 20.1: Calculating your nutrient percentages

STEP 1: HOW MANY TOTAL CALORIES DID YOU CONSUME FOR THE DAY?

_____

STEP 2: HOW MANY *FAT* CALORIES DID YOU CONSUME? _____

STEP 3: HOW MANY *CARBOHYDRATE* CALORIES DID YOU CONSUME? _____

STEP 4: HOW MANY *PROTEIN* CALORIES DID YOU CONSUME? _____

STEP 5: STEP 2 _____ ÷ STEP 1 _____ = _____.
NOW MULTIPLY THAT NUMBER BY 100. THIS IS THE PERCENTAGE OF FAT
CALORIES YOU CONSUMED. WRITE THAT NUMBER IN STEP 8.

STEP 6: STEP 3 _____ ÷ STEP 1 _____ = _____.
NOW MULTIPLY THAT NUMBER BY 100. THIS IS THE PERCENTAGE OF
CARBOHYDRATE CALORIES YOU CONSUMED. WRITE THAT NUMBER IN STEP 8.

STEP 7: STEP 4 _____ ÷ STEP 1 _____ = _____.
NOW MULTIPLY THAT NUMBER BY 100. THIS IS THE PERCENTAGE OF PROTEIN
CALORIES YOU CONSUMED. WRITE THAT NUMBER IN STEP 8.

STEP 8: COMPARE *YOUR* PERCENTAGES TO THE *RECOMMENDED* PERCENTAGES:

YOUR % FAT: _____   RECOMMENDED FAT: 20%–35%
YOUR % CARBS: _____   RECOMMENDED CARBS: 45%–65%
YOUR % PROTEIN: _____   RECOMMENDED PROTEIN: 8%–10%

How close were your percentages to the recommended
percentages (also referenced in equation 20.1)? Are any of them
way off? Well, now you know which of your major nutrients need

to be adjusted! You can head right back to your log to see the problem areas, and to start playing Twenty Questions:

- Is your carbohydrate intake out of control?
- Is your protein intake too high?
- What types of food is your protein coming from? (plant versus animal versus processed protein product)
- Is there a specific item that blows your protein intake out of the water? There is? Great! Is it something you consume regularly and need to reconsider (i.e. make your portion smaller, or eliminate it completely if it's a processed pile 'o crap food product)?

If your percentages are wildly off, head to Appendix C, where there's a long list of foods abundant in fats, carbs, and protein. All you need to do is start adding in some of the ones you're lacking (because our focus is to *add* healthy foods, right?!). For example, if you're low on fats, add some healthy high-fat foods. If you're high on fats, it means you're low on something else (carbohydrates, for example); try substituting some healthy high-carb foods for some of your high-fat foods. And always keep in mind that if you're having a hard time adjusting your percentages, it may be because of your ratio of plant, animal, and processed foods. Try adding more plant foods in place of some processed or animal foods.

Plant foods naturally have similar percentages to what is recommended for our bodies. As soon as you start steering away from plant foods and gorge on either animal or processed foods, shit gets wacky and you'll feel like you're pulling your hair out trying to get your percentages anywhere near accurate. Am I telling you never to eat anything that comes from an animal or a box again? Nope. I'm simply saying if you *base* your diets on those types of foods (and leave out foods like vegetables, fruits, legumes, whole grains, herbs, nuts, and seeds) this will be near impossible for you. Reason number 579 why I choose to consume a shitload of plant foods.

Will you have to do all of this calculating and logging every time you eat a meal? Why yes! Jeezus no, of course not. The moment you understand what types of foods you have to consume in order to stay near the optimal percentages, you can disarm your calculator and stand down—this shit will become second nature.

Moral of the Story:

To achieve optimal health, it's important to make sure everything you consume comes together to hit the recommended nutrient percentages. If you don't have ESP, I would recommend using a food logging site to assist you.

Chapter 21

Shit to Avoid like the Plague

I'm going to give you fair warning that this chapter is one huge-ass pile of nutrition bullshit that will most likely make you want to break your knuckles on a brick wall. Also, I feel like after this chapter someone should start handing out honorary nutrition degrees to you readers. So here we go: apart from the types of nutrients, as well as good or bad options we've been discussing, we're now going to discuss dangerous types of *chemicals* that can tag along. Many of them will, without a doubt, rip the shit out of your insides.

Let's start with the substances *added* to processed foods. These are called "food additives" (makes sense), and processed foods are usually far from healthy because of them. But, if you have a product to sell, and you want that product to travel across the world and sit in a grocery store for weeks (or months, or years) without wavering in taste or appearance, you have to add stuff to it to keep it dazzling and irresistible. Thus, additives are mainly used to increase shelf life and provide a more consistent "state" (e.g. it won't change consistency with different temperatures, or won't separate into different parts). This way, the product can look beautiful for years on end while it waits for its forever home.

Past longevity, additives can also be used to arouse our senses by enhancing the smell, flavor, color, and texture of a product.

They are there to put us in a trance, lure us in, and then slam us with addictive properties that will have us wanting more. High fives for an excellent sales tactic, but hey, FUCK YOU for the trickery! Many companies go to the end of the Earth to make their food appear better and last longer. And the FDA approves all of these additive-laced products that are no longer 100% food, because . . . WHY THE HELL NOT?!

Actually, it's obvious why. The food additive industry is quite the money-maker (which we know is the driving force behind all of this madness). The market value of food additives was $4.8 *billion* in 2012. That number is projected to reach $5.8 billion by 2018.[157] Let's face it—who the heck cares if a product is going to poison consumers?! The manufacturers will finally be able to purchase that island they've always wanted! Golf claps!

How do we know if we're consuming this toxic shit? You won't —unless you read the nutrition label, where they're conveniently listed. These d-bag additives can sometimes be listed as a simple "E" number (seen in table 21.1), which also means they've passed a series of tests by the European Food Safety Authority (EFSA), and therefore must be safe, right? Wrong.[158, 159] Numbers in food. What the fuck is happening? (Slams head down on table.)

Table 21.1. E Number Categories

Number Range	Category Description
E100-E199	Colors
E200-E299	Preservatives
E300-E399	antioxidants, acidity regulators
E400-E499	thickeners, stabilizers, emulsifiers, gelling agents
E500-E599	acidity regulators, anti-caking agents
E600-E699	flavor enhancers
E700-E799	Antibiotics
E900-E999	glazing agents and sweeteners
E1000-E1599	additional chemicals

The countries that don't use these numbers will instead just write out the additive's name (usually a long word that you will have a hard time pronouncing). There are hundreds upon hundreds of harmful additives being thrown into our "foods" and "beverages" before they are presented to us, and I will now lose my shit and bitch about some of them (all have been approved by the FDA at one point or another). I have selected the ones I get asked about most frequently, but there are gazillions more—and they are just as scary as these. If you're not pissed off at the FDA yet, just you wait. If you want to read more about any of the additives I'm about to discuss, you can head right to the FDA's website; they're all listed there for your convenience![160-162]

Before I start the bitching though, there's another category of chemicals I must mention. I like to call them "farm chemicals," and some of the upcoming substances will fall into this category. Sometimes foods (even whole foods that look healthy and untainted), or even livestock, have certain chemicals *attached* to them (e.g. pesticides, herbicides) or *injected* into them (e.g. antibiotics, hormones). The difference between farm chemicals and the previously mentioned additives, is that additives will be listed on nutrition labels, and farm chemicals won't. This is why it's imperative you learn about where your food was produced or manufactured.

Here we go. It's time to secure your storm shutters and head to the bunker, because we're about to face the destructive category-5 food industry hurricane head on. I'm about to describe some of the common additives or farm chemicals you may unknowingly be shoving down your pie-hole. Get comfy, kick back, and revel in the fact that you are most likely being poisoned on a daily basis. Especially if you live in the US, as most of these fuckers are banned in other countries. 'Murica!

Antibiotics

Antibiotics have been around for the greater part of a century, and let's face it; who *hasn't* had a good ol' dose of them at some point? Doctors were handing them out like lollipops in my younger years. This has led to a growing concern for their over-use, which actually leads to antibiotics that are no longer effective. Their effectiveness goes down the shitter because, over time, the bacteria that the antibiotics are supposed to kill become "resistant" to being destroyed because they've adapted to the antibiotics that are supposed to kill them. This can lead to disease of epidemic proportion, folks. It is estimated that three hundred *million* people will die prematurely by 2050 due to this antibiotic resistance if something doesn't change.[163] Holy schnikes.

How does this relate to our food? Well, decades ago it was discovered that if antibiotics were fed to livestock in "sub therapeutic" doses, they actually gained up to 3% more weight than their non-drugged counterparts. More meat equals more money! As a result, farmers far and wide started administering regular antibiotics to their livestock in order to plump them up (as well as to help combat the disease that started taking over their herds, caused mainly by their shitty living conditions). Today, more than *80%* of all US antibiotics go to livestock.[164]

How does this affect the animal products we eat? Great question, and it's one that should have been asked *before* farmers started infusing it into their animals. Here's the answer: we now have studies demonstrating that antibiotic-infested meat is making people sick. It starts with the animals acquiring bacterial infections (again, probably from most of their shitty living environments), and they can't get better because their bodies have become resistant to the over-administered-antibiotics. Flourish bacteria, FLOURISH!

Then, individuals who work with the livestock, as well as anyone who eats the bacteria-contaminated meat, can wind up with immortal bacteria in them.[165] The bacteria of course causes horrible sickness, and antibiotics can't come to the rescue for the same reason they didn't come to the animal's rescue. How bad is the problem? Every year, *two million* Americans will become sick, and *twenty-three thousand* of them will die.[164, 166] All because they consumed meat (or worked with animals) that contained antibiotic-resistant bacteria. But hey, at least the meat industry is profiting at our expense. .

Have I mentioned that animals that *weren't* cooped or caged, and were allowed to roam free *as intended,* got sick less (and thus didn't need a constant antibiotic drip)? Ask any conventional-turned-organic farmer.[167] They will tell you that their organic, pasture-raised farms produce healthier animals. If you're a meat-eater, all signs point to consuming meat from grass-fed, cage-free animals.

But, antibiotic dosing "has" to be done, according to Dr. Trisha Dowling, a pharmacologist—WEEE-OOO, WEEE-OOO, WARNING SIREN!—from the Western College of Veterinary Medicine. She states that "if you don't put [antibiotics] in the feed, and you wait until you get an outbreak of necrotic enteritis, you've got a lot of dead birds and you've lost a lot of money."[168] Well shit! Don't let the animals die! Let the *people* die instead! We would hate for you to lose money, Trisha. Hey, I have an idea, put your damn animals outside and let them live naturally, and then only give them antibiotics if you must. Or, not at all. Crazy idea, I know.

Thank goodness the FDA is listening. Well, not really (who am I kidding?!). In 2013 they issued a *voluntary* plan for the industry to phase out only *certain* antibiotics for livestock use.[169] Hey FDA, how many companies do you think are going to "voluntarily" reduce their paycheck? (Eye roll.)

Aspartame

Born in 1965, and known as "E951," aspartame is an artificial sweetener marketed to dieters and diabetics because it has *zero* sugar. Fuck yeah! Must be safe! This is the typical "market one good quality and disguise the rest" situation. And they sure did disguise the rest. Like how the original safety testing of aspartame on seven baby monkeys caused one of them to die, and five others to have grand mal seizures.[170] Basically, one monkey escaped unscathed. Good start, I'd say! Get that shit in the mouths of the

people, stat! And they did! And the people ate it, because it was
SUGAR-FREE.

Aspartame was originally sold under the name "NutraSweet"
(and then eventually "Equal"), and has been a controversial
additive since day one. In fact, it has been banned and "un-
banned" several times since its conception. Red flag much?! While
many reports say aspartame is completely safe "at current levels
of exposure" (because I'm sure they have a way of knowing
everyone's aspartame exposure), research shows otherwise.[171]
Aspartame accounts for 75% of all adverse reactions from food
additives—more than *all* of the other food additive reactions
combined.[172] Those reactions are: headaches/migraines, dizziness,
seizures, nausea, numbness, rashes, depression, irritability,
insomnia, hearing loss, vision problems, loss of taste, vertigo, and
memory loss.[173] Oh, and occasionally DEATH. So . . . nothing major.

And, in case you want to worsen, trigger, or cause brain
tumors, multiple sclerosis, chronic fatigue syndrome, mental
retardation, epilepsy, diabetes, heart attack, stroke, kidney
disease, lymphoma, Parkinson's disease, behavioral changes,
fibromyalgia, or birth defects (pregnant ladies, TAKE NOTE), then
you'll be happy to know aspartame might just do the trick![171-180]
What a multi-talented chemical!

Ooooh, and do you want to hear the "fun" stories about
airplane pilots who consume aspartame-laced products and then
either have blurred vision (to the point where they could no
longer read their instruments) or suffer seizures mid-flight?[181-183]
Think about *that* next time you're thirty-five thousand feet in the
air and have no idea what your pilots are shoving down their pie-
holes.

If all of that sounds pleasing to you, you should be thrilled to
know that aspartame can be found in over *six thousand* products
made specifically for YOU![184] Simply head down to your grocery
store and grab some diet sodas, breath mints, processed cereals,
drink powders, cough syrups, vitamins (especially children's
vitamins), processed desserts . . . the list is endless.

There are many regions or countries (e.g. Indonesia, Japan, Philippines, South Africa, and *all* of Europe) that are labeling or considering removing aspartame from food and beverage production completely.[185-189] Just not quickly enough, if you ask me. Perhaps we need to kill a few more monkeys?

Azodicarbonamide

Azo . . . what?! Azo-di-carbon-a-mide! Sounds *totally* natural and health promoting! How about we call it "Azo" for short, or "E927" if you're a numbers person. Little Azo is an "improving agent" mainly used to bleach flour and make bread products more irresistibly awesome (think breads, croutons, pie and pizza crusts, stuffing, etc.). That's not what it's mainly used for though; its prime purpose is to help shape and develop foamed rubbers and plastics (like yoga mats and shoe soles)! You may have read about a 2014 petition to have the folks at Subway Sandwiches remove Azo from their "fresh" (ha!) breads, which they finally agreed to do (but don't assume for a second that there aren't other chemicals hidden in those sandwiches).[190] You can bet your bottom dollar that most fast-food joints and bread companies are still shoving this shit into their burger buns and bread products.

The main issue with Azo is—wait for it—that it is a "risk to human health" (direct quote from the World Health Organization back in 1999).[191] Apparently it's a human asthmagen (causes asthma symptoms to develop) and a potential carcinogen. Seeing as though it can cause asthma and possibly cancer, it has been banned in Australia, New Zealand, and the whole European Union (for *years*). In 2004, the whole European Union even banned it as a *blowing agent* (meaning it couldn't even be used in "materials and articles intended to come into contact with [food]").[192] I guess Subway (and everyone else still using it) didn't get the memo.

Lastly, check this out: according to an article in the Chicago Tribune, if you're ever in Singapore the "use [of Azo] can result in up to fifteen years imprisonment and a fine of $450,000."[193] The good news is, if you need an Azo fix, you don't have **to** stroll the black market in Singapore, you simply need to head down to any mainstream US grocery store! Pick up any generic, highly-processed bread loaf, bun, roll, etc., and you'll see it listed in the ingredient list. Basically, any product containing flour should be checked for Azo. And, if it has it, the product should then immediately be fed to the nut jobs at the FDA who approved it. Let *them* be the subjects for a case study on Azo safety.

Butylated Hydroxyanisol (BHA) and Butylated Hydroxytoluene (BHT)

Oh my gosh, these names are brutal. What's the first sign that this shit shouldn't get near your mouth? You can't even pronounce the fucking words! Known as "E320" and "E321," BHA and BHT are chemicals used to preserve consumables for ridiculous amounts of time. You know, because it's natural for products to last for years on a shelf without sprouting mold. These fuckers are usually found in fatty foods like butter, processed meats, and baked goods, but can also be found in products like cereals, chewing gum, and beer. Most products I've seen that contain BHT deceivingly add the term "for freshness" on the label next to it, because they *know* they have to manipulate your mind in order for you to believe something with that name is favorable.

This gets more exciting though: these two fantabulous chemicals are also used in oil, rubber, jet fuel, petroleum products, cosmetics, and some medicines (including Zocor, the wonder-drug with a bazillion side effects discussed back in chapter 6). To make things even *more* thrilling, they're also flammable! Rock on! In case that isn't enough to make you want to steer clear of them, they also may promote cancer growth, as well as liver, thyroid, and kidney problems.[194, 195] "Here are your Zocor pills for your cholesterol issue. When you get cancer and organ failure from them, come back so I can give you more drugs that give you more problems." Righty-o, doc! Will do! High fives to Japan and most of Europe for banning these little shits.[196]

Bisphenol A (BPA)

BPA isn't a food additive or farm chemical, but rather a chemical added to food *containers* (e.g. soda cans, canned foods, plastic containers, plastic coffee cup lids), and therefore touches your food. I get a lot asked a lot of questions about BPA though, so I'm throwing it in here. It has actually been used commercially since 1957 and was known to cause health problems way before that.[197] Why is it in our food packaging? Your guess is as good as mine, since it's well known that BPA migrates into the foods or beverages we consume.[198] The outcome isn't child's play either. You're looking at an increased risk of obesity, neurological effects, adverse effects on the thyroid, increased risk of cancer, miscarriage, ovarian dysfunction, asthma, heart disease, and suppressed immune function, amongst many other fun ailments.[199-207] The shit will screw you sideways 'til Tuesday.

You should find it quite "interesting" then, that between 2003 and 2004, 93% of children and adults tested in a study had BPA in their urine—which certainly didn't crawl up there itself.[208] The chemical was being consumed in foods that had been enclosed in BPA-laced containers. It took nearly a decade to ban BPA . . . but only in baby bottles.[209] Not the *packaging* of baby formulas and foods—merely baby *bottles.* Because that makes sense.

Not only that, but since school lunches are generally pieced together from bulk food items stored in cans and plastic containers, school lunches are often riddled with BPA.[210] Just *one* school lunch could be toxic for your child.

Since BPA is still widely used in food storage containers, what do you think happens if pregnant women are unknowingly ingesting foods or beverages (e.g. canned beans or Starbucks coffees) that are encased in BPA-laced containers? They can significantly harm their unborn child, that's what.[211] Acidic, vinegary foods like tomatoes, artichokes, sauerkraut, beets, and pickles are the worst culprits. They will pull BPA out of a container more than other foods, so steer clear of them if they're canned or stored in plastic.

You can also steer clear of the following canned food *brands,* as in 2014 it was confirmed that they were all still choosing to contaminate their cans (and thus food) with BPA.[212]

Andersen's	Del Monte	Marie Callender's
Armour	Dennison's	Musselman's
Bar Harbor	Dinty Moore	Ocean Spray
Brooks	Duncan Hines	Old El Paso
Bush's	Goya	Progresso
Carnation	Green Giant	Rosarita
Casa Fiesta	Healthy Choice	Spam
Cento	Hormel	Valley Fresh
Chef Boyardee	Hunt's	Vancamp's
Chi-Chi's	La Choy	Wolfgang Puck
Clear Value	Manischewitz	World Classics

These aren't the only assholes poisoning us. There are several lesser-known brands still hiding this shit up their sleeves as well. And then there are plenty of companies that *don't* use BPA, because, quite frankly, THEY DON'T NEED TO.

It angers me to have to write this, because there is no reason this shit should exist anywhere *near* us, especially in close quarters to the stuff we're putting in our pie-holes. Yet health organizations world-wide say that a "low dose" of this shit is perfectly fine, and therefore it's okay to have low doses in our consumer products.[213] The only problem is that if we're completely surrounded by low-dose BPA-laced products, then that low-dose begins to add up, and becomes greater than a low-dose. It becomes a fucking disease-causing dose (and our level of disease speaks to that statement). Add that to the rest of the chemicals in which we're swimming—I mean drowning—and SHAZAM! We're all on a chemical highway to hell!

The not-so-good news is that at the end of 2014 the FDA revisited BPA safety, and yet again reassured the public that current levels of BPA were safe[214]. Their ninety-day toxicity study (which had more holes than a golf course) unfortunately didn't take the potential reactions with the kajillion other chemicals floating around in our food system into account, and also completely ignored the years of proof that the shit is dangerous. I guess that's easier than telling the multi-billion dollar can industry to change the way they make containers. Swept that one right under the rug, didn't ya, FDA?!

Hint: if you buy packaged foods out of glass jars instead of plastics or cans, you can avoid most of the BPA. Thankfully, over *thirty* European nations, China, Malaysia, and South Africa, have banned BPA (in varying degrees).[215] Clearly some people have their head screwed on straight.

Brominated Vegetable Oil (BVO)

BVO, or "E443," is an emulsifier—or something that stabilizes a mixture of ingredients so they don't separate from one another. Not only is BVO used in plastics, medications, pesticides, and flame retardants, but once again it is put in the food and beverage products we consume! Party in our mouths!

This flame retardant is found most commonly in fluorescent drinks like Mountain Dew, Fanta, Gatorade, and Powerade. But wait—a 2014 *Newsweek* article announced Coca-Cola's decision to remove BVO from all of their products (which includes Powerade) by the end of 2014. Don't get too excited though, they're replacing it with sucrose acetate isobutyrate or glycerol ester of rosin. Which are both clearly real fuckin' wholesome ingredients.[193, 216]

To make the party even more exciting, if you consume enough BVO you may get to experience memory loss, fertility problems, early puberty, thyroid problems, neurological impairment, tremors, fatigue, loss of muscle coordination, headaches, and eyelid drooping. BVO, you are bad-ass! Thankfully this little shit is banned in over one hundred countries, including India, Japan, and the whole European Union.[196] The US is, unfortunately, not on that list.

Calcium Disodium EDTA (EDTA)

EDTA is listed as "E385" on the good ol' list of food additives. In case you were wondering what "EDTA" stands for, it's Ethylenediaminetetraacetic acid. Let's say it together: eh-thil-eneBLAHBLAHBLAH . . . probably something you don't want to ingest. EDTA is a salt made from ethylenediamine, formaldehyde, and sodium cyanide.[217] It's used not only to preserve a food, but also to enhance its color, texture, and flavor. Because apparently, food doesn't look, feel, and taste good enough on its own.

Calcium disodium ethylenedia-minetetraacetic acid (ha! I just wanted you to have to try to pronounce that fucker again!) is hidden in everything from condiments to canned goods. When I was doing research on this little gem, I came across this statement on the popular WebMD website:

> EDTA is safe when used as a prescription medicine, as eye drops, and in small amounts as a preservative in foods. EDTA can cause abdominal cramps, nausea, vomiting, diarrhea, headache, low blood pressure, skin problems, and fever.

Huh? Do those sentences not totally contradict themselves, or is it just me? The same site then went on to say that EDTA can make heart problems worse, interact with blood sugar, cause low calcium, potassium, and magnesium levels, and cause liver problems (including hepatitis), kidney problems, and seizures.[218] That's after it said EDTA was safe in small amounts in food. Great, but who is regulating how much each person consumes? Surely not everyone eats the same amount of EDTA-spiked food? No thank you, I'll pass. As will Australia, where it's banned. Good on ya, mates!

Caramel Coloring

Also known as "E150," caramel coloring is a brownish artificial food coloring that has been around for decades. You can find it in hundreds of products, but here are some of the popular ones:

beer	chocolate	preserves	pickles
breads	cookies	gravy	sauces
cake batters	cough drops	ice cream	dressings
chips	donuts	liquor	soda

First things first. Why the fuck do we need to change the color of our foods and beverages in order to enjoy them? Are we so screwed in the head that we can't simply enjoy foods and beverages in their natural state? Secondly, since we *do* find it necessary to enhance the colors of our foods, why the heck are we choosing a diarrhea-brown color?!

The scary part is that this caramel coloring can come from a wide variety of sources, like wheat and milk. What happens, for example, if someone with a soda addiction also has a wheat or dairy allergy, and unknowingly consumes caramel coloring in all of the soda they guzzle? I'll let you do the math on that one (unless you couldn't get through the math in the first section, then don't hurt yourself).

In January 2014, a consumer report on caramel color came out linking it to cancer. Long story short, because of the link to cancer, instead of completely banning it (which would clearly be the intelligent thing to do), products that have over a certain amount of it are simply required to have a warning label about it. The cutoff amount the California Office of Environmental Health set as an "acceptable" level placed consumers at a 1 in 100,000 risk of getting cancer if they consumed the product. Excuse me? If it causes cancer, nobody should be consuming it! Period! That "1" in 100,000 is going to be pretty pissed off when they discover that they were the lucky bastard whose luck ran out.

Furthermore, I guarantee there are people out there consuming a heck of a lot of different diarrhea-brown-colored products, which increases their risk of disease even more. On top of that, some drinks have been tested and were found to have *over* the amount considered safe anyway, so clearly someone is throwing the rulebook out the window. I'm not going to name any names though (ehh hemmm, Pepsi products. Oops). Oh, and the only state that regulates this crap is California. Apparently the rest of the US doesn't give a shit about who gets cancer.[219]

Carrageenan

Carrageenan, or "E407," is an additive extracted from a type of red seaweed. Sounds natural and healthy, right? Right! That's why many companies choose it over other additives. It's mainly used to stabilize or thicken processed consumables. It's most commonly found in products like ice cream, baby formula, beer, toothpaste, cheese, yogurt, non-dairy milks, lunch meats, canned soups, and frozen meals. It's even found in *organic* versions of those foods, since seaweed can be organic. The only problem is that red flags are being raised over connections to more and more diseases (including cancer) due to carrageenan's inflammation-causing abilities one it becomes a processed, degraded food additive.[220-224] It's still unclear whether or not it *causes* diseases, but it is well known to cause *inflammation*, which can lead to hundreds of diseases. Let's put it this way: I'd rather stir my separated coconut yogurt prior to pie-holing it, than consume another yogurt being held together by carrageenan. It doesn't need to be there. It is the lazy-man's additive.

Food Dyes

I don't know about you, but bright-colored foods and beverages scare the shit out of me. I *know* those fluorescent products include some chemical concoction to make them look like Rainbow Brite shat all over them. Why are they "necessary"? Because the color of food can influence the perceived flavor of something. Meaning, if you take artificial grape gum (which has no real "grape" in it . . . shocker!) and then dye it purple, more people are likely to believe it actually *tastes* like grape.[225] Several food dyes are commonly used in the US (derived from petroleum, if you were wondering), most of them having some sort of detrimental effect on us. The most commonly used are:

yellow 5 (E102)   citrus red 2 (E121)
yellow 6 (E110)   green 3 (E143)
blue 1 (E133)   red 3 (E127)
blue 2 (E132)   red 40 (E129)

If you're wondering where Yellow 1–4 disappeared to, they've all been banned (along with Red 2, Red 4, Red 32, Orange 1, Orange 2, Violet 1, and several more). I'm totally convinced that they got those yellow dyes right the fifth and sixth time though.[158, 162]

Carol Potera, a writer for several health and science journals, states that "nine artificial dyes approved in the United States likely are carcinogenic, cause hypersensitivity reactions and behavioral problems, or are inadequately tested."[226] Great. Chances are, any processed food or beverage product that has a distinct bright "color" to it, has a food dye in it. In fact, around fifteen million pounds of artificial food dyes are pumped into US foods every year (mainly kid's products, because kids LOVE color), even though most of them are considered to have health risks.[227] And what about pills like Aleve (a.k.a. naproxen) that are blue in color? Blue 1 and Yellow 6, that's what. How about Advil (a.k.a. ibuprofen) gel caps? Red 40 and Yellow 6. Let's numb your pain and grow some tumors! All of this artificial color shit is dumb as fuck because there are numerous natural foods (e.g. beets, paprika, turmeric, blackberries) that can be used to dye food if someone feels the need to consume brightly-colored products.

Food dyes are not safe, period. It has been determined that as little as 30mg of food dye can cause health issues.[228] Let's see how quickly this could add up:

1 serving Cap'n Crunch's Oops! All Berries Cereal	41.0mg
1 serving Kraft Macaroni & Cheese	17.6mg
1 serving Kool-Aid Burst Cherry Drink	52.4mg
1 bag of Skittles	33.3mg
Grand total of food dyes	144.3mg

As stated above, only *30mg* of this shit can start to cause behavioral problems in a child. If they consumed those listed products between breakfast and lunch (which many kids do), they would have ingested almost *five times* that amount IN ONLY A FEW HOURS. Sorry to fuck with your insides, little Johnny, but EAT UP!

Shit, merely *one* bag of skittles can cause behavioral problems! Imagine *chronic* ingestion of this shit, day after day, after day. You have to wonder how many tragic events (e.g. school shootings, stabbings) could have been avoided if those kids weren't fed fluorescent-colored products that are *known* to affect their behavior (on top of all of the other additives they're also consuming, of course). Let's give a standing ovation to Norway, Finland, Austria, France, and the United Kingdom, where these fluorescent fuckers are banned.[196]

Glyphosate

Glyphosate is a farm chemical, and the main ingredient in the commercial weed-killer "Roundup." It is the Hitler of herbicides and is sprayed on most commercial food crops. This allows crops to grow freely and not be taken over by weeds. Bam! More money in the pocket! This shit is absolutely *everywhere*, and has become the most widely used weed killer for its assassin-like killing power.[229] To date, over 18.9 *billion* pounds of glyphosate has been dumped on our food (globally).[230]

If this weed killer is so strong and murderous, how are the crops not killed off as well, you ask? GREAT question! You see, the original manufacturer of the weed-killer also came up with a genetically modified "super seed" designed to withstand the powerful weed-killing poisons. "Want a super seed that will survive anything and allow you to grow more crops for more money? Buy the so-called 'Roundup Ready' seeds and spray them with Roundup—both of which we manufacture and sell!" Genius.

Who's the creator of this money-making spray-and-seed combo? Mighty Monsanto, who happens to be number one on my shit list. They are a chemical company that has invaded our food system (along with others like Dow, Syngenta, and DuPont), and genuinely care more about their pockets than our health. They are willing to bribe anyone and everyone to support their product, do not offer any transparency to their product safety, and are tearing apart our world faster than you can say, "I'd rather not sprout tumors, thanks."

To support my hate for them, you should know that in the past, Monsanto has concocted many similar "safe" products like Agent Orange, DDT, and PCBs, all which have been banned for their extremely harmful effects on humans and the environment. Agent Orange was the chemical used in the Vietnam War that caused *millions* of horrendous birth defects and health issues (even to the US veterans who dumped the chemicals). Guess what? Agent Orange happened to be an herbicide as well—and was once deemed safe. Hey, I know, let's trust that Roundup is totally safe, and then spray it all over our food! Monsanto, you're an asshole.

Roundup was obviously never meant to be a nutrient. Roundup should be nowhere near our food. Unfortunately, not only is it all over our food, but also in the air and ground water, where it spreads far and wide to unknowing habitants of this planet and affects *everything*. In fact, Roundup was detected in 70% of household drinking water in the US, and is finding its way into our bodies. It's in our urine (the US has levels ten times higher than found in Europe), and in our breast milk.[231, 232] Yes, lactating mothers are unknowingly feeding their innocent babies a horrible, destructive chemical. Roundup is fucking everywhere.

Why should we care? This asshole of a chemical has been linked to infertility, cancers, GI disorders, Parkinson's, birth defects, Alzheimer's, and autism spectrum disorders.[233, 234] In fact, in 2015, the World Health Organization declared that glyphosate "probably causes cancer."[235] When they say "probably," by definition they mean there's sufficient evidence in animal tests to show that glyphosate causes cancer, yet only *limited* evidence in human tests.[236] A few more studies on humans, and glyphosate will get the carcinogenic stamp of approval—just you wait. Or, we can take Philippe Grandjean's word— the professor of environmental medicine at the University of Southern Denmark—

who suggests that, "when we see that other mammals get cancer from glyphosate, we must assume that people who are exposed to the substance can also develop cancer."[237] No shit.

In fact, glyphosate exposure specifically *doubles* your risk of getting lymphoma, the very cancer my step-mother succumbed to.[238] And as we mentioned earlier in the "Malnutrition Costs What?!" section, pregnant women living near glyphosate-sprayed crops are 60% more likely to have an autistic child than pregnant mothers living elsewhere.[239] SIXTY-FRIGGIN'-PERCENT! Take a guess how much autism spectrum disorders have increased in the past two decades. 5%? 20%? 75%? Not even close. There has been somewhere between a 1,500%–6,000% increase in autism spectrum disorders in the last twenty years, even though we have information like this.[240] SOMEBODY PLEASE FUCKING LISTEN!!! Do you even know if *you* live near a glyphosate-sprayed (or any harmful herbicide-sprayed) crop field? You could be getting poisoned as we speak. Close those windows! Ah, screw it, it's going to be in your water supply anyway.

Roundup, glyphosate—whatever the fuck you want to call it— has always spelled "disaster," yet many people are still trying to fight for its use and safety. They suggest it's our only answer to producing enough food for the world's population (which is incorrect on so many levels). "The more food we grow, the more autistic, tumor-filled mouths we'll feed!" I'll let you guess who's doing the fighting. The people making the money off of the "Roundup Ready" crops, of course (sorry if I didn't give you enough time to guess). Those folks don't give *two shits* about us consumers once they've pillaged our pockets. Their money runs *deep,* and they have the means to pay off anyone and everyone they need to, in order to keep their chemical business alive. And that's exactly what they do.

Thank goodness some countries, like Argentina, Brazil, Mexico El Salvador, The Netherlands, Denmark, Russia, and Sri Lanka, are getting their shit together and realizing that "glyphosate herbicide should be banned" since it's making people die horrible, prolonged deaths.[241, 242]

High Fructose Corn Syrup (HFCS)

HFCS flew on to the shelves in the 1970s and never looked back. It's a liquid sweetener derived from corn, and since corn is one of the most genetically modified food products, this means that HFCS is most likely genetically modified. And if it *is* genetically modified, then chances are it's also doused with a nice dose of the murderous glyphosate we previously discussed. It's used in everything from baked goods, to dairy, to canned fruits, to baby formulas, to sweetened beverages.

Dr. Mark Hyman is an eight-time New York Times bestselling author, family physician, international leader in his field, and dedicates his life to **eradicating** chronic illness. On his website he states that the dangers of HFCS include: obesity, fatty liver, liver failure, diabetes, heart disease, cancer, dementia, tooth decay, and more. He also states that the presence of HFCS is a good indicator of whether or not a food or beverage is "poor-quality, nutrient-poor [and] disease-creating."[243] Basically, if something has HFCS in it—while it may be cheap—you can be sure as shit that it's not going to promote your health.

Monosodium Glutamate (MSG)

MSG, otherwise known as "R2D2" . . . just kidding—I wanted to see if you were still awake! *"E621"* is a flavor enhancer that tricks the brain into believing whatever you're eating is a billion times more fantastic than it actually is. Companies that produce shitty food products that don't have much flavor can throw a little MSG in there and call it a day. Suddenly their cheap, nutrient-depleted, bland-as-fuck foods explode with addictive flavor. Our brains then get tricked into thinking something tastes better than it actually does, we consume the shit out of it, and keep coming back for more.

Unfortunately, this comes at a price: brain damage. Yes, BRAIN DAMAGE. MSG is a known neurotoxin. The brain-destroyer also causes obesity, eye damage, headaches, fatigue, disorientation, depression, numbness, burning, tingling, chest pain, difficulty breathing, nausea, rapid heartbeat—shall I continue? The shit is fucking *toxic*. Therefore, after discovering that MSG was extremely damaging, companies put their smart pants on. They started calling MSG by other names so they wouldn't have to remove it and could still improve the taste of their product(s). Thus, you can't purely keep your eyes peeled for "MSG" or "Monosodium Glutamate." You must also look for the following terms as well, and know that these ingredients are most likely MSG in disguise.[244]

autolyzed yeast	monopotassium glutamate
calcium caseinate	sodium caseinate
gelatin	textured protein
glutamate	yeast extract
glutamic acid	yeast food
hydrolyzed protein	yeast nutrient

There are several more ingredients that most likely contain MSG (e.g. "natural flavors," "soy protein isolate," "citric acid"), but there's no way of knowing for sure (and the manufacturer certainly won't tell you). For that reason, if you don't feel like getting brain damage, eat some real damn food that doesn't have a long list of food additives attached to it. You'll also want to stay away from the following products, since they all contain hidden forms of MSG—at least in the US (this list is *not* conclusive).[245]

Doritos	Kraft products
Pringles	most protein powders
Marmite	Campbell's Soups
Ramen noodles	Lipton Soups
Boar's Head cold cuts	Progresso Soups

I know what you're thinking ("oh *shit!*"). Time to clean out your pantry and fridge, please and thank you.

Natural Flavors

Any time you see the term "natural," "natural flavors," or "natural flavoring" on a product, you can guarantee it's a marketing ploy, simply because the word "natural" sells. What exactly *is* a natural flavor though? Fruit extract? Veggie extract? I think it's time we unveiled the origin of these "natural" flavors. The US Code of Federal Regulations defines "natural flavors" as:

> The essential oil, oleoresin, essence or extractive, protein hydrolysate, distillate, or any product of roasting, heating or enzymolysis, which contains the flavoring constituents derived from a spice, fruit or fruit juice, vegetable or vegetable juice, edible yeast, herb, bark, bud, root, leaf or similar plant material, meat, seafood, poultry, eggs, dairy products, or fermentation products thereof, whose significant function in food is flavoring rather than nutritional.[246]

Did you get that? That's their way of saying that "natural flavor" is a blanket term for fucking *anything* found naturally occurring on this planet. This should truthfully be a game changer, because it could literally mean horse shit. Or seal scrotum. And, believe you me, manufacturers are getting their natural flavors from some pretty fucked up places.

Furthermore, if you've been paying attention, you previously learned **that** the term "natural flavors" may also indicate the brain damaging MSG, so right there it should be an indicator to avoid them. Just for funsies though, let's talk about where some of the most common "natural" flavors come from.

- Shellac. Sometimes termed "confectioners glaze" or "resinous glaze," this natural flavor is actually made from the secretion of the beetle-like lac bug and is mainly used to coat candy and glaze donuts. So yes, next time you eat jellybeans, Junior Mints, Milk Duds, Raisinettes, or a glazed donut, please understand that you're also eating bug discharge. The splooge is also sometimes added to juices and wines. Who knew that bug jizz could taste so wonderful?! Oh, and yes—it's also the same "shellac" used as wood and fingernail polish.

- Cystine (or L-Cystine). This natural flavor is a dough conditioner derived from human hair . . . or possibly duck feathers. It's mostly found in breads and baked goods, and most people get super excited when they see it listed as an ingredient, because it's part of a protein, and PROTEIN IS GOD. Ever stop to think where that protein may have come from? Quack, quack.

Last, but not least, my favorite:

- Castoreum. This would be the natural flavor from (drum roll please), a beaver's anal gland secretion. I'm not making this up. It's used to manufacture vanilla, strawberry, and raspberry flavors. Let that sink in. The last time you ate something vanilla, strawberry or raspberry-flavored that contained "natural flavors," it most likely had secretions from a beaver's anal gland. This isn't a joke. My question is, who the fuck discovered this?! Did someone actually get the bright idea that anal ejaculate would help flavor food and then spend their days testing out different anal secretions before declaring, "AH HA! Let it be the *beaver's* anal gland that shall flavor our food!" WHAT. THE. FUCK. This seriously rates a ten on my weird-shit-o-meter.

Let's revisit the fact that real, whole food already *has* flavor. The only reason "natural flavor" is included in a product, is if it is so fucking processed that all of the *real* flavor has been sucked out and the company needs to make it somewhat palatable for consumers. What about vegetarians or vegans who unknowingly ingest a "natural flavor," assuming it's something derived from an herb or fruit, and instead wind up eating bug secretions or duck feathers? And what about the products that merely contain "flavor," rather than "*natural* flavor"? What the fuck is *that* shit?

What it boils down to, is that if I'm going to eat something vanilla flavored, I WANT TO FUCKING SEE "VANILLA" LISTED IN THE INGREDIENTS.

Nitrates and Nitrites

The "Nit" brothers refer to a group of chemicals usually used to preserve meats (think deli meat, sausages, bacon, hot dogs, etc.), and include:

E249, or potassium nitrite

E250, or sodium nitrite

E251, or potassium nitrate

E252, or sodium nitrate

The first sentence you'll find in the US Environmental Protection Agency's report on Nitrates and Nitrites is, "nitrates and nitrites are chemicals used in fertilizers, in rodenticides, and as food preservatives." Read that again. The same chemicals used to kill rodents are used to preserve our food. Righty-o. Makes about as much sense as a trap door on a canoe. Nitrates and nitrites are naturally occurring in feces though—and we know "natural" is good—so that should make you breathe a huge sigh of relief.

The same report mentioned above then goes on to explain that these chemical additives can lead to coma and death in children, and cancer in adults.[247] So riddle me this, Gilligan: WHY THE FUCK IS THIS FUCKING FUCKED UP SHIT IN OUR FOOD??! Don't try to preserve your food people, just fucking eat it when it's fresh (or freeze it) and then go buy some more. Holy heck, what a concept.

Potassium Bromate

You may have heard the term "bromated flour" before, as potassium bromate (or "E924") is generally used to "improve" dough by making it whiter and thicker, and by allowing it to rise higher and be "fluffier." It's also sometimes used in fish paste, as well as the malting of barley (for fermented beverages). In a perfect world, the companies using this crap hope that it oxidizes (or "burns off") during the cooking process. At least that's what's *supposed* to happen. If it doesn't completely burn off, and there's some left in the food (which happens), the shit *will* give you cancer. This is probably why it has been banned in the whole European Union, Canada, Nigeria, Brazil, South Korea, Peru, Sri Lanka, New Zealand, Australia, and China. Guess where it hasn't been banned? You betcha—the good ol' US of A. At least California somewhat has its shit together and requires a warning label on any product containing it.[195, 196, 248]

Propylene Glycol (PG)

There's nothing "PG" about propylene glycol, or "E1520." In fact, this little gem is often used as a lubricant on condoms! Bow-chica-wow-wow! It doesn't stop there; this multi-faceted liquid food additive is also used to help de-ice planes (i.e. it's used as anti-freeze). I'm still not done: it's also used in animal feed, plastic laminates for bath and kitchen wear, industrial soap, engine coolant, and also as a solvent in many pharmaceuticals (it's in Motrin and other popular pills).

Isn't this guide about nutrition though, you ask? Have no fear, PG's talent extends even further! When it comes to food, PG is generally used as a humectant, which is something that "holds water" and keeps the product moist. You'll find it in items like sodas, beer, and salad dressings. You know what, I'm not even going to research the health risks (that's a lie, I already have). I'm simply going to take an educated guess that if a chemical can de-ice a plane, lube a condom, and laminate my countertops, I don't want to fucking eat it.[249]

Ractopamine

First off, I'd like to point out how naturally delicious and mouth-watering "ractopamine" sounds. Secondly, if you've ever consumed meat that wasn't certified organic (in America, at least), you most likely have—unknowingly—consumed ractopamine. What is this delectable gem? It's a "growth promoter" for livestock, manufactured by—dah, dah-dah—a *pharmaceutical* company looking to make some money! Basically, unlike hormones and antibiotics which are given to animals from an early age in the livestock process, ractopamine is fed to animals *just prior* to their slaughter, to force them into a last-minute protein explosion (i.e. their muscles grow, producing more meat). Bigger chicken thighs! Ginormous steaks! MONEY!

Unfortunately, the ractopamine can linger in the meat, and anyone who eats that meat is subjected to eating ractopamine. This is yet another example of a money-making scheme that focuses solely on profit and takes *zero* note of the fact that we're eventually consuming this shit (and what the repercussions are). It should be a red flag that the workers who handle ractopamine must wear impermeable gloves and a mask. Wouldn't want to get that shit on your skin—or even worse, inhale it.

Ractopamine is marked as "not for use in humans," yet is used in around 80% of US cattle and pig operations (because who cares if it fucks *them* up, right?).[250] It has fancy-schmancy names to make farmers believe they're buying something incredibly special for their beloved pets: it's labeled as "Paylean" for pigs, "Optaflexx" for cattle, and "Topmax" for turkeys. It's like the animals have their own little supplement bulk-up program! Cute!

What are the side effects of ractopamine? Well, "shockingly," there are hundreds! Where should we start . . . in animal studies you will see side effects such as reduced fertility, anorexia, tachycardia, heart attack, birth defects, bloating, respiratory disorder, pneumonia, lameness, behavioral disorder, diarrhea, frothing at the mouth, skin lesions, aggression, lethargy, stiffness, and, drum roll please . . . death! That's purely *animal* side effects though. We don't care about them—they're merely a disposable commodity, right? (Insert sarcastic tone.)

It *has* to be better in human studies. Why else would it be allowed in our food? Just you wait. *Human* side effects noted from ractopamine are: respiratory disorder, circulatory disorder, heart disorder, nausea, dizziness, pain in the limbs, fever, headache, chest pain, weakness, nose bleeds, loss of senses, itching, sinus inflammation, anemia, coughing, spasm . . . the list goes on.[251-254] Sounds like a bloody country song! It's estimated that since 1999 over *seventeen hundred* people have been "poisoned" by ractopamine-contaminated pig meat alone.[250] It probably makes sense then, that ractopamine is banned in approximately 160 out of the 196 countries in the world.[255] Not only is the US still using it, it's using it *a lot*. Go big or go home, right?!

Thank-fucking-goodness people are starting to take note (including other countries who have banned the import of ractopamine-contaminated meat from the US).[256] In fact, in 2013 the FDA was actually sued by the Center for Food Safety and the Animal Legal Defense Fund for its non-transparency on ractopamine use.[257]

Now some may argue (just like with everything else), that the level of ractopamine in meat is "insignificant," and we have nothing to worry about. Wait a second though—how much ractopamine-contaminated meat are you eating? And how can anyone tell you the amount you're eating is safe if they don't know how much you're eating? Even more importantly, how can they tell you it's safe for consumption when they're only referring to it as a *single* chemical reaction rather than what happens when it mixes with the fifty million other chemicals you're probably also ingesting? The answer is they can't tell you it's safe, because, like everything else, there's no way to test the safety of ractopamine and its infinite reactions with the other chemicals in your internal environment. Testing ractopamine on its own, and then saying it's safe in small quantities on its own is a big, fat joke. Except I'm not laughing.

Recombinant Bovine Growth Hormone (rBGH)

You don't have to be a genius to realize that this is a hormone that makes something grow. Not to be confused with "BGH," which naturally occurs in cows, this made-in-a-lab version vastly increases a cow's milk production, thus increasing profit for farmers. Brilliant! What *haven't* they thought of?!

The synthetic hormone was approved by the FDA in 1993, but has actually been around since the 1970s. "Surprisingly," it was originally produced by none other than the chemical company, Monsanto. Since then, it has been banned in many nations, thus also banning the export of US milk that contains it.[258] Smart people around the world simply want to drink milk, not milk pumped full of unnecessary (and potentially harmful) shit.

Speaking of harmful shit, what actually happens if a cow over-produces milk? Ask any woman who has ever breastfed and over-produced. IT FUCKING HURTS LIKE HELL. It feels like a fifty-pound bowling ball is trying to hatch out of each boob. (Gentlemen, feel free to substitute "testicle" for "boob" to get an idea of what I'm talking about). That shit happens in lactating moms *naturally*. I can't imagine what it would feel like if someone forced me to produce even *more*. I'd probably pull a Van Gogh and rip my own tits off.

"They're just cows" though, so they're none-the-wiser, right? They probably can't feel their lead udders as they stretch further and further towards the ground (that's a joke for all of you animal-rights activists out there who just started penning death threats to me). Of course they can fucking feel it!

Furthermore, with the unnatural over-production of milk comes some horrendous side effects (e.g. mastitis, udder infections), which leads to a build-up of pus in their milk. Yes, *pus*. That well-known yellowy goop that seeps from infected wounds is in your rBGH-laced milk. Don't worry though! The dairy industry has figured out that they can get the pus levels down to an "acceptable level" by administering antibiotics to their cows (please see "Antibiotics," at the beginning of this chapter). An *"acceptable"* level of pus?? That's a joke, right? Nope. Folks, I dare you to go Google "cow mastitis" and check out some images of what your milk might be rubbing shoulders with. Right now. Go. I double dog dare you.

That's simply what happens to the *cows*. What happens when *humans* drink the hormone, pus, and antibiotic-filled milk, you ask? GREAT question! Most seriously, it poses "serious risks of breast and prostate cancer."[259-261] Meh. Who cares. At least the diary industry is providing more milk to more people. What a great service. We should thank them.

Now imagine the impact this shit has on little *children* who start to drink hormone-disrupting milk from a young age. Besides the diseases mentioned above, I'm going to make a bold statement here and suggest that this growth promoter has a huge influence on the fact that kids are going through puberty at a younger age every year. A few decades ago, a girl showed signs of breasts around age 15. Today, 10% of white girls, 23% of black girls, and 15% of Hispanic girls have developed breasts by age 7.[262] I don't think I could spell "boobs" when I was 7. At this rate, by 2030 we're going to see boobs in our sonograms.

The only people or organizations I can find that say this shit is safe is Monsanto, Eli Lilly and Company (the folks that purchased the business from Monsanto, and currently profit from it), or farmers that use it. Yet organizations like the United Nations and European Commission have ruled it completely unsafe for human consumption and have been putting out warnings since the late 1990s.[259, 263] I genuinely want to know who is doing the horizontal tango with the folks over at the FDA to get them to keep this shit on the "a-okay list."

Long story short, if you're going to consume dairy, do yourself a favor and consume non-rBGH dairy (in other words: organic dairy). That means you won't consume the cancer-causing growth hormone, which also means there won't be copious amounts of pus and antibiotics floating around in it either. Gosh, my mouth is watering! Nope, sorry, that was vomit.

Sulfites

These are some of the first known food additives, and have been around since the 1500s. Well, gee golly gosh they *have* to be good if they've been around for THAT long! Shit, no. They're just stubborn fuckers that won't go away.

The term "sulfites" (sometimes spelled "sul*phi*tes") actually encompasses the following group of additives:

E220 sulphur dioxide

E221 sodium sulphite

E222 sodium bisulphite

E223 sodium metabisulphite

E224 potassium metabisulphite

E225 potassium sulphite

E226 calcium sulfite

E227 calcium hydrogen sulfite

E228 potassium bisulphite

These vintage beauties are found mainly in dried fruits and wine (a perfect pairing), and are used as a preservative. They also naturally show up during fermentation though, so anything that is fermented will naturally have *some* level of sulfites. However, *adding* sulfites as a preservative is the issue at hand, as sulfite additive reactions affect about 1 in 100 people (usually asthmatics). When I say "effect," I mean cause anything from chronic skin and respiratory problems, to death. Perhaps those "asthmatics" aren't actually "asthmatics." Just a thought.

Get this: the FDA has banned sulfites from being sprayed on fresh, whole foods, and in the same breath has also ruled that any processed foods containing sulfites must be labeled. Makes total sense; ban from one type of food, and allow it with labels in another. That's not confusing. Why not simply get rid of the shit (like Australia has)? Ohhhh right—because then our dried fruit wouldn't last on a shelf for seventeen years.[61, 264-268]

Trans Fat

Trans fats were discussed back in chapter 16, and I'd like to reiterate their danger here. They are nothing less than silent killers. If you can remember, they are most commonly hidden in processed products like fast foods, baked goods, chips, coffee creamer, microwave popcorn, and frozen pizzas. Without warning, they will creep up on you and shred your insides as if trying to destroy the evidence that they were ever there. There has been concern about their safety since the early 1900s, and in 1994 a study concluded that:

> Because the consumption of [trans] fats is almost universal in the United States, the number of deaths attributable to such fats is likely to be substantial. Federal regulations should require manufacturers to include trans fatty acid content in food labels and should aim to greatly reduce or eliminate the use of [trans] fats.[269]

Guess what, here we are several decades later and those little fuckers *still* aren't banned! The FDA now currently recommends that people "keep trans fat consumption as low as possible by limiting foods that contain trans fats formed during food processing" (just fucking ban them, you asshats!). Why the recommendation? It was shown *years* ago that trans fats were estimated to cause somewhere between 30,000 and 100,000 deaths *annually* in the US.[270] Say WHAT?! Mmmm hmmm. And they're still in our fucking food! I'm talking *everywhere* in our fucking food. They're not purely linked to death; they are now also linked to heart disease, stroke, diabetes, and cancer. They are murderous little bitches. However, so is the FDA if they're the ones approving them. Yeah, I went there.

It is widely assumed that trans fats will be completely banned in the near future (don't hold your breath). Until then, you need to be weary of all processed foods. Even "innocent" foods like Girl Scout cookies; delectable, mouth-watering, at-the-door-of-every-house-in-America Girl Scout cookies. Yup, once full of trans fats, they finally listened to the growing concerns and reduced the synthetic fat in their treats. Since 2006 they have claimed "zero trans fats" on their products. But, wouldn't you know it—those little tasty fuckers *still* contain trans fats, but are flying under the allowable 0.5g radar that was mentioned in chapter 16. Fuckwads. Why on earth would you want to play "I'm going to poison you with little cute cookies" with millions of Americans? Why not be safe and get the shit out of your fuckin' cookies? Or, I know, how about you teach kids about nutrition and health and show them how to sell something other than fuckin' *cookies*.

Let's solute the following countries that have the light on upstairs, and have either full bans or harsh restrictions on trans fats: Argentina, Australia, Austria, Brazil, Canada, Denmark, Iceland, Sweden, and Switzerland.[99, 114, 271-276]

* * *

Now that we've survived that chemistry lesson, I have one final question for you: WHAT THE BLOODY FUCK IS ALL OF THIS FUCKING SHIT DOING IN OUR FOOD?! I'm going to lose my voice if I keep shouting (but at this point it's involuntary). Food should *fuel* us, not fuck us up. We should feel like we have the energy to fight lions after eating a meal, not take a nap or slip into a coma. Seriously though—talk about corporate-sponsored genocide. If you're not saying, "crikey Dick, something isn't quite right here," and giving a ginormous middle finger to the FDA, pharmaceutical, and chemical companies for corrupting and invading the system that's supposed to *nourish* us, please start this chapter over. Our "food" is highly contaminated. What is even more concerning is there are thousands of more unnecessary or harmful chemicals (in numerous countries) surrounding our foods that aren't even mentioned here.

I'll reiterate: it seems as though most companies who get their chemicals approved as "safe," do so purely by testing that *one* chemical in a simple, controlled environment, and don't take synergistic effects into account. The FDA may approve a certain chemical because, by itself, it's safe when exposed to a single human cell. Or, because a rat living in an extremely controlled environment doesn't immediately die from it. What they don't take into account is the fact that no one has simple one-chemical reactions in their body, nor is anyone limiting their chemical exposure to the recommended amount. Do you know the "safe levels" of the chemicals you ingest?? No, because you probably don't even know you're ingesting them.

Chances are, most people have a long list of chemicals inside themselves, all interacting together at once, and no one knows what that combination will do. Unless someone is studying every synergistic effect between the thousands of chemicals added to our foods, they can't say whether those chemicals are safe in our bodies. The notion that someone will only consume *one* specific "safe" chemical *and* stick to the recommended amount of that "safe" chemical, when they have no understanding of that limit, is absolutely absurd. Yet chemicals are approved based on that very notion.

Our food system has become utterly polluted, and we have become sick and miserable. It would be foolish to believe the two weren't related. To understand what I'm talking about, go pull out some of your packaged, processed "food" products (e.g. condiments, yogurt, cheese, bread, canned goods, crackers, spreads, beverages, pills, oral hygiene products), and count how many non-food ingredients you're ingesting. Remember, each additive *on its own* can cause ailments like cancer, diabetes, liver disease, thyroid disease, and ADHD. Mix them all together, and who knows what they can cause (maybe a world-wide, genocidal disease storm?). People are unknowingly eating themselves sick. Thus, at this point, you are no longer allowed to be confused about where all of this disease comes from, because the majority of it comes from our food system. Eat up, buttercup.

Next time you buy a food or beverage product (or pills, or oral hygiene products) that are either non-organic, or come in a package, and you wonder what the long list of chemical ingredients are, do your fucking research before purchasing it and putting it in your mouth. Or, better yet, simply buy certified organic whole foods and products, because how else are you going to avoid the farm chemicals that don't even show up on ingredient labels?

Thankfully, many countries are starting to ban certain additives, but unfortunately many US organizations and companies are way too fucking stubborn to see past their paycheck. Rather than wait for harmful chemicals to be banned, we need to avoid them. It's actually quite a simple concept: if you eat non-processed, whole, organically grown foods—which you can then concoct into any processed food you'd like in the safety of your own kitchen—you don't need to worry about any of these horrible chemicals anyway! I realize that's much easier said than done, but that's what this book is here for: to help you with the journey.

Moral of the Story:
Consumer products are littered with toxic chemicals—whether they're processed foods, restaurant foods, or whole foods that have been sprayed. If you don't want to grow third nipples (or get sick in general), you do your research and keep contaminated foods out of your fuckin' pie-hole.

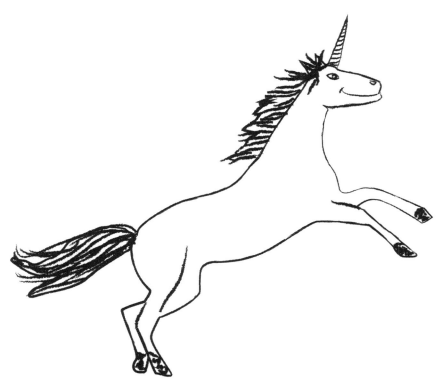

Well Done! You've made it half way!
Who needs another ribbon...
when you can have a shiny UNICORN?!

Chapter 22

Let the Games Begin!

Now that we've had an absolute hoot talking about some of the poisonous shit that's thrown in our food, let's play a little game! Think of this as a reward for the chemistry and math that you've been subjected to (you're welcome). Listed here are some of the most popular consumer products available. Your goal is to guess what these items are, solely based on their ingredients (good-fucking-luck). Then, once you discover how "awesome" they are, DISPOSE OF THEM (if you happen to have any).

Let the Games Begin.

Mystery Item #1a	Mystery Item #1b	Mystery Item #1c
carbonated water	carbonated water	carbonated purified water
HFCS	caramel color	cane sugar
caramel color	aspartame	caramel color
phosphoric acid	phosphoric acid	food acid
natural flavors	potassium benzoate	Flavour
	natural flavors	
	citric acid	
	caffeine	

It's kind of hard to tell what something is when there isn't much of anything real in it (other than those "natural" flavors! ha!), right?

Meet Coke (left) and Diet Coke (middle). We'll get to the right column in a second. Coke is chemical water. In case you forgot, the majority of those ingredients were all discussed earlier as shit to avoid like the plague. It's *Coke* and *Diet Coke* for fuck's sake — clearly something that's not being widely avoided. Heck, Coca-Cola has been the longest continuous corporate sponsor of the Olympic games![277] Be like an Olympian! Drink Coke! Get fucked!

Are you on the edge of your seat about the mystery item on the right? That's coke sold in *New Zealand*, where high fructose corn syrup and non-purified water apparently aren't desired. Don't get me wrong, it still doesn't make Coke a healthy option, but my point is that many harmful ingredients aren't often needed in consumer products. Many companies who distribute internationally often change their ingredient lists to conform to the regulations in that country, which means it is 100% possible for these companies not to stop serving up harmful shit to us.

Mystery Item #2	
sugar	soy lecithin
gum base	aspartame
corn syrup	acesulfame k
dextrose	hydroxylated soy lecithin
natural and artificial flavors	yellow 5
glycerol	BHT "to maintain freshness"

Oh heck no. Do *not* take away my chewing gum! That's right, this is gum, and I'm not going to take anything away from you — *you're* going to take it away once you realize what you're putting in your mouth. If you can explain *right now* what all the above ingredients are (refer back to previous chapter if you'd like), and why they're safe for you to put in your mouth (regardless if you swallow them or not), then by all means, continue to chew that shit. As long as you're making an educated decision about it, there's nothing I can do to stop you.

By the way, this was Wrigley's Juicy Fruit gum—you know, the kind everyone assumes is healthier for them simply because it has "fruit" in the title (wow, look at all the fruit listed in the ingredients). This is all about common sense, folks. Gum doesn't naturally grow somewhere; gum—especially sugar-free gum—is a man-made potion of harmful chemicals. I don't care if you chew gum once a week. Remember, it's all of the "little" things you do that add up to one big chemical clusterfuck in your body. Chewing on a sweaty jock strap would be healthier.

Mystery Item #3	
beef	sodium phosphates
water	sodium diacetate
corn syrup	flavor
salt	ascorbic acid
potassium lactate	extractives of paprika
dextrose	sodium nitrate

Now, the "beef" may have been somewhat of a hint, but I bet you still couldn't guess that this chemical concoction is a good ol' American hot dog (Oscar Mayer brand, to be exact)—served at every BBQ and ball game in the US. Who doesn't like sharing chemicals with friends?! Sharing is caring! Unfortunately, caring could mean cancer. Next time you go to grab a ground up meat-and-chemical stick (hot dog, sausage, whatever)—which is also probably wrapped in a chemical-filled bun, topped with chemical-filled condiments—please take a second to consider what you're putting in your pie-hole.

Mystery Item #4	
corn	tomato powder
vegetable oil	lactose
maltodextrin	spices
salt	yellow 6
cheddar cheese	yellow 5
whey	red 40
monosodium glutamate (MSG)	lactic acid
buttermilk	citric acid
romano cheese	sugar
whey protein concentrate	garlic powder
onion powder	skim milk
corn flour	red and green bell pepper powder
natural and artificial flavor	disodium inosinate
dextrose	disodium guanylate

How much crap can one pack into a product? Apparently, as much as they'd like! These would be nacho cheese-flavored Doritos. They have to be one of the most popular brands in America, and are available world-wide. The ingredients listed above are US ingredients. They, like Coke, have different recipes for the different countries they export to. But hey! At least there's red and green bell pepper powder in there! Doritos for the win!

Mystery Item #5	
American cheese	salt
water	sodium phosphate
milk fat	sorbic acid
sodium citrate	vitamin D3
calcium phosphate	

Either you stopped reading, or you clearly noticed that this was American cheese (Kraft "Deli Deluxe" brand—deluxe piece 'o shit, if you ask me). If I had a dollar for every time I got asked what was "wrong" with cheese, I'd be funding the mission to Mars. *This* is what is wrong with cheese (well, this isn't *all* that's wrong with cheese, but we'll save that for the next chapter). Unless you're making your own, or you purchase from a local organic farmer, *this* is what's shoved into your cheese (along with any hormones and antibiotics that were previously pumped into the cow, and aren't listed on the label). Contrary to popular belief, cheese isn't awesome simply because it contains calcium and protein. You know what else contains calcium and protein? Poop.

Mystery Item #6a	Mystery Item #6b
carbonated water	carbonated water
sucrose	citric acid
glucose	taurine
citric acid	sodium citrate
taurine	magnesium carbonate
sodium citrate	caffeine
magnesium carbonate	acesulfame k
caffeine	aspartame
inositol	inositol
niacinamide	niacinamide
calcium pantothenate	calcium pantothenate
pyridoxine hcl	pyridoxine hcl
vitamin B$_{12}$	vitamin B$_{12}$
natural and artificial flavors	xanthan gum
colors	natural and artificial flavors
	colors

Mmmmmmmm—nothin' says lovin' like paying a high price for caffeinated, sweetened, chemical water. These items are Red Bull (left) and Sugar-Free Red Bull (right)—the most consumed energy drinks in the world. I've never had one, so I can't even *begin* to imagine the orgasmic taste that must flow from those cans. I *do* remember a "fun" time back in my early twenties though, when my then-boyfriend consumed a whole lot of Red Bull and we got to spend the night with a bunch of cool doctors and nurses in the emergency room. What a party *that* was! Those ingredients are not wonderful vitamins your body "needs" in order to stay energized.

If you consume *real* foods made up of *real* vitamins, you'll have all of the energy your little heart desires. Wings-schmings; I'm fine with my fucking *cape,* thank you very much.

Mystery Item #7	
water	riboflavin
modified food starch	durum flour
salt	sodium bicarbonate
flavoring	sodium acid pyrophosphate
monosodium glutamate	yeast
caramel color	soy protein concentrate
corn syrup solids	salt
autolyzed yeast extract	caramel color
disodium isonate and guanylate	flavoring
xanthan gum	sodium tripolyphosphate
salt	dextrose
hydrolyzed soy protein	spice
sugar	citric acid
monosodium glutamate	corn
flavor	potatoes
caramel color	mono- and diglycerides from vegetable oil
vegetable juice concentrates	disodium dihydrosphate
extracts of paprika	sodium bisulfite
dried whey	citric acid
water	BHT
mechanically separated chicken	soybean oil
pork	salt
beef	sugar
water	potassium chloride
rehydrated onions	maltodextrin
soy flour	natural flavor
caramel color	magnesium carbonate
bleached wheat flour	calcium chloride
niacin	magnesium chloride
reduced iron	calcium carbonate
thiamine mononitrate	

I did not make that list up. This is a Banquet microwave dinner: a lovely, mouth-watering salisbury steak meal. And when they say "steak," they apparently mean "mechanically separated chicken, pork and beef."

Some of these awesome ingredients are listed multiple times due to the fact that each "food" in the box needs to be enhanced or held together. By the way, this is purely supposed to be steak, potatoes, and corn. Oh, and the lovely tag-line on the box is "Child **Hunger** Stops Here." Of course it does! If you feed this crap to your child they will die, and then they won't be hungry anymore! Kill the child, stop the hunger!

Mystery Item #8	
lemon juice from concentrate	sodium sulfite
sodium benzoate	lemon oil
sodium metabisulfite	

Oh goodie! Something doesn't have a list of ingredients as long as Aunt Ethel's prescription list! Hmmmm, something is still fishy though. Wouldn't you assume that something boldly labeled "100% Lemon Juice" front and center on the label would only contain, oh, I don't know . . . lemon juice? Nope.

Mystery Item #9	
unbleached enriched flour	calcium sulfate
water	dough conditioners
high fructose corn syrup	mono- and diglycerides
canola oil and/or soybean oil	calcium propionate
yeast	azodicarbonamide
gluten	ascorbic acid
sea salt	soy lecithin
whey	

Fuck this shit. You know how I make bread? I mix flour, water, and yeast and call it a day. If I really want to live on the edge, I throw in some honey and fresh rosemary. What the fuck is all of that shit doing in a loaf of bread?!

Mystery Item #10	
water	sodium citrate
sugar	monopotassium phosphate
dextrose	modified food starch
citric acid	glycerol ester of rosin
natural and artificial flavor	blue 1

This lovely train wreck comes from a Gatorade Sports Drink. Can you tell what flavor it is? Of course not. They've used beaver ass or who-knows-what-else to "naturally" flavor this potion and then logically label it "Grape." I want to know who the geniuses were that convinced *athletes*, of all people, that *this* was what should fuel their bodies?! Answer: the people with the money! If you want to be a top athlete, *don't* drink sports drinks. If you *are* a top athlete, *stop* endorsing this shit so that every up-and-coming athlete who wants to be like you will stop reaching for it.

Mystery Item #11	
sugar	natural flavor
corn flour blend	blue 2
wheat flour	turmeric color
whole grain oat flour	yellow 6
oat fiber	annatto color
soluble corn fiber	blue 1
partially hydrogenated vege oil	BHT
red 40	

The first problem here is that the first ingredient is "sugar." The second problem is that Kellogg's thinks they're so fucking smart for putting the word "fruit"—sorry, *"froot"*—in a cereal title so parents feel better about giving it to their kids. Here we have the technicolor, and wildly scrumptious Froot Loops (which are all the same flavor, by the way). Good thing they didn't spell "fruit" correctly, or I would have actually thought there might have been fruit in there. Fueling kids with chemicals is such an awesome idea. No really, I wonder why kids are struggling in school when they're eating shit like this.

Mystery Item #12	
phenol	glycerin
red 40	purified water
flavor	sodium saccharin

This is an interesting one. Even though it's not meant to be consumed (it actually tells you to spit it out on the label), I'd take an educated guess that most people don't realize they're supposed to spit it out. Let me introduce you to throat and cough spray: Chloraseptic Sugar-Free Cherry Flavor (hold on—where were the cherries listed?). When was the last time you sprayed your throat down with cough spray and then spit it out? Or, did you just keep spraying the shit out of your throat because that numbing relief and cherry "flavor" made you want to vigorously indulge? Riddle me this: If your throat is red and raw, do you want to spray some chemicals on it that temporarily "soothe" it by merely making it go numb? *Or,* do you possibly want to have a honey, ginger, and lemon tea that actually *does* soothe and heal your throat rather than simply making it numb? It's your call. Please head to your medicine cabinet and throw out anything that isn't natural that you could potentially put in your pie-hole. There are ways to make natural versions of every harsh chemical remedy out there. I know this because I make them and fill my house with them.

Mystery Item #13	
stannous fluoride	flavor
glycerine	sodium lauryl sulfate
hydrated silica	sodium gluconate
sodium hexametaphosphate	carrageenan
propylene glycol	sodium saccharin
peg-6	polyethylene
water	xanthan gum
zinc lactate	titanium dioxide
trisodium phosphate	blue 1

You probably put this in your mouth every day. Most likely *multiple* times per day. That is, if you have "good" oral hygiene. Hello, Crest Pro-Health Toothpaste! It's nice to meet you and your healthy-sounding, "pro-health" self.

Even if you spit your toothpaste out, you still ingest and absorb these chemicals. Especially if you use the python-sized amount seen perfectly perched on toothbrushes in advertisements (you only need a pea-sized amount to clean those pearly-whites . . . but then you wouldn't go through your toothpaste fast enough, and sales would decline). You can probably now understand, why I make my own toothpaste ("YOU FUCKING HIPPIE!"). I discovered that even the "natural" toothpastes still have toxic ingredients in them, which I'm not willing to take a risk on. Call me a "hippie," call me "extreme," or call me a *genius* for eliminating more chemicals from my body while at the same time saving money! Cha-ching!

Mystery Item #14	
tobacco	diammonium phosphate
water	ammonium hydroxide
sugars (sucrose and/or invert sugar and/or high fructose corn syrup)	cocoa and cocoa products
propylene glycol	carob bean and extract
glycerol	natural and artificial flavors
licorice extract	

The wacky tabacky! In my opinion, people who smoke cigarettes need counseling. They *have* to know there's a good chance it will kill them, and anyone who wants to kill themselves is suicidal, severely depressed, or insane. Fucking hell, please don't smoke. This is quite possibly my biggest pet peeve. If you smoke, you are asking for cancer *and* you are also putting everyone around you at risk for cancer—actually, not only cancer, but heart attack and stroke as well.[278, 279]

Basically, you have a death wish if you smoke. What you don't have, is the right to give everyone around you a death wish. Yet, there are thousands of *non-smokers* who die every year from breathing second-hand smoke. That's right—listen up all of you fuckers out there smoking in the vicinity of others (or in any public space): you are irrefutably increasing someone else's risk of dying a slow, painful death. Children, pregnant women, fetuses *inside* a pregnant women, someone's dad, someone who already quit smoking . . . everyone. Who gives *you* the right to cut someone else's life short? Stop being so fucking selfish.

My husband has a saying for when he sees someone smoking in a public place: "I don't fart in your face, so don't smoke in my space." I'm waiting for him to force a nasty fart in someone's face one of these days. It *will* happen. I'd take a good fart inhalation over cigarette smoke any day though, because it's not going to make me die a slow, painful death (unless it's one of my husband's rippers, then that's debatable). I hereby release the rights to the above quote and give you permission to not only use it, but also to fart in everyone's face who blows smoke in your space. Tip from a pro: eat a bunch of curry first.

Mystery Item #15	
norgestimate	pregelatinized starch
ethinyl estradiol	blue 2
lactose	yellow 10
magnesium stearate	

Oh boy, am I going to get shit for this one. Feast your eyes on oral contraceptives (i.e. birth control). Yes, I'm going to go here. I pride myself by saying that I have never shoved an oral contraceptive down my pie-hole. The first time I ever found out about what they actually did (i.e. they stop a woman's natural build-a-baby process), I thought, "how the fuck does *that* sound okay?!" It's common sense people: something that completely shuts down one of your bodily processes is NOT OKAY, will have a long list of side effects, and can in no way be good for you.

But, they're an *excellent* money-maker for pharmaceutical companies! Let's get them in the hand of *every* young woman on this planet! Not only do they make it harder for women to conceive, but oral contraceptives are also being linked to more and more health issues with every passing year. For instance, Ortho Tri-Cyclen's insert states right on it that "an increased risk of [heart attack] has been attributed to oral contraceptive use." They also have a loooooong list of less-than-fun side effects, including increased risk of liver, breast, and cervical cancer.[280-282] Going further, a 2014 study suggests that long-term oral contraceptive use effects the grey matter in your *brain*, thus effecting learning and memory.[283] Hey, why not?! All of that kind of sounds better than pushing a baby through a vagina, right?

Be smart, use your common sense, and put the shit in the trash. Be smart about sex if you don't want to conceive (this doesn't mean that you need to stop having sex). Simple as that. I've done it, and so can you. For those of you who take oral contraception to minimize menstrual symptoms or manage other ailments: put your big girl panties on. Then, remember that the cleaner you eat, the more regular you will be with your cycle, the less ailments you will have, and the less PMS you will experience. My PMS completely disappeared when I climbed to the top of the Nutrition Spectrum. No cramping, no bloating, no bitching. No excuses; get rid of the shit. Men, this goes for you as well; don't think for a second that a male birth control pill won't be lining pharmacy shelves in the near future. Don't you dare even consider it.

That was a fun game, eh? How did you do? Did you recognize any of those popular consumer products filled with shit that isn't food? Can you see how all of this shit would accumulate if you constantly ate contaminated foods? Did you go to your pantry and medicine cabinet and do a purge of all things harmful? It's quite disheartening that this is the "food" being presented to us.

From grocery store items (e.g. ketchup, salad dressing, yogurt, bread), to restaurants and cafes (e.g. Applebee's, Olive Garden, Outback Steakhouse, IHOP, Denny's, Panera Bread, Starbucks, Subway), nothing is safe. They all use products contaminated with harmful shit. Don't assume anything is safe until you've done your research—even if they promote themselves as being healthy. To illustrate what I mean, I have one more mystery item (well, three versions of an item)—this time from a restaurant—to throw at ya.

Mystery Item #16a	Mystery Item #16b	Mystery Item #16c
potatoes	potatoes	potatoes
canola oil	canola oil	vegetable oil
soybean oil	butylated hydroxyanisole (BHA)	dextrose
hydrogenated soybean oil	citric acid	
natural beef flavor	polydimethylsil-oxane	
citric acid	dextrose	
dextrose		
sodium acid pyrophosphate		
salt		
tert-butylhydroquinone		
citric acid		
dimethylpolysil-oxane		

French fries. Those are all versions of fucking FRENCH FRIES, because it's apparently impossible to make them purely out of potatoes these days. Not only are they all versions of fries, but they also come from the *same* restaurant. Not that I would ever step foot in this place, but they are some of the most famous fries on Earth—from the golden arches themselves: McDonald's. Why three versions? Some countries are using their fucking brains more, that's why. There are actually a lot more than three versions—I just don't want to write a whole book on McDonald's. Is the suspense killing you yet? Okay, okay—in the left column are the ingredients in McDonald's fries found in the US, in the middle column are the ingredients in McDonald's fries found in New Zealand, and in the right column are the ingredients in McDonald's fries found in the UK. Interesting, eh? When was the last time your fries came with an ingredient list *that you read*? If you answered "I don't eat fast food," then give yourself a pat on the back, you champion. Unfortunately, it's not just fast food; if you eat out, chances are you *will* eat extra shit without knowing it. Generally more if you live in America.

Another problem arises though, because even if you eat out, hunt down a label, and determine that the ingredients in your desired dish are on your "okay" list, you won't necessarily be safe. Take the McDonald's french fry example. Even if none of those listed chemicals were added to those fries as they were being made, what about all of the farm chemicals that those potatoes were sprayed with down at the field before they even made it to the golden arches? McDonald's sure as shit isn't using *organically grown* potatoes. Those bitches are guaranteed to be covered in herbicides and pesticides, unless we trust that they thoroughly wash their produce . . . with something that won't leave more chemical residue on the food. Suddenly, you have fries that may cause cancer, disrupt your hormones, and hinder brain development. Mmmmm, "I'm lovin' it!"

* * *

There you have it—*some* of the dangers lurking in the shit we put in our pie-holes (there are thousands more). In everyday life, if you *know* something is dangerous, you steer clear of it, right? If you put a loaded gun to your head, you won't pull the trigger (at least I hope you won't), because you *know* it can kill you. Why the heck then, would you put something in your pie-hole that you *know* could kill you (albeit a slow, painful death)?! For the love of God, stop pulling the trigger!

Our food system is laced with harmful crap, and the consumer is usually completely unaware. What makes things worse, is that food companies and food establishments have gotten pretty good at playing the game. They'll get Olympic Athletes to endorse things like sports drinks and fast food so we don't think twice about consuming them. For fuck's sake, McDonald's was one of the *main* sponsors of the 2012 Olympics! Now every child, person, and athlete around the world associates McDonald's with success, and believes it's okay to fuel themselves with some of the worst "nutrients" out there.

There are some pretty gnarly tactics being used in the food marketing game, and I tell you what: they're turning me into a fire-breathing dragon. It's imperative that you start to question these sales tactics and really understand the meaning (or lack of meaning) behind them. For instance, non-organic, non-fresh apple slices were added to McDonald's Happy Meals (sorry to shit on you so much, McD's, but you kind of ask for it). Parents now somehow justify the safety of that *whole* happy meal for their child, simply because they have soggy, chemical-covered apples hanging out next to them—which the child rarely touches anyway. And McDonald's somehow ends up being placed on the healthy train because they're doing their part to provide healthy food to kids. It's a load of bull.

There's another tactic that drives me crazy, and it involves bread. We know whole grain bread is healthier than refined white bread (or if you didn't know, then now you do), right? How are companies using this to their advantage? They are dying their white breads brown—usually with the harmful caramel coloring we previously learned about—to make them look more natural. They then conveniently call them something like "wheat" or "9-

grain." How much wheat does it have? Is it *whole* wheat? What are the "9 grains"? Just because it has "9 grains" doesn't mean it doesn't also have fifty chemicals. We saw what bread contains—just head back to mystery item number nine. Make your own bread if you must eat bread. It's about as easy as baking gets.

Another great tactic came with "Coke Life": a version of Coke's famous cola that arrived in 2014. It comes in a green bottle, because "green" is associated with health, sustainability, and peace. While it may boast fewer calories and sugar than standard coke, it's still full of the standard harmful chemicals. Yet, if you put a "healthier" version of something on the market, it presents another option for consumers to flock to. "Sweet! I can justify my soda habit now because there's a healthier version!" "Healthier" does not mean "healthy," please go find your smart pants, because they must have fallen off.

Speaking of Coke, my husband purchased a bottle of L&P on our latest trip to New Zealand. L&P stands for "Lemon and Paeroa." If you haven't heard of it, you're probably not from New Zealand. L&P is in every store in New Zealand, and Kiwis are damn proud of this "homemade" drink of theirs. Since the 1940s, L&P has been pumped out to the public. Unfortunately, it's no longer the same product it was decades ago. You see, L&P used to be made with *actual* lemon and *actual* carbonated mineral water from the little town of Paeroa. Somewhere along the way, the company sold out to Coca-Cola. Do you want to take a stab at what the ingredients are now? I can tell you for certain there's no longer any lemon in that drink.[284] Here is a list of the current ingredients:

carbonated water	flavour
sugar	mineral salts (504, 500, 170)
food acid (330)	colour (150d)

That's a *long* way off from the original mineral water and lemon mixture, and also a long way off from being healthy. In a nutshell, Coke saw a successful product and wanted it (you gluttonous cow, Coke). They bought out the original owners, and found ways to make the product taste similar (or "better"), yet without costing as much. Now we have L&P as we know it today—a complete chemical blow out. This is how consumer products go down the shitter: companies are consistently trying to produce food cheaper to make more money. The consumer usually has no clue something has changed so drastically, assumes the product is still what it appears to be, and continues to buy it because they have trust in the food system. We will now have a moment of silence for all of the Kiwis who are mourning the loss of their national drink.

(Begin silence.)

(End silence.)

All in all, you can't simply assume something is good for you, or that it actually contains what it's assumed to contain simply because it's been presented as safe. The titles thrown on packaged foods these days are a fucking joke. A can of "corn" doesn't only contain corn. "Ginger ale" may not contain ginger. "Bacon Bits" might not contain any bacon. Minced garlic contains whatever is needed to keep that garlic "fresh." Fruit-flavored Jell-o contains— you guessed it—zero fruit. Everyone is playing games. Big fucking mind games. And this fire-breathing dragon is sick of it.

Thankfully, you're starting to educate yourself. And once you do so, you can start to avoid all of the disease-causing, toxic shit and just eat real, untainted food. We, as consumers, simply need to put our brain and reading skills to use—and I'm going to assume that if you've made it this far into the book, you're at least at a third grade reading level.

Moral of the Story:
Don't ever assume consumables are safe;
the food industry's toxic roots run deep.

Chapter 23

Controversy

At any given moment there are usually a handful of nutrition topics being pulled back and forth between good and evil. You know, topics that if mentioned to a group of people, half will chant, "fuck no! That shit will kill you!" And the other half will shout, "heck yes! That shit is the fountain of youth!" Dah, dah, dah—controversy!

First off, let's face it, "knowledge" changes over time. What was once considered safe may not actually be safe anymore—like smoking cigarettes and painting your walls with lead paint. Thus, unless you're open to the idea that "knowledge" may evolve, you might find yourself in a rough spot. Holding on to something that isn't safe anymore simply because you grew up on it or your family business depends on it will not get you far in this ever-shifting world. Similarly, automatically writing something off for the sole reason that someone random deemed dangerous won't get you anywhere either. Clean the slate, do your research, and try not to be swayed by your family business, your personal trainer, your health magazine, or the industries themselves. Or me. I mean it—I cleaned the slate, did my research, and formed my own beliefs based on that research. I want you to do the same.

I'm happy to get you started by offering my findings and opinions on some of the latest controversial forerunners. As always, my opinions are based on personal experience and a shitload of scientific research. Take them as you'd like, but if you find yourself questioning *any* of what I'm about to discuss, the logical thing to do would be to go out and research the topic(s) yourself (reputable, third party sources, remember). Suit up, nutrition warrior—we're about to venture into the daunting world of controversy.

Genetically Modified Organisms (GMOs)

In the first ten years of genetically engineered ingredients . . . being introduced into our food supply (1997-2007), there was a 265% increase in the rates of hospitalization related to food allergic reactions. Correlation is not causation, but it begs the question: Are we allergic to food or what's been done to it? It merits investigation, and at the very least, the labeling of these genetically engineered ingredients. —Robyn O'Brien, the "Erin Brokovich of the Food Industry"

I can't even begin to understand why GMOs are controversial. I feel like they should be on everyone's shit list (you'll soon find out why). But is it the actual genetic modification, or the chemicals that go hand-in-hand with GMOs that should be a worry?

We've already touched on GMOs a bit. They are the human-built "super seeds" (or "mutant seeds") to which we referred in the previous chapter when we discussed the herbicide "RoundUp" (which contains the awesomely-fabulous, and ever-so-destructive ingredient glyphosate). These genetically engineered seeds (which grow into crops) are specially designed to have an increased immunity to herbicides like glyphosate. With this genetic alteration and enhanced immunity, farmers can spray the shit out of their crops, kill encroaching weeds, and not affect the stuff we're eventually going to consume (or so they say). This obviously leads to increased production and more Cubans and Bugattis for the high-rolling CEOs.

The leader of GMO production is the chemical company Monsanto, who, as we already learned, also conveniently

manufactures the harmful weed killer Roundup. They consider
their genetically modified seeds to be "Roundup Ready," meaning
their seeds are capable of thriving, even after being doused with
Roundup. Therefore, you can buy their mutant seeds *and* their
weed killer, and grow a shit load of crops.

As my good buddy Robyn O'Brien states (we've never met, but
let's pretend), "[GMOs are] a brilliant business model for a
chemical company: food crops are engineered by the chemical
company to withstand their chemicals. It drives revenue." She's
right. They rake in the dough from all sides. It's brilliant. But only
in the most twisted, sadistic sense.

Robyn also argues that genetically modified foods aren't
produced by *food* companies; they're produced by *chemical*
companies. I completely agree, and, in my not-so-humble-opinion,
believe they have no business in our food system. What also
doesn't sit well with me is that since the introduction of these
genetically modified foods, food allergies have skyrocketed. We're
talking a 400% increase in child allergies alone.[285] As Robyn
admits, "correlation is not causation" (meaning that simply
because two things seem to be associated, it doesn't mean one
causes the other)—but I don't give a shit in this instance. It's
common sense: we fuck with our food, our food fucks with us.

The controversy with GMOs then, is that some people say
they're safe (generally the folks profiting from them), and some
people say they're harmful (generally the folks who care about the
health of society and the environment). Either way, there's great
confusion about whether or not the actual seeds or the chemicals
attached to them are doing the damage. The other controversial
part about GMOs is that they're not labeled, so even if you made a
decision on whether or not you wanted to consume them, it's hard
to know how to avoid them.

We'll soon discuss some good tips on how to spot a genetically
modified product or ingredient (it would be nice to possess
Superman's x-ray vision right about now, but we can't have our
cake and eat it too, now can we). Just for your reference though—

before we become GMO-spotting supersleuths—let's take a look at some of the companies that are regularly using GMOs. Table 23.1 depicts a small selection of them (and some of their famous brands) that knowingly use, and thus support, genetically modified products in their consumables.

Table 23.1. Companies using GMOs in consumables

Company	Brands	
Campbell's	Healthy Request	Pace Foods
	Bolthouse Farms	Pepperidge Farms
	Wolfgang Puck Soups	
Cargill	Truvia Sweetener	Nature Fresh
	Shady Brooks Farms	Good Nature
Coca-Cola	Vitamin Water	Minute Maid
	Smart Water	Honest Tea
	Dasani	Odwalla
	Nestea	Vitaminenergy
Con-Agra	Orville Redenbacher's	Healthy Choice
	Hunt's Organic	
General Mills	Nature Valley	Larabar
	Fiber One	Gold Medal Organic
	Cheerios	Food Should Taste
	Cascadian Farms	Good
	Muir Glen	
Hain-Celestial	Earth's Best	Soy Dream
	Spectrum Organics	Walnut Acres
	Garden of Eatin'	Fruiti di Bosco
	Rice Dream	Celestial Seasonings
Heinz	Bagel Bites	Tater Tots
	Heinz	TGI Friday's
	Ore-Ida	Wattie's
	Smart Ones	Weight Watchers
The Hersey Company	Almond Joy	Whoppers
	Milk Duds	York Peppermint
	Mounds	Patties
	Reese's	

Table 23.1. (*continued*)

Company	Brands	
J. M. Smucker, Co.	Smuckers	Carnation
	Jiff	Hungry Jack
	Folgers	Life is Good
	Pillsbury	Natural Brew
	Dunkin Donuts	Santa Cruz Organic
Kellogg's	Kashi	Bear Naked
	Muslix	Morningstar Farms
	Nutrigrain	Gardenburger
Kraft	Snapple	South Beach
	Triscuit	Boca
	SnackWell's	Nabisco
Merck	Clarinex	Proventil
	Fosamax	Sinemet
	Gardasil	SingulaiR
	MMR Vaccine	Vytorin
	Nasonex	Zocor
	NuvaRing	
Nestlé	Pure Life	Gerber
	Pellegrino	California Pizza
	Perrier	Kitchen
	Poland Spring	Sweat Leaf Tea
PepsiCo	Sun Chips	Ocean Spray
	Aquafina	Tropicana
	SoBe	Quaker
	Harvest Crunch	Naked Juice
	Dole	Sabra
Starbucks	Evolution Fresh	Tazo
	Seattle's Best	Teavana

Here's the kicker: not only do these companies *use* GMOs, but they also often donate thousands (sometimes *millions*) of dollars toward anti-labeling campaigns to *stop* GMO labeling and to keep consumers in the dark. Why pour so much money into *not* labeling something? Um, because they know their products wouldn't bring in as much revenue if people knew the truth—and revenue is what matters. Thus, I hate to break it to you (that's a

lie), but even if a large company has an organic spin-off brand
(e.g. General Mills and their Gold Medal Organic brand), buying a
product of that organic brand means you are giving the larger
company money to then turn around and lobby to keep GMOs
hidden in our consumables. Well, shit.

What's interesting, is that GMO supporters—who cite
hundreds of studies supporting the fact that "GMOs are just as
safe as organically grown or conventional foods"—may not
realize that almost every single study published on GMOs comes
directly from the GMO-producing companies (e.g. Monsanto).
That's like a cigarette company doing a study on cigarettes and
telling us they're safe—and then us believing them. Finding
independent studies, by people *without* ties to the GMO industry, is
like trying to find a Big Mac in a Whopper haystack. They are one
in a million. This is due to the dumb fucking intellectual property
rights put into place by companies like Monsanto. These rights
prohibit outsiders from doing research on their products without
their approval (and guess how often that happens).

This means that GMO companies can tailor studies in order to
make the public believe something. It also means they can pick
and choose which studies they publish, and can contort, alter, and
hide whatever the fuck they want within them. If you know about
science and research, you know just how important it is to have
independent researchers (i.e. outsiders) studying products in which
they have no stake. Thus, I trust GMO safety studies about as far
as an armless man could throw them.

What I *do* trust, are stories from the multitude of farmers
(without ties to the GMO industry) who have seen firsthand how
the use of GMO crops has affected their livestock and the people
living in close proximity to their production. They are putting
their hands up to tell their stories after turning away from GMO
feed. After switching back to *non*-GMO feed, they suddenly see
livestock with reduced diarrhea and stomach inflammation. They
see healthier animals that need less medicine. They report *higher*
milk production, more live births, and less birth defects. Basically,

animals are much healthier and *more* productive if they're fed the non-fucked with version of their food.[234, 286-293]

It doesn't stop at animals. Argentina is the world's third-largest producer of genetically modified soybeans, and since the "large-scale introduction of Roundup Ready soy beans" infiltrated their country, both cancer and birth defects in humans have *skyrocketed:* "Residents and doctors in soy producing areas began reporting serious health effects from glyphosate spraying, including high rates of birth defects as well as infertility, stillbirths, miscarriages, and cancers."[294] I guess that's one way to deliver birth control to your nation—this shit probably has a greater success rate than condoms! Many of the long-term effects from Roundup can take ten to twenty years to show up. By then, Monsanto (and the other asshole chemical companies that have infiltrated our food system) will have made their billions and moved to Mars.

The difficult part is that I hear people making statements like: "but we need to make a living," and "our farm runs on GMOs!" You know what also makes a pretty penny? Robbing banks. But that doesn't make it the best option. "We need to make a living" is never the right answer when it comes to a product that could be endangering the people who consume it, or the environment around it. Everyone *needs* to make a living. We just need to be smart about how we go about it. And we're far from that.

Speaking of being smart, there are currently over sixty countries that have either significantly restricted, completely banned, or initiated labeling laws of GMOs due to their reputation.[295, 296] Not one or two, but *sixty-five*:

Australia	Bulgaria	Ecuador	Hungary
Austria	Cameroon	El Salvador	Iceland
Belarus	China	Estonia	India
Belgium	Croatia	Ethiopia	Indonesia
Bolivia	Cyprus	Finland	Ireland
Bosnia &	Czech	France	Italy
Herzegovina	Republic	Germany	Japan
Brazil	Denmark	Greece	Jordan

Kazakhstan	Mauritius	Saudi Arabia	Switzerland
Kenya	Netherlands	Senegal	Taiwan
Kyrgyzstan	New Zealand	Slovakia	Thailand
Latvia	Norway	Slovenia	Tunisia
Lithuania	Peru	South Africa	Turkey
Luxembourg	Poland	South Korea	Ukraine
Malaysia	Portugal	Spain	United
Mali	Romania	Sri Lanka	Kingdom
Malta	Russia	Sweden	Vietnam

Either all of those countries are wacked on crack, or the people making the decisions in America (and other countries that still engage in GMO production) are complete asshats. I'm going to go with the latter, and here's why: 91% of Americans want to label consumables that contain GMOs. This means that pretty much everyone either wants to know what they're putting in their pie-hole, or they have a concern about GMO safety (and I'm guessing the other 9% either don't have a clue what GMOs are, or directly profit from them).[297] Yet, not only are we still pumping our foods full of GMOs (about 80% of processed foods in America have GM ingredients), but there's also no federal law on labeling them.[298] *And*, since people who use or grow genetically modified crops *know* that GMOs are a controversial commodity, most of them don't have any desire to volunteer to label them. Why would they?! "They're trying to make a living!" They *know* their sales will drop if their products don "I'm produced in a lab and am slathered with damaging chemicals" labels.

America is pumping out GMOs faster than I can say, "tumor." But wait—what happens when an American company with genetically modified-laced products wants to export to one of the previously-listed countries that has red-flagged them? They quite easily label their products as having GMOs! Yet, when they sell those same products to Americans, they will omit that little fact. Even better, sometimes GMO-selling companies wind up having *two* versions of their products: a genetically modified version that they can sell to the US, and a non-genetically modified version that they can ship off to countries that have completely banned GMOs.

It's insane. Instead of slapping a simple label on a product, lobbyists are doing everything they can to *stop* GMO labeling in America. In fact, in the first six months of 2014 they spent over $27 *million* in their efforts. That was almost triple what they spent in *all* of 2013.[299] Hmmm, I wonder how much a label would cost. Things are heating up, and someone is sweating in their panties (sweat motherfuckers, SWEAT!). They're spending whatever it takes to keep us in the dark, and there could only be one reason why. Just label the fuckers and call it a day, you wacky tyrants!

Nearly every processed food would have to be labeled though, because, as mentioned previously, 80% of processed foods have something genetically modified hiding in them. Since I clearly love making lists, below is a list of some common ingredients you may find in your consumables. All of which generally come from genetically modified food.[300]

Aspartame (a.k.a. *AminoSweet, NutraSweet, Equal, BeneVia, E951*)	cyclodextrin
	cystein
baking powder	dextrin
canola oil (rapeseed oil)	dextrose
caramel color	diacetyl
cellulose	diglyceride
citric acid	erythritol
cobalamin (vitamin B_{12})	Equal
colorose	food starch
condensed milk	fructose (any form)
confectioner's sugar	glucose
corn flour	glutamate
corn masa	glutamic acid
corn meal	glycerides
corn oil	glycerin
corn sugar	glycerol
corn syrup	glycerol monooleate
cornstarch	glycine
cottonseed oil	hemicellulose

high fructose corn syrup (HFCS)
hydrogenated starch
hydrolyzed vegetable protein
inositol
inverse syrup
inversol
invert sugar
isoflavones
lactic acid
lecithin
leucine
lysine
malitol
malt
malt syrup
malt extract
maltodextrin
maltose
mannitol
methylcellulose
milk powder
milo starch
modified food starch
modified starch
mono and diglycerides
monosodium glutamate (MSG)
Nutrasweet
oleic acid
phenylalanine
phytic acid
protein isolate

shoyu
sorbitol
soy flour
soy isolates
soy lecithin
soy milk
soy oil
soy protein
soy protein isolate
soy sauce
starch
stearic acid
sugar (unless specified as *"cane sugar"*)
tamari
tempeh
teriyaki marinades
textured vegetable protein
threonine
tocopherols (vitamin E)
tofu
trehalose
triglyceride
vegetable fat
vegetable oil
vitamin B_{12}
vitamin E
whey
whey powder
xanthan gum

Fucked. Up. An ingredient like "vitamin E" can look fantastic to the untrained eye. However, that vitamin E is probably not be the naturally-occurring substance you believe it to be. Spoiler alert: real food naturally has vitamin E in it; it shouldn't have to be added and listed on an ingredient label. Basically, if you're eating processed, packaged foods, you're guaranteed to be eating GMOs—and even worse, the harmful chemicals attached to them.

Avoiding GMOs gets tricky though, because even if you're in a country where GMO production doesn't take place, it doesn't mean they're absent. The *import* of GMO ingredients may still be happening under your nose. For example, in New Zealand (where there is no genetic engineering of food), any food imports— whether they be whole foods or processed foods—should be checked for genetic modification (good luck if they're not labeled). To add to that, just because something is "made in" a country that doesn't produce genetically modified foods (e.g. "made in New Zealand"), it doesn't make it safe. It can still be pieced together with mutant ingredients imported from overseas. I told you it was nearly impossible to know how to avoid **this** shit.

Which foods do those ingredients generally come from? The top culprits are sugar beets, soy, cotton, canola, and corn.[301] Therefore, if you're buying anything derived from those commodities (or products containing them), and they're not certified "organic" or "non-GMO verified," you can almost *guarantee* they're genetically modified and smothered with toxic, herbicidal (genocidal?) chemicals.

Here's where the manipulating gets even worse: even if something is genetically modified, or contains genetically modified ingredients, it can deceitfully be labeled "100% natural." And, of course, all companies who use GM ingredients choose to slap that word on their products because consumers flock to it like magnets. Does manipulating the DNA of cells in a lab sound natural to you? It's not something that happens on its own in nature, so yeah . . . liar, liar, pants on fire.

In the big scheme of things, even with the lack of published studies, it's hard to argue that GMO production isn't butchering us, our livestock, and the environment. Who knows if it's the gene-altering or the chemicals that go hand in hand with production that are making us sick (I'll bet my left lung it's the chemicals like glyphosate). Either way, I'd rather not test my luck and instead choose to grow my own food with organic seeds, or buy whole, non-processed foods that are clearly certified "organic" or "non-GMO." Or, I purchase products from my local farmer's market that I *know* are grown locally and organically. I also try not to live near major GMO farms (i.e. near the chemicals that could rain down on me)—it's just not worth the risk. Can we all do our best to ignore genetically modified foods, let them shrivel up and die, and get back to eating untainted food? Please?

Soy

Pop Quiz! What starts with an "s," ends with "oy," and is one of the most genetically engineered crops on the planet? Hint: you just read about it in the GMO section. As of 2011, approximately 94% of American soy crops were genetically modified).[301] That doesn't leave much room for "untainted" soy (don't get out your calculators—it leaves 6%). Therefore, when most people state that you should steer clear of soy, which version do they mean? Probably neither, because they don't know the difference.

Like everything else though, soy is not harmful unless you eat the wrong kind, prepare it the wrong way, or inhale it like it's going out of style. In fact, organically grown, untainted soy has many fantastic benefits in the ways of preventing disease and boosting your nutrient intake. It's simply a chore to find.

One of the biggest concerns I hear about soy is that it will give you breast cancer. Not only has soy has been falsely linked to breast cancer in the past (mainly because a component of soy acts similarly to the "female" hormone estrogen), but people also assume that if you eat a lot of soy, you grow woman parts. Thus, for you soy-haters out there who think men who consume soy will turn into women, I can assure you my husband has not grown a vagina yet. In fact, people who eat soy (including breast cancer patients and survivors) may *improve* their health by including organic, non-GMO soy in their diets.[156, 302] Since only 6% of soy falls into that category (in the US anyway), you'll have to don some war paint and hunt that shit down!

The best way to examine soy is to study certain Asian cultures that, for centuries, have used it as a staple in their diet. One study illustrated that Chinese females have a significantly *decreased* risk of breast cancer with soy consumption.[303] A similar finding was discovered in a study on Japanese women.[304] Furthermore, soy has also shown to *decrease* menopausal symptoms and guard against heart disease.[305] A review of fourteen trials that evaluated thyroid function and soy consumption showed that the "findings provide little evidence that . . . soy foods . . . adversely affect thyroid function."[306, 307] Thus, "hypothyroid adults need not avoid soy foods." Oddly, patients with thyroid problems are often told to avoid soy (which kind, who knows). Hmmm.

How about osteoporosis—another ailment that concerns people when they weigh up soy? Once again, soy consumption will not cause brittle bones.[308-310] Soy sounds *horrible*; stay away from it! (*Insert sarcastic tone.*)

Where the fuck does all of the soy fear come from?! Welcome to the Western diet, which mainly consists of genetically modified, or highly processed soy "products." It now becomes a whole different game. For instance, did you know that many harmful food additives—including the ones we discussed in the "Shit to Avoid like the Plague" section—are derived from genetically modified soy? You *should* know, because many of them were listed in the previous GMO write-up. Check your food labels for some of the following additives:

artificial flavors

citric acid

emulsifiers

flavors

lecithin

monosodium glutamate (MSG)

natural flavors

protein isolate

soya (or soja, or yuba)

stabilizers

textured soy flour

textured soy protein

textured vegetable protein

thickening agents

vegetable gum

vegetable oil

vegetable paste

vegetable protein

vegetable starch

There's a good chance that many of those ingredients came from genetically modified soy, have a layer of chemicals on them, and will therefore have a negative effect on your health. Thus, I'll argue that it's not *soy* that's harmful, but it's the way some of the food company asshats have processed soy or shoved it into every nook and cranny of every processed food product out there. It also doesn't help that people assume meat substitutes (e.g. soy sausages, veggie burgers) to be healthier than meat, when in reality they're merely processed, chemical-filled piles of crap. Or, even worse, people unknowingly buy foods like tofu and tempeh thinking they're doing a good thing. Yet, unless they're buying *organic* versions void of harmful chemicals, they're instead only harming themselves.

Therefore, if you want to eat soy, do so. Just make sure you choose organic, non-GMO soy that hasn't been highly processed and pumped full of shit. Try some certified organic, fermented soy as well, which offers a whole other array of fantastic benefits. Experiment with options like organic miso soup, or tempeh. Steer clear of non-organic, highly processed soy foods and meat substitutes that will contain GMOs and a plethora of other nasty ingredients. *Those* are the soy products to avoid.

Gluten

The gluten controversy exploded onto the scene around 2010, and has been pissing me off ever since. I'd estimate that about 90% of the people I encounter who limit or avoid gluten have *no* clue why they do so, *or* what gluten even is. I have been "enlightened" by declarations like, "gluten is a grain," "my body can't digest it," "my trainer told me not to eat it," or the best one yet: "I'm going to get celiac disease if I eat it!" You're fucking killing me, folks.

Gluten is a protein. Wait what?! A *protein*?! Well, shit I change my mind then! It can be found in grains like wheat, barley, and rye (because remember, plant foods do, in fact, have protein). Some people can't process this protein properly. Enter celiac disease: an autoimmune disorder defined by an allergy to gluten.

This means that anyone with celiac disease will have an inflammatory response if they consume gluten. Similar to there being no point in avoiding peanuts if you don't have a peanut allergy, there's no point in avoiding gluten if you don't have celiac disease. People who can process gluten just fine, do exactly that: they process gluten just fine. For that reason, I'm sorry to tell you that you're missing out on a whole lot of wonderful gluten-filled foods if you decide for no reason whatsoever to cut gluten out.

How do you know if you have celiac disease? What you don't do, is diagnose yourself. Instead, you go see a professional and either do an elimination diet, or have certain invasive tests done (e.g. blood work, endoscopy). Or, see if you experience some of the following symptoms on a regular basis:

anemia	infertility or miscarriages
arthritis	joint pain, stiffness, or swelling
bloating	mood swings
chronic fatigue	mouth sores or ulcers
confusion or brain fog	pale skin
depression or anxiety	pale, mucus-covered poop
diarrhea or constipation	short temper
dizziness or vertigo	skin rashes
hair loss	stomach pain
headaches or migraines	thyroid dysfunction
heavy or painful periods	weight loss

If you experience many of those symptoms on a regular basis, and you eat grains like wheat, barley, and rye on a regular basis (or processed foods like breads and pastas, which usually contain wheat), you may want to get checked for celiac disease. Remember though, those symptoms can also be caused by a boatload of other issues, so don't freak out just yet. If you *don't* regularly have those symptoms, then you probably *don't* friggin' have a problem consuming gluten!

Unfortunately, people who don't see a doctor are frequently diagnosing themselves as having a "gluten intolerance" without actually having any clue what that actually means. "Gluten intolerance" (or "sensitivity") means that someone hasn't been diagnosed with celiac disease, yet they get symptoms of the disease. It's usually a self-diagnosis, and it's usually phony. Several professionals can attest that you either have celiac disease, or you don't. There's no "in between."[311] Just like you don't "kind of" get cancer or "kind of" have a heart attack.

For people who *actually* suffer from celiac disease, this is truly a bummer, mainly because they are missing out on some wonderful foods. I know people who can't consume gluten, and I have seen the frustration first-hand. However, only about 1% of the US population actually suffers from celiac disease, yet around 30% of the population want to eat less gluten (do we need to get out the calculators see the issue there?).[312] So what happens? Suddenly there are gluten-free foods bursting onto the food scene faster than shit starts to stink. Ahoy! Another fantastic money making scheme! Companies are throwing the title "Gluten Free!" on their products to increase sales because they know it's the latest craze— even when products are naturally gluten free in the first place. Gluten free fish! Gluten free carrots! Gluten free forks! Ugh.

It is estimated that, by 2016, gluten-free food sales in the US will hit $15 billion.[312] Cha-ching! Holy heck. *Please* don't be fooled as all food companies scramble around making gluten-free versions of their current products, because it *will* happen (it *is* happening). Profit, profit. Profit. Gluten-free profit!

For people who *can* eat gluten, let me tell you why you shouldn't do away with it. First and foremost, it has been proven time and time again that whole grains are not a threat to health— contrary to what most trendy blogs will tout. In one scientific review on wheat and health, the author noted:

> Five major recent scientific reviews addressing the impact of cereal consumption on health and disease concluded that the consumption of whole grains, of which globally most widely consumed is wheat, generally exerts positive effects on health, thus recommending increased intake of whole grain for the general public, in exchange for refined foods.[313]

Did you catch that? People who don't have celiac disease should eat *more* whole, untainted grains to reap the health benefits. Here's where it gets tricky once again. Whole, unrefined grains are hard to come by, and tell a whole different story than the stripped-down, nutrient-depleted, fucked-up grains that are in the majority of the packaged, processed products on the market today. It's the fucked-up, refined, processed grains that are most likely to fuck you up.[314] By consuming whole, untainted grains, you can actually look forward to benefits like improved weight management, reduced incidence of type 2 diabetes, and reduced incidence of heart disease.[315-317] Yay! If this weren't true, the whole country of Turkey (which has an extremely high intake of wheat-based foods) would be in one downward chronic disease and celiac spiral.[313] Guess what, they're not.

Let's make sure we're on the same page. You should be reaching for *whole*, unrefined grains like wheat (including spelt), oat, barley, brown rice, rye, millet, amaranth, teff, buckwheat, and quinoa (some of those are actually seeds, but are eaten like a grain). You should also not be giving two shits if there's gluten in them. Unless, of course, you have been diagnosed with celiac disease. Steer clear of the shitty, refined, run-of-the-mill supermarket processed products like flours, pastas, and breads that are usually full of additives, stripped of all of their nutrients (and then fortified with other "vitamins"), or they're brown because they've been dyed with cancer-causing caramel coloring to trick you. Make your own damn flours, pastas, and breads, from whole grains.

If you haven't heard of half of those wonderful health-promoting whole-grains listed above, that's fine. First off, you're not alone. Most people haven't heard of them, because most people reach for the fucked up versions of processed pastas and breads. Second off, it's never too late to learn. Start searching for recipes with those whole, organically grown grains (some are gluten free and some aren't . . . and who really cares which are which?!). Then go *buy* the whole, organically grown grains (bulk bins are a great place to start), and recipe the shit out of them.

Why organically grown grains? Conventional grain (mainly wheat) farmers spray the shit out of their crops to aid production. What do they spray with? Our little buddy glyphosate, a.k.a. Roundup, which has—drum roll please—officially been linked to the cause of celiac disease.[318] Shocker! It's not the bloody grain (or wheat, or gluten) that will screw you sideways, it's what's been *sprayed* on the grain. This is why people can sometimes eat wheat (with no chemical residue) and feel fine, and other times eat (chemical-covered) wheat, and feel their insides exploding. This is also why people, who can't eat wheat in America, travel to other countries (that *don't* spray with glyphosate), and can suddenly, "miraculously" eat wheat. Are you seeing the pattern yet? Eat untainted food, folks. If it has been fucked with (or doused in chemicals), it will most likely rip you apart.

Fish

Wait, "fish" is controversial? Yup—and it was controversial even *before* the Fukushima plant decided to pollute the Pacific with its nuclear waste. Over the past decade, fish has become a widely debated food source. People started to cut it out of their diets without knowing why. The main two reasons people did this, were 1) mercury levels, and 2) factory farming. Let's hit mercury levels first.

Mercury is a chemical element that ends up in our environment from the burning of fossil fuels and other industrial systems (like power plants). This mercury travels through the air until it is rained down into water sources far and wide (and that shit can travel *far*). What lives in the water? Fish, of course! The mercury is usually first absorbed by tiny bacteria or plankton. Then the fish eat the bacteria and plankton, and BAM! We have mercury-contaminated fish. Then *we* consume the fish and unknowingly consume a byproduct of the mercury (called methyl mercury), which—drum roll please—also happens to be a neurotoxin.

Remember, a neurotoxin is something that screws with your nervous system (which includes your brain), and can lead to ailments like impaired memory, intellectual disabilities, dementia, neuropathy (which can lead to weakness and balance issues), myopathy (muscles that don't function properly), and epilepsy. All stemming from the polluting of our environment. I feel like the human population is not winning at the game of life.

How much mercury is in our environment? How much is in the fish? How much is safe? *Great* questions! On average, about 5,500 metric tons of mercury finds its way into the environment every year.[319] That's more than twelve *million* pounds per year (or five-and-a-half million kilograms). That amount, my friends, is why the World Health Organization considers mercury to be one of the top ten chemicals of "major public health concern."[320]

That certainly doesn't mean *all* mercury is winding up in the fish supply. It also doesn't mean all fish have the same level of contamination. It works on a tiered system, meaning the little predators (like sardines and crayfish) usually have less mercury in them than the large predators (like swordfish and shark). Not only do those large predators eat the contaminated bacteria and plankton, but they also eat all of the smaller, contaminated fish.

I'm not going to talk about exact contaminations in parts-per-million (ppm) here, but I *will* make a list of common commercial seafood for you.[321] The most contaminated are on top, and the least are on the bottom (if you're a super-nerd and want to know specific ppm, you can head straight to the FDA's list).[321]

Mercury Contamination in Seafood

(highest)	tile fish
	swordfish
	shark
	mackerel (king)
	bass (Chilean)
	tuna (albacore; canned, fresh, frozen)
	halibut
	snapper
	bass (striped, black, saltwater)
	cod
	lobster (northern/American)
	lobster (spiny)
	mackerel (pacific)
	trout (freshwater)
	crab
	haddock (Atlantic)
	mackerel (Atlantic)
	crawfish
	catfish
	squid (a.k.a. calamari)
	salmon
	tilapia
	oyster
	shrimp
	clam
(lowest)	scallop

In a nutshell, if you're eating lots of seafood from the *top* end of that list, you are consuming more mercury than someone who eats fish or seafood mainly from the *bottom* of the list. To put things into perspective though, tuna (which is high on that list) has, on average, a mercury level of 0.25ppm. A flu shot has a mercury level of 51.0ppm (that's over *two hundred times* the contamination of the tuna). Also, the flu shot is *injected* into the body, which becomes much more potent than something ingested.

Thus, if you're going to fear mercury in fish, I better not see you getting the flu shot.

If you *are* concerned, and your brain hasn't been fried by the flu shot yet, use it. Avoid fish high on the fish food chain (especially if it comes in a can—that way you can also avoid the BPA). Instead, eat fresh fish (and other seafood) lower on the food chain (i.e. smaller predators), and even then do so sparingly.

Here's a trick though: if you *do* choose to eat fish, there are other foods you can eat that will help capture the mercury and draw it out of your body (they are full of insoluble fiber, which pulls waste out of the body). These are foods like hemp protein, peanut butter, strawberries, cilantro, and cacao powder.[322] Eat them when you eat seafood, and voila! Adios, mercury (well, some of it).

Now that we understand mercury contamination a bit better, let's talk about the other main concern when it comes to eating fish: factory farming. Factory farming is the production of a species outside its natural environment. It means the fish (or any other farmed species) usually don't get to "roam free" as they normally would, they don't get to eat what they would normally eat, and they are packed in so tightly they start to suffer from injury and illness. Many different types of fish are farmed, and there are various degrees of shittiness when it comes to their environments. Then there are *wild* fish that are plucked from their natural habitat and have eaten, grown, and flourished as intended.

Let's pretend for a second that *you* get put in a cramped cage and bump shoulders with a thousand other people who are rubbing their infected parts on you and sneezing shit in your face. You're also only getting fed a special "feed" so you grow bigger, and are having dyes pumped into you so you look healthier. Take a wild stab at whether or not you're going to thrive in that environment. Well, neither do the farmed fish in this instance (or anything else factory farmed, for that matter). Factory farmed fish—because they are not allowed to thrive in their natural environment—wind up being less nutritious, and contain more contaminants from their environment and feed.[323]

In case you're wondering, the "feed" is commonly an unnatural concoction of grains, antibiotics, dioxins (which can cause cancer, developmental, and reproductive problems amongst other ailments), PCBs (which were banned in 1979, but still showing up, and can cause cancer as well as immune, reproductive, nervous, and endocrine system ailments), and anything else the farmer feels like chucking in there.[324-326] If we eat factory-farmed fish, we eat all of that shit. I'd also bet my life savings that the grains the fish are munching on are not the whole, certified organic variety we discussed either, which means they may also come bearing farm chemicals, like glyphosate.

Past the mercury levels and factory farming, we can't ignore the fact that fish still contain cholesterol and saturated fat like other meats do (both of which are associated with heart disease). All in all, if you choose to eat fish, your best bet is to buy a wild, low-on-the-totem-pole variety, and then eat it sparingly. Or, if you're pregnant or a child growing a brain, perhaps choose to avoid fish altogether.[320, 327] Unless, that is, you're craving an abundance of peanut butter-and-cilantro-covered strawberries.

If you buy fish from a restaurant, don't hesitate to ask them if it's wild. If they answer "I don't know," then it's not. If you want a nice pocket guide (US only, sorry) that will tell you what fish to purchase depending on where you live, check out Monterey Bay Aquarium's Seafood Watch Guide.[328]

Or, if you don't like fish, don't eat it. Again, we don't need certain *foods*, we need *nutrients*. Like everything else, the nutrients found in fish can be found elsewhere. If you're on the "plant protein promotes health and animal protein promotes disease" wagon, then shit, your decision should be easy. To be honest, the less people who eat fish for a while, the better. If you haven't heard, the world's fish supply is on its way out, with 75% of the fish population either maxed out or over-exploited. Fish are knocking on the door of extinction.[329, 330]

Eggs

This is a difficult topic for me, mainly because I can't wrap my head around the fact that an egg was "pooped" out of a chicken, and that I could be eating the beginning of a goopy embryo. I ate eggs while growing up, but now, when I consider what I'm eating, I kind of gag. I'm not here to tell you about my dry-heave capabilities though, so let's discuss why eggs made the controversial list.

Eggs have been on-again, off-again for decades. The moment they were found to be high in cholesterol, they were doomed.

"Eggs will increase your cholesterol!"

"Eggs will clog your arteries!"

"Egg whites are okay, but that yellow shit will kill ya!"

I have heard all of it a million times. Let's break it down and take a closer look at some of the research done on eggs—specifically their cholesterol content—to see whether those statements hold any water.

First off, it has been proven time and time again that dietary cholesterol (i.e. the cholesterol that you *eat*) is *not* a big factor in raising blood cholesterol levels—which is a concern because high cholesterol levels can lead to heart disease and stroke, among other ailments.[331-334] This is why, in 2000, after years of scrutiny, eggs were suddenly deemed "okay" by the American Heart Association.[335] Furthermore, eggs have several other good qualities we can cheer for—like vitamins, minerals, and disease-fighting carotenoids. Therefore, without cholesterol being an issue, they jumped up high on most nutritionists and dieticians "good" lists.

On the other hand, it has been proven time and time again that dietary cholesterol *does* have a negative effect on your cholesterol levels. Say what? Hello, controversy. There are articles that show that cholesterol *doesn't* negatively affect health, and articles that show that it *does*.[336-342] However, it might also be helpful to know that approximately 90% of research on dietary cholesterol is funded by the egg industry.[343] Something smells sulphery. This little fact led to a massive corruption lawsuit, because dietary egg recommendations were literally being paid for. Boom! More controversy! The 2016 lawsuit cleared things up by stating that:

> Abundant scientific evidence shows that cholesterol is a significant contributor to cardiovascular disease, the leading killer of Americans. The DGAC's [Dietary Guidelines Advisory Committee's] recommendations are part of a 20-year attempt at a cholesterol image makeover based on research funded by USDA's egg promotion program and designed specifically to increase egg consumption regardless of the health risks that may result from unlimited cholesterol ingestion.[343]

The lawsuit was successful, and cholesterol recommendations were changed to the following: "individuals should eat as little dietary cholesterol as possible."[344] And since dietary cholesterol can only be found in animal foods (like eggs), that now puts eggs on the back burner. Where does that leave us? I mean, eggs are the staple of most breakfasts in the western world. How the fuck are humans going to survive without their goopy chicken embryos?!

It may not be the *cholesterol* in the eggs that's causing the fiasco though. From what I have read, human cholesterol levels have more to do with the amount of animal *protein* one eats, rather than cholesterol (evidence of this dates back almost a century).[345-350] We'll talk about this specific issue a bit later on, but either way, eggs contain animal protein *and* cholesterol, so things aren't looking good for Humpty Dumpty. Most (non-corrupt) studies on eggs and dietary cholesterol can agree that people at risk of cardiovascular disease should steer clear of dietary cholesterol entirely, while "healthy" people are okay to consume it *if* they stick to the recommended cap of 300mg per day.[351] But since everyone's definition of "healthy" is different, and since we don't need to consume cholesterol anyway, who the fuck knows what that means.

And guess what—one egg has anywhere between 175mg and 275mg of cholesterol, depending on who you ask. Have *two* eggs (which most people do—some I know have *six* eggs at one sitting), and you're already over the cholesterol limit without even taking into account any *other* cholesterol-laden foods you may be eating that day. In my case (regardless of my gag issue with eggs), I'd rather get the nutrients eggs have from sources that *don't* have cholesterol, and let my body produce its own. But again, that's just me. I don't care how many "good" qualities eggs have; if there's one potentially harmful quality, I'm walking away.

Speaking of harmful qualities, several studies have linked *minimal* egg consumption (we're talking a couple eggs per *week*) to prostate cancer—excuse me *"lethal"* prostate cancer (meaning subjects actually died).[352] One study was done on almost twenty-eight *thousand* men over about a fifteen-year period. During their follow-ups, it was determined that the men who had consumed only 2.5 eggs *per week* had an 81% increased risk of prostate cancer compared to the men who ate less than a half an egg per week.[353] That's mind blowing—especially since I know several people who regularly eat two to three eggs in one *meal*, several times per week. If you assume that by not having a prostate you're safe, um, how do I say this nicely? Pretty please, don't be a fucking idiot. If eggs can screw up a prostate this much, do you think there *might* be a chance that they could screw up other organs?!

If you answered "yes," you're right! Past prostate cancer, egg consumption (as few as 1.5 eggs per *week*) is also linked to colon, rectal, and bladder cancers.[354-356] You can't claim to not have *those* organs! Studies also show that people who consume higher quantities of eggs wind up with 19% increase in their risk for heart disease. Or, if you're a diabetic, that number jumps to an 83% risk for heart disease.[341] People who eat higher quantities of eggs also wind up increasing their risk of diabetes by 68%.[357] Or, if we're talking about *gestational* diabetes (i.e. diabetes during pregnancy), women who consumed higher quantities of eggs (before *or* during pregnancy) had between a 77% and 165% increased risk.[358]

Unfortunately, I've mentioned these statistics to people and they *still* want to eat twelve eggs per day (especially if they're working out—"gotta get that protein"), mainly because the egg industry has done a damn good job convincing them that eggs are one of the best sources of protein and cholesterol need not be worried about . Unfortunately, *something* in eggs clearly is destructive (my guess is that's it's the animal protein).

And then there are those who think that by consuming "better" versions of eggs—which mainly has to do with how the chickens were raised (either pasture-raised, or caged)—makes them suddenly healthy. Not the case. Sure, if you cage or contain an animal and treat it differently than it would normally live, it's going to turn out to be different, but all versions of eggs still contain cholesterol and animal protein no matter how you look at them.[359-362]

But I know that some of you love to live on the edge. And if that's the case, it's imperative you eat eggs from *pasture-raised* chickens that were allowed to roam free and feed on untainted nutrients, and then try to eat them sparingly. At least then you'll have *reduced* your risk of disease. Please, please, please steer clear of the caged chickens. You know, the ones that are fed arsenic-laced, wheat-based feed, and are pumped full of hormones and antibiotics to enlarge their breasts and keep them "healthy" to increase sales.

Dairy

I was recently getting a sports injury checked out at a doctor's office in New Zealand. In their medical offices, they have this set-up called "Health TV" which, according to the website, is there to have a "major impact on patient's lives, through health-related education."[363] I'm assuming they're going for a positive impact, but after my experience I realize the impact had more to do with revenue than anything else.

As I waited for over forty long-ass minutes in the waiting room, I heard the following message on repeat: "Milk is the richest form of calcium for the diet!" I shit you not I used all of my powers to not go dismantle the TV from the wall and politely crush it to smithereens with my super-human strength. "The *richest* form of calcium"? What does that even mean? What makes something "rich"? Surely they know other foods actually have more calcium than milk, right? Were they even talking about the amount? OH WAIT, I get it—they must mean that milk comes from the *"richest"* industry, and therefore gets to plaster their annoying ads everywhere for people to unknowingly get brainwashed. That has to be it. Smart choice of words, diary industry.

This "crucial" message gets delivered to the public simply because the dairy industry paid for it to be there—even though it really has no meaning. It's just 100% enticing. And, since it's in a *doctor's* office, the message seems much more valid and vital to people. The dairy industry is one of the best marketing geniuses out there (and have so many people tucked in their back pockets—including doctors—it's insane). They know "that patients are more receptive to receiving health information and acting immediately on it, at a time when they are waiting to see their health professional."[363] Thus, it's the perfect time to advertise and make up some deceptive statement about milk being "rich." *This* is why the dairy industry has been successful—not because it's a nutrient powerhouse.

Before I carry on, let's reminisce about the fact that I come from Vermont, where you're in the minority if you haven't hand-milked a cow. In addition, my sister's family runs a dairy farm near the town in which I grew up. Nevertheless, while I clearly have dairy connections, and while I was once a dairy-milk-smuggling, cheese-addicted child, I have researched the industry immensely and now cross my fingers that I'm not disowned by my home state or my family when I deliver the following *rich* message (see, I can throw the word "rich" wherever the fuck I want as well).

If you're old enough to remember the dairy movement ("Milk: it does a body good!"), then you'll remember that dairy milk advertisements were plastered everywhere, and it was "imperative" you drank it in order to have strong bones and not break hips. It was incessantly promoted because it was of close relation to human milk, and had this incredible nutrient called "calcium," which, when consumed, would grow people into fierce, indestructible bone warriors. It was its own food group, and it was vital to your survival that you included it in every meal. This, my friends, is another marketing ploy. Nobody "needs" milk (or dairy). Broken record in 3 . . . 2 . . . 1 . . . you don't need certain *foods*, you need certain *nutrients*, and you can decide wherever the fuck you get those nutrients! Believe it or not, calcium exists elsewhere! Like, *lots* of elsewhere. The dairy industry tried to make it seem otherwise, however.

It was well known a century ago that strong bones and teeth are full of calcium. When that fact hit the public—BAM!!—the dairy industry jumped on it. They started waiving their hands enthusiastically, and shouted to the world that their products were *full* of calcium, and therefore it was imperative that everyone consumed dairy to fight off brittle bones and weak teeth.

The only problem is there isn't research to back this up. In actuality, instead of making everyone stronger, the *opposite* effect took place: the countries that started consuming more dairy started having the *most* hip fractures (which is an indicator of weak bones, or osteoporosis).[364-367] Huh? How is this possible? Well, we obviously know that dairy comes from cows, and therefore contains animal protein. What you might not know is that animal protein, much more so than plant protein, causes the body to become "acidic," and in order to buffer, or offset, that acidity, the body pulls calcium out of the bones (because calcium is a great buffer).[368-372] Oops. Thus, the more dairy you consume (or all animal products, for that matter), the more calcium you'll pull out of your bones to buffer the acidic environment you've created, and the weaker bones you will have. This is something that is widely known and easily measured by noting the amount of calcium excreted in one's urine. The people who consume more dairy excrete more calcium, which, of course, comes from their bones.[372-376] Snnnaaap! There goes another hip.

If you're concerned about your calcium intake, there are ways to get it that are much "cleaner." Ways that don't weaken your bones, don't cause osteoporosis, are less processed, and are healthier than drinking dairy milk from an animal that's potentially been pumped full of shit. This is why I choose to drink certified organic almond milk, which actually has more calcium than dairy milk, is void of any potential hormones and antibiotics, does *not* leach calcium from my bones, and can be made by grinding whole almonds with water in my own blender.

Yet we don't hear about other milk or calcium options because the other industries purely don't have the funds behind them to market the shit out of their products like the diary industry does. There are *many* types of milks out there (e.g. almond, coconut, rice, soy, oat). There are also plenty of *foods* that contain calcium (e.g. broccoli, beans, leafy greens, kale, almonds). Figure this nutrition shit out, and you won't have to worry about calcium.

Over the years, due to this insurmountable "need for dairy," the dairy industry exploded into the mass-produced, unnatural farming system that it now is, and has left the end product tainted. How else were they going to keep up with the demand from consumers who were tricked into thinking they needed it in the first place?

Like everything else though, not all dairy is created equal. There *are* dairy farms that didn't follow suit. They let their cows run free, graze on the food nature intended (i.e. grass), and milk them as they're ready. Alternatively, there are the dairy farms that feed their cows the "feed" they were never meant to eat (which is usually full of GMOs), pump them full of hormones and antibiotics to keep them big and "healthy" (go back to the "Shit to Avoid like the Plague" chapter if you need a hormone and antibiotic refresher), and force them to produce as much milk as their able, as quick as possible. I'll let you guess which method is the healthier option.

The truth is, if you eat dairy products that came from a cow that was pumped full of GMO-laced feed, hormones, and antibiotics, you're going to be consuming those things as well. Michael Pollan, who has penned some kick-ass books on food, once said that "you are what you eat eats."[377] He meant if you're going to eat something (mainly animal products), you sure as shit better know what *that* thing ate as well, because you're also going to wind up consuming whatever crap has been previously consumed by it. Contemplate *that* next time you're chunkin' on some cheese. What did that cow eat? Or, better yet, what did that cow have injected into it?

With the growing concern about dairy, recommendations have been plummeting over the years (unless you talk directly to the dairy industry, then holy shit—DRINK UP BEFORE YOU BREAK A HIP AND DIE!!). One of the latest food guides—entitled "The 2011 Healthy Eating Plate"—was put out by Harvard's School of Public Health. For the first time in history, a food guide actually recommended "limiting" dairy, and even chastised previous recommendations for supporting the interest of the heavily-funded dairy industry:

> The (previous) guidelines' recommendation to increase the intake of low-fat milk and dairy products seems to reflect the interests of the powerful dairy industry more so than the latest science. There is little, if any, evidence that eating dairy prevents osteoporosis or fractures, and there is considerable evidence that high dairy product consumption is associated with increased risk of fatal prostate and maybe ovarian cancers.[378]

You've heard that message before, right? (Sigh.)

Going further, a 2014 study on nutrition and cancer had several outcomes that lead to multiple dietary recommendations. One of them was "limiting or avoiding dairy products to reduce the risk of prostate cancer."[156] This is because men with the highest dairy intakes had about double the risk of total prostate cancer, and up to four times the risk of metastatic or fatal prostate cancer than those who consumed minimal dairy.[379-382] I don't know about you, but if dairy—merely two glasses of milk a day—can lead to prostate cancer, then I'm pretty sure I'd rather take the "avoid" route (even if I don't house a prostate) . . . which brings us back to the connection between eggs and prostate cancer. If you regularly consume eggs *and* dairy, your prostate may be royally screwed.

If you think you're safe because you don't have a prostate, keep reading. There are numerous studies that point to the link between dairy consumption, and mortality and disease. There are also numerous studies that demonstrate the lack of connection between dairy and reducing bone fractures.[383-385] The studies actually demonstrate that the *more* dairy you consume, the more likely you are to become diseased or die. I know what you're thinking, but who the heck is going to put their hand up and spread that message?! How does a world which relies heavily on the dairy industry suddenly switch to considering dairy to not be so beneficial? I'm seriously asking, because I don't know the answer. I'm also putting my hand up and spreading that message.

I have spoken to friends in the dairy industry (oops, red flag right there) about these concerns, and after rattling off a bunch of facts to me on why dairy is so important (or that dairy milk is something like 95% genetically similar to human milk), it still just doesn't make sense to me. Regardless if you consume certified organic dairy milk void of the hormones, antibiotics, and whatever else is pumped into the cows, there is still a giant elephant in the room: dairy milk is the *breast milk* intended for, and genetically formulated to nurture, an animal that will eventually be one thousand to two thousand pounds.

Back in the '90s, a doctor by the name of Norman W. Walker was on to something when he compared human milk (which he labeled "mother's milk") to cow's milk:

> The chemical constituents of mother's milk are intended to nourish the child . . . so that its bone structure will develop eventually to what will be needed for a mature individual whose weight will be, say, 125 to 175 [pounds]. Cow's milk, on the other hand, contains 300% more [protein] than does mother's milk, and is intended to grow the calf to a maturity of about [1,500 pounds].[386]

Call me bat shit crazy, but that doesn't add up to me, regardless if it's certified organic, "clean" milk. That cow (or chinchilla, or camel, or honey badger—anything that lactates) should be lactating to support its *young*—not to support another species, much less the *adults* of another species. No wonder little eight-year-old Lola has sprouted boobs and seven-year-old Cindy-Lou is already menstruating. They're nursing from a cow! Let's open this can of worms, shall we?

We have somehow justified nursing from a gigantic, dissimilar animal (and well into our adulthood), when nursing is generally intended for infants (and between animals of the same species). That's what we're doing—we're *nursing*—regardless if you're sucking directly from a cow's teat, or have weaned yourself to a bottle or glass. If you consume dairy, you are nursing from a cow.

This is why I find it totally bizarre that most people will dry-heave at the thought of drinking another *woman's* breast milk, which is actually intended for humans (well, *infant* humans at least). I bet the thought of making a nice, creamy cheese from a woman's breast milk would repulse most (mmmmmm . . . boob cheddar), yet we find it "okay" to gulp down milk and cheese that comes from a ginormous cow (that I'm assuming doesn't have great hygiene habits), with vastly different protein and hormone levels. Pretty soon we'll be reaching for cow semen when we can't get pregnant. That's a joke, folks. Honestly though, it makes more sense to canvass your neighborhood for lactating mothers next time you run out of milk.

Moral of the story: the breast milk that another animal produces specifically for its (GINORMOUS) offspring may not be the best option for us. We can't continue to consume something simply because it's been consumed for years and because there's a huge, filthy rich industry behind it marketing the crap out of it—even if they produce cool commercials and have advertisements in doctor's offices. We need to look at the full picture here.

All in all, I recommend doing some real research on dairy if you're still in the "dairy is golden" boat. If you *are* going to consume it, for fuck's sake, please switch to certified organic dairy that comes from a farm that lets their animals live like cows, without pumping them fill of harmful chemicals. At least then you're taking the "better" option. As always, take note of how it makes you feel. Dairy milk, cheese, yogurt, ice cream, etc., all makes me feel like crap, but I only realized this after I eliminated it from my diet and then binged on cheesy nachos one day. I suddenly felt bloated and "clogged," which is a bummer because I *love* cheese. I would seriously eat a whole block of Vermont Cabot cheddar right now if it really did do my body good.

Okay, so perhaps I *did* eat a small block of cheese recently . . . and guess what happened? I wound up with sore, aching boobs — something I hadn't felt since high school when it had been a regular menstrual symptom for me (and when I regularly ate dairy). I took the hint, stopped eating the cheese, and the throbbing boobs disappeared (well, only the throbbing part). I love magic.

* * *

What it boils down to, is that when it comes to "controversial" nutrition topics, you have to make sure you've done your research first. Hopefully you'll use reputable sources (i.e. don't get your facts from the same industry you're researching, because *of course* they're going to back their products and not say a negative peep). Genetically modified, highly processed soy hot dogs are *not* the same as certified organic soy tempeh. You cannot compare certified organic dairy to factory-farmed hormone, antibiotic-filled dairy. Wild fish and farmed fish are nutritionally different. Personally, if I'm going to choose to eat something controversial (which I do on the rare occasion because I'm about as perfect as a three-eyed fish), my moral compass always points to "what's more natural" when choosing "the best" option.

If you find yourself confused about a specific food, there are questions to ask yourself:

- Did this food exist in this form a long time ago, or have we fucked with it in some way?
- Do I feel fantastic when I eat it?
- Is it whole or minimally processed without a lot of shit added to it?
- Does research suggest it's good for me, regardless of what the industry says?
- Does my common sense tell me this food is good (or bad) for me, regardless of what Negative Nancy down the road is preaching?

Before you scoff a whole food group simply because there are a whole lot of people "blogging" about it, do your research and ask yourself those questions. It would be a shame to cut out highly nutritious food from your diet purely because you haven't educated yourself properly. Likewise, it would be a shame to devour another food that is highly damaging to your system purely because that food's marketing plan is clever and wide-spread and all of the cool kids are consuming it.

Moral of the Story:

When making a decision on whether or not to incorporate a controversial product into your diet, do not take the advice of the industry you are questioning. Talk to people *outside* that industry. If you speak to someone *in* the industry about whether or not their product is safe and beneficial, it's like asking a car salesman if they think you look good in a Lamborghini.

Chapter 24

Buying Organic

Fact: all food used to be organically grown. There was a time, before pesticides, herbicides, fertilizers, and food additives, that all foods were grown and consumed untainted. Well, at the most they might be tainted with dirt or bird shit, but I'd welcome both over the crap that has become normal to slather on our food these days. You heard me: I would rather eat *bird crap* than herbicides, pesticides, food dyes, artificial sweeteners, or any other shit deemed "safe and edible" by the powers that be. What are now known as "elite, trendy, only-for-the-rich-and-famous organically grown foods," were once simply considered "foods," and *everyone* ate them.

Now that all of this crazy, toxic, non-food shit has infiltrated the food system, we have to somehow categorize which foods contain the shit, and which foods don't. The backwards part about this is that somehow the wonderful, natural, untainted foods became the category that had to put their hand up, go through testing, and be labeled as untainted, or "certified organic." While all of the foods that have additives, attached farm chemicals, or are genetically modified *don't* have to go through the painstaking process of paying for labels—they simply add harmful chemicals, play with DNA, and call it a day. In addition, since the harmful food and beverage products *don't* have warning labels, and are often mass produced and cost less, people wind up flocking to the very products that they should be avoiding. Bass ackwards.

This becomes ridiculously unfair to the farmers and growers that have not changed their practices (i.e. they're still simply growing real, untainted foods). They suddenly have to go through lengths to label their foods as something they have always been. This is mind-boggling—especially when they haven't changed anything or done anything wrong. If it were up to me (can it be?), I would make every non-organic consumer product bear a label that read: "This product is not natural. It may be genetically modified, and comes bearing chemicals. When we say 'chemicals,' we're talking about *harmful* chemicals that will reenact Hiroshima in your gut."

I'm not joking. I want that label on all non-organic foods—and I want the non-organic companies to have to dish out the money for them. Then, we can hang a big-ass sign over the organic foods that simply reads: "Real Food."

We've already discussed the fact that food allergies and certain diseases have skyrocketed since harmful additives and GMOs have tainted our food system. Therefore, I have no problem stating that I don't believe it's the food and beverages we're eating that are causing certain diseases to skyrocket—I'd be willing to put all of my chips on red that it's what's been *added* or *attached* to those foods and beverages that are destroying us. I also believe the only people who will refute that statement are the people and companies profiting from, or connected to, non-organic foods.

Let's explore some cool facts about organics. Crops that aren't doused in chemicals are much safer to consume (for instance, they reduce the risk of diminished IQ in children).[387-390] As a specific example, one report—which reviewed 343 separate studies—showed organic crops to have 48% lower levels of the toxic heavy metal cadmium (classified as a potential neurotoxin and carcinogen), and four times less pesticide residue than non-organic crops.[391] Furthermore, if any of you readers are men and are struggling to make babies, you may want to know that men who consume the most pesticide-smothered crops have about a 50% lower sperm count than those who consume the least.[392] For those reasons alone—unless you enjoy consuming harmful chemicals and heavy metals, and reducing the IQ of your children (if you're even able to have any)—you'll want to do your best to eat organically grown foods.

This means that foods have to have the "organic" stamp of approval to get the green light, because even if you choose something "innocent" like pureed baby food you're not safe. Yes, non-organic baby foods have been tested, and yes, they contain pesticides.[393] According to the American Academy of Pediatrics, "evidence demonstrates associations between . . . pesticides and pediatric cancers, decreased cognitive function, and behavioral problems."[394] Babies are getting cancer and having cognitive and behavioral problems at the hand of the food industry. Bloody brilliant. I need my heart rate to come down before we continue.

Think *that's* bad? Check this out: non-organic potatoes (the number one consumed vegetable in America) were found to contain *thirty-seven* different pesticides.[393, 395] Thirty-friggin-seven chemicals on *one* vegetable. Imagine what a whole plate of vegetables would contain! The chemicals on the potatoes included carcinogens, neurotoxins, and developmental toxins, by the way. Bravo, America, brav-o. Fries with that?

It seems we need to eat organic or get sick. Furthermore, beyond the argument that non-organic foods contain a bunch of extra shit we shouldn't want to get near our pie-holes, you may also hear the argument that "organic foods are no more nutritious than conventionally-grown foods." False. There are plenty of studies showing otherwise. The people who argue that organically grown and conventionally grown foods are nutritionally the same are not looking at the whole picture (they usually only focus on the larger nutrients: fats, carbohydrates, and protein). As an example, organically grown crops have significantly higher antioxidant levels, sometimes up to 69% more than non-organic crops.[391] Antioxidants strengthen your ability to fight infection and disease, so we can't say that organically grown foods are the same if they carry a crapload more antioxidants. Therefore, not only are organically grown crops chemically *inferior*, but they are also nutritionally *superior*.

By purchasing certified organic products (or by growing your own foods from organic seeds), you can avoid consuming the genetically-modified, nutritionally-depleted, and chemical-filled evil cousin versions of natural foods, thus decreasing your risk of disease. Finding the certified organic foods can be tricky though. Your best bet is to visit your local farmer's market or organic grocer, or simply grow your own. Alternatively, you can see if there is an organic Community Supported Agriculture (CSA) program in your area, which provides a way of working with local farmers to support local agriculture (you usually pay a flat rate and receive regular deliveries of in-season foods).

If you *do* choose to buy store-bought, certified organic products, you may need to do some further research. This means scoping out the company that produces them. Remember how I said that food companies were smart and would do anything to sell their products? Well, in recent times it seems as though everyone started using organics as a marketing tool to suck more money out of consumers. You'll now find not-so-healthy companies coming out with "organic" spin-off brands of their shitty products. You'll also find that larger corporations are buying up the smaller, organic companies, and making them part of their fucked-up food and beverage scheme. These large companies are generally the same folks that spend billions trying to keep us in the dark regarding what's hiding in their products.

For instance, the Coca-Cola company owns the organic brands Odwalla and Honest Tea, which have both been hugely successful.[396] Most consumers buy them assuming they're buying something fantastic, when in fact they're merely supporting the Coca-Cola company and its mission to put destructive products on the shelf of every store and restaurant across the planet. When they give money to Coca-Cola, Coca-Cola will then turn around and use that money to lobby against food labeling and our right to know what's in our food. Thus, not only should you buy certified organic foods and products, but you should buy them from companies that 100% support organic production, support the consumer's right to know what they're eating, and at the same time don't produce a bunch of other shitty foods. These are generally smaller, local companies that grow or source local crops. They are usually *not* the companies that spend billions sponsoring the Olympics or plastering ads on the sides of buses.

So clearly, in my opinion, you shouldn't support companies that sell a whole bunch of shitty products, and at the same time try to suck more money out of you by tempting you with a higher-priced product that's labeled as "organic." Thus, for your reference, table 24.1 provides a list of some of these larger, shit-producing companies that own smaller, well-known, organic spin-off companies.[396] You know, just so you can know who you're *really* buying from.

Table 24.1. Large companies with stakes in organic brands

Company	Spin-off Brand
Campbell's Soup Company	Plum Organic
	Bolthouse Farms
	Wolfgang Puck
Coca-Cola	Honest T
	Odwalla
	Green Mountain Coffee
General Mills	Lara Bar
	Food Should Taste Good
	Cascadian Farms
	Muir Glen
	Annie's
Kellogg	Kashi
	Bear Naked
	Morningstar Farms
M&M/Mars	Seeds of Change
Nestlé	Sweet Leaf Tea
Pepsi	Naked Juice

These organic spin-off brands from non-organic companies are everywhere—even in "health food stores" that feel they're doing a good deed by stocking organic foods. Furthermore, since these organic brands are being governed by larger I-don't-give-a-shit-about-your-health companies, you'll still find harmful chemicals like BPA lurking in their packaging (Wolfgang Puck, for example). Organic soup soaked a toxic container! I'll take three!

Thus, once again it's imperative that you become educated, so you know what brands to look for and purchase (when in doubt, simply flip the product over and read the fine print, as it should state what larger company actually produces it). Or, as I commonly say to my clients, "if they can make it, so can you." If there's something you love, that you can't buy locally and organically grown, *make it* from your own organically grown ingredients. Heck, you may find yourself with a local booming business.

I wish it were that simple, but there's more (holy shit, I know). Purely because something is labeled as "organic," and even comes from a local company, does not automatically mean it's safe. Take organic sugar, organic maple syrup, organic honey, etc. You clearly can't go around consuming a bunch of organic sweeteners all day if you want to be a crime-fighting superhero—even if they're *organic* sweeteners made in your back yard. Use your brain. Ask yourself if an organic-labeled product will *promote your health*. Don't consume it simply because the company paid to have an organic label slapped on it. At this point, you should be smarter than that.

The good news is that more and more people *are* actually buying certified organic foods and products, and not only in the US. All over the world (e.g. France, Australia, China, Canada, Mexico, the UK), organic sales are booming.[397-400] The US alone showed an 11% increase in organic sales between 2011 and 2012.[401] Fantastic news! But, wait—how do we know these organic sales are from "true" organic companies, and not companies like Coca-Cola with shitty organic spin-off brands? Answer: we don't. Thus, while the interest in organics is getting stronger, we need to shift that interest toward "real" organic companies, and not the major non-organic companies slurping up more money via their organic spin-off brands.

One topic I also want to revisit is that "natural" does not mean "organically grown." Some non-organic companies are trying to "cheat" their way into consumers' hands by boasting that their products are "natural," which is often confused with "organic." Companies are using that term an obnoxious amount, and we've already discussed the fact that it means nothing. Remember, "natural" foods can be genetically modified, and can also contain extras like herbicides and pesticides. Remember: real foods shouldn't have to make claims about being natural. When was the last time you saw an orange with a sign near it boasting its naturalness? If you see a claim on a package—specifically a "natural" claim—chances are it's actually the opposite. And it, in no way, means it's organic.

Lastly, although it may be beyond the scope of this guidebook, I'm going to mention it anyway: buying organic can help save the planet by reducing greenhouse gasses, supporting more species, and building carbon-storing soils.[402] If you're not familiar with those terms, please read a 2013 report by the United Nations entitled "World Investment Report 2013: Global Value Chains: Investment and Trade for Development." The report states that switching to an organic way of farming may not only mitigate climate change, but may also help solve world hunger.[403] Well, shit—let's do *that*.

Moral of the Story:

If you don't eat organic, you *will* be giving your insides a chemical-bath. Invest in your health, save yourself, and save your planet by eating as many organically grown foods as you're able.

SECTION IV

Variety is the Fuckin'
Keystone of Nutrition

Chapter 25

Variety

Thank effin' goodness we're past that last section—it was sucking the life out of me. It's seriously horrifying how fucked up our food system has become, and how much of our food isn't, in fact, food at all. If you made it through all of that info with a newfound hatred for highly-processed food, harmful food additives, chemical companies that have invaded our food system, and companies willing to do anything to get your dollar in their pocket, then you're right on track.

To recap, in the last two sections we've discussed how much to eat (*amount*), as well as which foods and beverages to choose or not choose (*type*). The next, and final, component of the Nutrition Triad is *variety*. Without variety it's impossible to get all the nutrients your body needs, and you *will* wind up malnourished from an incomplete, random supply of nutrients.

What I'm saying is that you can eat the right *amount* of calories, and choose the right *type* of foods, and still be unhealthy. Oh for fuck's sake, this is getting ridiculous. Hang in there—there's beer and chocolate at the end of this book! Sorry, I'm lying, but you've come this far, so one foot in front of the other, nutrition warrior!

For example, spinach is a healthy, nutritious food that provides some awesome, kick-ass, ailment-fighting nutrients. Nevertheless, if you eat 2,000 calories of spinach every day, you may be getting the right *amount* of food, and choosing a healthy *type* of food (and are probably dating a skinny chick named Olive Oil), but you're not going to get the *variety* of nutrients your body needs. You see, while spinach provides a high level of *some* awesome nutrients, it's lacking in several others. Sorry, Popeye.

It's extremely easy to believe your nutrition habits are fantastic simply because you have the *amount* and *type* of your nutrients in line. In fact, I have people come to me regularly who consider their diet brilliant, yet aren't seeing results. I quickly discover that they *do*, in fact, get all of their nutrients from good sources, but they are totally missing out on some key nutrients due to their lack of variety. Those deficiencies will creep up on them and cause their bodies to shut down and start sprouting the common signs and symptoms of malnutrition listed back in chapter 4.

Holy shit this is getting complicated, right!? WRONG. We make "eating" complicated for ourselves not only because are we stubborn with our bad habits, but also because we have tunnel vision on the millions of shitty food-and-beverage-like products or diets being presented to us, rather than real, whole, seasonal, healthy foods. If you want to remind yourself what "real" foods are, please check out Appendix B, where you'll find a long list.

Therefore, in this section we will discuss what happens when you lack the variety of nutrients your body needs, leaving you with a deficiency. You will begin to see how important it is to focus on variety, and why so many people suffer from so many different ailments these days—even if they make healthy choices. *Then* you'll realize how easy it would be to fix everyone's ailments, if they actually knew how to use their g-d pie-holes!

Moral of the Story:

Simply counting calories and eating the right types of foods won't get you in your superhero suit. Add *variety* to the mix, and— SHAA-BAM—you'll be fighting superhero crime in no time.

Chapter 26

The Mighty Macros

We defined macronutrients back in chapter 15, and now we're going to dive in a little deeper. Because, what we didn't discuss is what happens when the foods you choose don't provide the right *ratios* of macronutrients (i.e. the foods you're choosing aren't varied enough). Basically, all hell can break loose.

Nobody wants their body to break loose, so let's do our best to get this right. I previously mentioned that macronutrients had the following caloric sweet spots:

- 20%–35% of your calories should come from fats
- 45%–65% of your calories should come from carbs
- 8%–10% of your calories should come from proteins

Those numbers are based on *science*, not trendy diet blogs. They're also ball-park figures for the average adult, so if you give a shit about long-term health (and not simply weight loss), you'll try your best to snuggle up to them. I've been getting cozy with those percentages for years (including as an athlete), so I'm an advocate. Back in chapter 20 you should have noted what *your* typical percentages were after logging your food. If you didn't, well then fuck—this chapter won't be much fun for you. PLANT THAT STUBBORN ASS IN A FOOD LOG AND DO IT!

As far as percentages go, please keep in mind that when a macronutrient is either "high" or "low," it's in reference to their sweet spots. Meaning, a diet with 40% fats would be considered a *high*-fat diet, but a diet with 40% carbohydrates, would be a *low*-carb diet. Both have the same percentages, but in relation to what those percentages *should* be, one becomes "high," and the other becomes "low." *Capisce?*

Let's pause for a second to reminisce about the fact that hitting the ideal percentages becomes a piece of (organic) cake if you eat a plant-based diet. Again, this is because the make-up of plant foods (when eaten in a wide variety) is pretty on par with what our bodies need. The more processed foods and animal foods you consume, the more you may stray from those percentages (you'll most likely enter the world of the high-protein, low-carb diet). I'm not talking about a periodic tuna steak or egg. I'm talking about you folks who regularly reach for "protein" (meat, cheese, yogurt, eggs, powders, bars, etc.) when you're hungry, thinking it's the healthy option. Basically, those of you who don't regularly reach for veggies, fruits, legumes, whole grains, herbs, nuts, and seeds, are in for a challenge.

Most people who come to me (even the ones who *think* they eat healthy) hover somewhere around 35% fats, 35% carbs, and 30% protein. Even Steven! In reference to the guidelines, however, that would be a high-protein, low-carb diet, and chronic intake would send them plummeting towards Diseaseland at the bottom of the Nutrition Spectrum. Since most people wind up on this path (generally from failing to consume enough health-promoting plant foods), let's discuss what happens if your percentages go haywire.

High-Fat Diets

A high-fat diet occurs when your fat consumption soars over 35% of your total calories. These diets usually arise from too many fatty processed foods or animal foods, and are typically high in calories (thus usually contribute to weight gain and obesity). It's extremely hard to consume a high-fat diet from plant foods, as long as you're eating *whole* plant foods. One could guzzle a bucket of olive oil—which is clearly not a whole food—to hit a plant-based, high-fat diet, but um, gross. If you want to consume a high-fat diet, get ready for certain types of cancer, heart disease, and diabetes.

Low-Fat Diets

A low-fat diet—one with less than 20% of its calories from fats—usually means that someone has been hoarding processed, refined carbs (see "High-Carbohydrate Diets"), which are high in sugar and low in fat. Eating this way often leaves you feeling hungry since processed high-carb foods are nutrient-void and lack the filling fiber (think chips, sodas, white pastas, white breads, etc.). When you're always hungry, you tend to over-consume, and we know what that means. Low-fat diets also cause dry skin, poor body temperature regulation, extreme mental fatigue, and loss of menstrual cycle (don't be tempted, ladies).

High-Carbohydrate Diets

High-carb diets—a diet with more than 65% of calories from carbs—are usually full of refined, sugary, processed food, which also means they lack health-promoting foods. You're guaranteed to be malnourished on this type of diet, because as the amount of sugar (or crap in general) you eat increases, the amount of vitamins and minerals you eat decreases. Thus, diets high in the "bad carbs" (e.g. refined breads, pastas, flours, cookies, chips, soda, sugar) can lead to weight gain, diabetes, and tooth decay.

But wait—is it possible to consume a diet high in "good" carbs? Most "good" carbohydrates (whole plant foods like vegetables, fruits, whole grains, herbs, and legumes) are busting with fiber, so you'll probably wind up feeling like a stuffed turkey before that ever happens. However, if you *do* manage to consume too many good carbs (gobble, gobble), and thus too much fiber, it can cause hard stools, gas, and bloating. You'll feel the opposite of sexy and it will be time to grab the elastic-waist pants.

Low-Carbohydrate Diets

Low-carb diets are diets that provide anything less than 45% of calories from carbs. Since carbohydrates are our number one energy source and provide dietary fiber, these diets immediately lead to symptoms like fatigue and constipation. In addition, since nutrients like vitamins, minerals, antioxidants, and phytonutrients are all found in carbohydrate-rich *whole* foods, you're guaranteed to be deficient in many important nutrients if you send your carbs packing. But that's not all: low-carb diets are shown to adversely affect and even destroy blood vessels.[404] They also usually mean high-protein diets (see below). It's the low-carb, high-protein diets that are fucking up most people who don't know how to use their pie-holes, so TAKE NOTE.

High-Protein Diets

Since we don't need much protein to start with, these diets (anything over 10% protein) are fairly easy to consume if you're not a plant eater. They're abundant in developed nations where people try to consume endless protein because they consider it the "safe" nutrient. Not only do they pack it in like they're about to hibernate for a year—but the protein they choose is generally *animal* protein. These diets will put you at risk for ketoacidosis, kidney disease (including stones), osteoporosis, heart disease, cancer, gout, and many, *many*, MANY other ailments. Furthermore, high-protein diets usually mean low-carbohydrate diets, so you can also factor in all of the ailments mentioned in the "low-carbohydrate" paragraph above. Someone needs to throw protein off its high-horse and I'll be damned if I'm not the one to do it. FUCK OFF YOU HIGH-PROTEIN DIETS!!

Low-Protein Diets

It is rare to find low-protein diets in developed countries since, 1) we don't need much of it anyway, and 2) everyone seems to be hypnotized by products that boast their high-protein content. However, if you *do* consume less than 8% of your total calories from protein (which you'll find more in *developing* nations), it puts you at risk for diseases like marasmus and kwashiorkor. Never heard of them? That's how rare low-protein diets are.

* * *

The big concept here is that it is pretty darn crucial for you to consume the right percentages of macronutrients so your body gets what it needs, and can function as intended. Stay alert however, because while something like a Big Mac may have the right percentages of fats, carbohydrates, and protein (I have no idea if it does because I don't come within a city block of that shit), it obviously won't provide kick-ass nutrients. Thus, it is crucial you don't forget everything we've discussed up to this point in terms of the *types* of food that should make up your diet to fulfill your fat, carbohydrate, and protein requirements. Check out Appendix C if you want to learn more about the macronutrient percentages in certain foods and how to make corrections if your percentages have gone haywire.

Before we move on, we should revisit poop. Yay! Why the hell not?! We already discussed how checking out your number ones and twos can be a good indicator of hydration status, but guess what?! Poop can also be a great indicator of whether or not you're getting the right *nutrients* in your diet! Finally, you have a good reason to talk shit with your friends!

What *is* poop? I mean, everyone knows that they poop, but do they really know what the point of pooping is, and what poop is made of? Not usually. Poop is essentially the waste, or non-digestible part of what we consume. It can tell us a lot about how well we're eating or digesting (and if we're close to hitting our macronutrient ratios). Hence, why I wanted to provide you with some dookie information to help you identify changes you may need to make. Give me a "P"! Give me an "O"! Give me another "O"! Give me a "P"! What's that spell?! POOOOOOOP! Hopefully spelling the word out makes this less uncomfortable for you. Poop.

First off, poop should be shaped like a submarine—minus the rudder and propeller (although *that* would be talent). It should also usually sink to the depths of your porcelain sea. If it *doesn't* resemble Red October, continue reading and consider making adjustments. Keep in mind, I'm talking about *consistent* poops. I'm not talking about a one-off runny turd after a night of cheap beer and vindaloo.

Rabbit Poo (little hard pellets)
You probably need to eat more fiber so your poop doesn't sit in your colon for so long. Fiber only comes from plants (e.g. beans, veggies, whole grains), so graze away! Diets high in protein (usually animal protein) can result in rabbit poop as well, as the protein is usually taking the place of the fiber in the diet.

Technicolor Poo (discolored or tar-like)
Poop should be brown. If it's anything other than brown (and you're not on supplements, meds, or recently ate a bucket of beets), then you should go see a medical professional, as it could mean a variety of things. But hey, pretty poop!

Diarrhea (more water than poo)
You're either sick, increased your fiber intake too quickly, or are hoarding processed protein supplements. Get better, keep drinking fluids so you don't dehydrate yourself, and don't binge on fibrous foods or shitty protein supplements.

Italian Poo (appears greasy and likes to float on water)
You're most likely not absorbing fats properly (from something like celiac disease), or you have too much fat in your diet (usually bad fats). Decrease fatty food consumption (especially oily, fried high-fat meats), and then go talk shit with your doc.

Sandpaper Poop (hard and dry)

You're probably dehydrated, over-medicated, or eating too much dairy (the main culprit in my experience). And you're most definitely in tears from the grating of your turd-hole. Seek water and try reducing dairy (and then get healthy so you can toss the meds).

The Worm (thin and long)

This doesn't have to do with diet so much. It's possible—but not definite—you may have some sort of obstruction, especially if you have been pooping worms for a while on a regular basis. Don't freak out, but go have someone peep up your worm hole.

The Disappearing Act (heaving, heaving, aaaaand . . . nothing)

Constipation sucks. You're probably dehydrated, eating too much calcium, too little magnesium, or too little fiber. Increase water, magnesium rich foods, and fiber slowly, or you'll end up with diarrhea (see previous). Remember, pooping shouldn't feel like childbirth or give you a brain hemorrhage.

The bottom line (get it, "bottom" . . . tee hee) is: pooping should be easy. If it's a chore, makes you cry, bleed, burn, or wish you hadn't eaten those twelve tacos, change something. For instance, don't eat twelve tacos.

Moral of the Story:
Getting the optimal percentages of macronutrients in your diet is key. Your body will respond with health and happiness, and a whole lot of beautiful, submarine-shaped poos.

Chapter 27

The Mini Micros

After the big guns (a.k.a. *macro*nutrients), come the little guns: *micro*nutrients. These are smaller nutrients such as vitamins and minerals—which we will attempt to get from real food, right? Right.

Later in this chapter you will find two long, intricate tables filled with information about these smaller nutrients. Don't attempt to read all of the information now, or even worse, attempt to memorize it. Use the tables as a *reference*. Understand that they offer examples of ailments caused **by** certain micronutrient deficiencies—deficiencies that show up when there's a lack of variety in your diet.[405-415]

These deficiencies—or not having enough nutrients—equate to malnutrition. Therefore, you can peruse the thrilling tables to help figure out which nutrients you may need to consume to help fix a malnutrition issue. Alternatively, if you have plenty of time on your hands and want to be horrified by the many ways nutrient deficiencies can destroy you, you can read the tables word for word. Then head to Appendix D for more information on which foods contain which micronutrients, you bloody over-achiever.

What didn't I include in these tables? I chose not to include toxicity information (i.e. having *too much* of a nutrient). I did this for a couple of reasons—mainly because you are much more likely to be nutrient-deficient than overflowing with nutrients (due to our fucked up, nutrient-depleted food system). The only nutrient I regularly find that people have a toxicity of is sodium—due to shitty, processed foods that are swimming in salt. If you don't eat shitty, processed foods anymore, the salt problem will fix itself.

I don't want you to think that toxicities shouldn't be of concern though. "The more the merrier" doesn't work when it comes to nutrients. Sometimes certain vitamins and minerals can have quite a negative effect if they're over-consumed. For instance, if you consume a lot of zinc, it can affect the way your body absorbs copper, therefore causing a copper deficiency. Excess iron may leave you with a manganese deficiency. There are many more examples like this, so stop pumping yourself full of random vitamins and minerals for shits and giggles. If you don't need them, they can do more harm than good. First find out if you need them, and then attempt to get them from real food.

What I also didn't include in the tables were the millions of "minor" ailments like oily skin, mood swings, weight gain, dark eye circles, etc., because I wanted to make way for the more serious ailments (and also because if this book gets any longer I might stick a fork in my eye). Please realize that if vitamin deficiencies can cause so many *serious* ailments, the *minor* ones they cause are endless.

Lastly, I also chose to skip information like Recommended Dietary Allowances (RDAs), Adequate Intakes (AIs), and Estimated Average Requirements (EARs)—basically the exact amount of each nutrient you should be ingesting. Why? Many of these numbers are inaccurate, and have actually been set at a level the Food and Nutrition Board and Institute of Medicine feel *optimistic* people can ingest—not what people actually *need* to ingest. Furthermore, similar to calories, no one can tell you *exactly* how much of a nutrient you should be having. And the recommendations usually vary by country anyway!

Basically, I don't want to overwhelm the shit out of you any more than you may already be. For example, if I told you to make sure you got 700mg of phosphorus (and not from a pill), would you know how to do that? Probably not. Thus, we're going to forget about those numbers and try to simplify things. If, while exploring this chart, you realize that you don't eat any of the foods listed next to "phosphorus," try eating more foods that contain phosphorus. Simple.

Keep going. You may stumble upon another group of foods that your rarely consume ("shit, I don't eat any of the foods listed next to vitamin A!"). What should you do? EAT SOME OF THEM. See how they affect you. It may be a case of simply not realizing you were experiencing symptoms of a deficiency, and a little experimenting might prove helpful ("HOLY SHIT I CAN SEE AT NIGHT NOW!"). It's a trial and error process, but it works. Best of all, it doesn't involve lots of confusing numbers, or calculations of (inaccurate) recommended nutrient intakes.

Please realize that these lists are not exhaustive. Not only do they not include every ailment for a certain nutrient deficiency, but they also don't list every single food that has each nutrient either. Therefore, if you feel you don't eat enough vitamin A-packed foods, and you don't see any vitamin A-packed foods listed here that you'd be keen to try, do some research and find some that you *would* like to try. There are so many wonderful foods in this world, and chances are you haven't tried half of them. For now, simply skim through the chart and get a feel for how it works. And get excited! Many of the ailments you may be experiencing could go "POOF" if you discover what to shove down your pie-hole!

Disclaimer: Please remember there is a long list of reasons why someone could experience an ailment. A nutrient deficiency is merely *one* of them (the main one, in my opinion). Furthermore, you don't need to exhibit *every* sign listed by a vitamin deficiency to have that deficiency. Everyone reacts differently. Lastly—and I can't stress this enough—please don't diagnose yourself with every form of cancer as you scroll through the tables. You are *most likely* experiencing certain symptoms because of malnutrition. This chart does not diagnose problems. It simply provides examples of what *could* be out of whack in your diet. Don't go bat-shit crazy while reading it.

Please also realize that these ailments listed have not been *proven* to be caused by deficiencies (nothing in science is ever proven). Some symptoms and diseases have a higher correlation than others, and let's put it this way: it certainly won't hurt you to eat some whole foods. Go get 'em tiger; see you on the flip side.

Table 27.1. Vitamins, food sources, and signs of deficiency

Vitamin	Healthy food sources	Signs of deficiency
vitamin A	paprika, dried basil, peppers, dandelion greens, cayenne pepper, carrots, sweet potatoes, spinach, dried parsley, butternut squash, leafy greens	night blindness, total blindness, decreased growth rate, poor bone health, increased risk for respiratory and diarrheal infections, increased susceptibility to cancer, acne, red or white acne-like bumps (on cheeks, arms, thighs, and buttocks), accelerated aging
vitamin B$_1$	pecans, sunflower seeds, sesame seeds, pine nuts, dried cilantro, poppy seeds, dried sage, macadamia nuts, yeast, pistachios, tuna fish	anxiety, loss of appetite, anorexia, upset stomach, fatigue, constipation, dry eyes, chest pain, poor sleep, depression, weight loss, irritability, confusion, memory loss, muscle weakness, beriberi, enlarged heart
vitamin B$_2$	yeast, ancho chills, paprika, wheat bran, dried cilantro, wild Atlantic salmon, almonds, sesame seeds, dry roasted soy beans, sun-dried tomatoes, mackerel	ariboflavinosis, cancer, heart disease, sore throat, inflammation and cracked corners of the mouth, swollen tongue, scaly red rash on face, head and torso, neurological and developmental disorders, normochromic and normocytic anemia

Table 27.1. (*continued*)

Vitamin	Healthy food sources	Signs of deficiency
vitamin B3	cooked yellow-fin tuna, cooked chicken/turkey, cooked pork chop, green peas, sunflower seeds, avocado	pellagra, pigmented rash, dermatitis, vomiting, diarrhea, constipation, headache, bright red tongue, dementia, cracked corners of the mouth, loss of memory, neurological symptoms, fatigue, amnesia, poor concentration, depression
vitamin B5	rice bran, wheat bran, caviar, avocados, sunflower seeds, liver, sun-dried tomatoes, wild Atlantic salmon, mushrooms	irritability, restlessness, fatigue, apathy, malaise, headache, sleep disturbances, nausea, vomiting, muscle cramps, staggering gait, fatigue, insomnia, depression, numbness and tingling in feet, upper respiratory infections,
vitamin B6	wheat bran, rice bran, chili powder, paprika, pistachios, garlic, liver, wild Atlantic salmon, yellow-fin tuna, sunflower seeds, molasses, sesame seeds, hazelnuts	microcytic anemia, water retention, convulsions, diabetes, heart disease, blood pressure issues, diarrhea, neurological disorders, dermatitis, carpal tunnel syndrome, premenstrual symptoms, dementia, tingling or numbness in hands and feet, allergies, asthma, weakened immune system
vitamin B7	wild Alaskan salmon, avocados, mushrooms, cauliflower, nuts, raspberries, bananas, leafy green veggies, liver	dermatitis, alopecia, central nervous system abnormalities, hair loss, hallucinations, dry eyes, paresthesia, conjunctivitis, dry scaly skin, cracking in the corners of the mouth, red swollen and painful tongue, loss of appetite, fatigue, insomnia, depression, lethargy

Table 27.1. (*continued*)

Vitamin	Healthy food sources	Signs of deficiency
vitamin B9	beans, lentils, spinach, broccoli, cos or romaine lettuce, asparagus, avocado, mango, pomegranate, oranges	pellagra, poor red blood cell production, cardiovascular problems, megaloblastic anemia, tingling or numbness in hands and feet, neural tube defects (anencephaly, spina bifida)
vitamin B12	bacteria (residing in animals) is the only organism that produces natural B12. Therefore, most animal foods are a good source of B12. If you find a plant food that has vitamin b12 listed, it has been added.	pernicious anemia, tingling or numbness in hands and feet, uneven gait, memory loss, dementia, hair loss, cognitive changes, paranoia, depression, loss of concentration, visual disturbances, loss of taste and smell, insomnia, disorientation, cracked corners of the mouth, sore tongue, impaired bowel and bladder control, infertility
choline	cauliflower, cod, broccoli, amaranth, quinoa, spinach, kidney beans, peanuts, almonds, cooked brown rice	fatty liver, liver damage, brain fog, memory problems, decreased focus, insomnia, nerve and muscle problems
vitamin C	red/green chili peppers, guava, bell peppers, fresh thyme, cauliflower, fresh parsley, broccoli, kale, mustard greens, brussels sprouts, papayas, kiwi fruit, oranges, strawberries	follicular hyperkeratosis, petechiae, bruising, hair loss, coiled hairs, inflamed and bleeding gums, joint pain, perifollicular hemorrhages, joint effusions, impaired wound healing, shortness of breath, swelling, sjorgren syndrome, weakness, fatigue, weak immune system, , heart disease, depression, cancer

Table 27.1. (*continued*)

Vitamin	Healthy food sources	Signs of deficiency
vitamin D	the big ball of fire in the sky!	lung disease, diabetes, rickets, osteomalacia, osteoporosis, bone pain, stunted growth, muscle pains or weakness, high blood pressure, frailty, early puberty, pregnancy complications, allergies, increased inflammation, congestive heart failure, heart disease, seasonal affective disorder, night blindness, reduced immunity, certain cancers, cognitive decline, depression, multiple sclerosis, dementia, rheumatoid arthritis
vitamin E	cooked spinach, shrimp, almonds, avocados, roasted sunflower seeds, cooked squash or pumpkin, broccoli	nerve degeneration in hands and feet, chronic kidney disease, hair loss, hemolytic anemia, psoriasis, chronic pain, muscle weakness, chronic fatigue, poor bone health, chronic infection, depression, night blindness, neurological disorders, ophthalmological (eye) disorders, susceptibility to cancer and heart disease, decreased sexual performance
vitamin K	dried basil, dried sage, dried thyme, spinach, fresh parsley, broccoli, kale, green onion, brussels sprouts, cabbage, prunes, asparagus	inadequate blood clotting, bruising, hemorrhages, increased risk of bone fracture

Table 27.2. Minerals, food sources, and signs of deficiency

Mineral names	Healthy food sources	Result of deficiency
calcium	dried basil, dried thyme, sesame seeds, flax seeds, almonds, watercress, curly kale, bok choy, pak choi, okra, broccoli, green beans	reduced bone mass, fractures, osteoporosis, muscle cramps (mainly in toes, calves, backs of legs, and feet), joint aches, increased cholesterol levels, nervousness, brittle nails, rheumatoid arthritis, tooth decay, sleep disturbances
chloride	sea salt, rye, seaweed, tomatoes, lettuce, celery, olives	hypochloremic metabolic alkalosis, growth failure, blood in the urine, anorexia, irritability, lethargy, gastrointestinal symptoms, weakness, hypokalemia, increased plasma renin metabolic hyper–aldosteronism,
chromium	onions, tomatoes, brewer's yeast, oysters, whole grains, potatoes	anxiety, racing heart, lightheadedness, anxiousness, muscle weakness, chronic fatigue, mood swings, weight loss, impaired glucose tolerance, neuropathy
copper	liver, oysters, lobster, squid, sesame seeds, cocoa powder, cashews, sunflower seeds, roasted pumpkin seeds, sun-dried tomatoes, hazelnuts, dried basil	anemia, immune and cardiac dysfunction, nerve damage, confusion, fatigue, muscle weakness, impaired coordination, impaired wound healing, depression, altered sense of taste

Table 27.2. (*continued*)

Mineral names	Healthy food sources	Result of deficiency
iodine	dried seaweed, cod, baked potato, shrimp/prawn, baked turkey breast, cooked navy beans	hypothyroidism, goiter, stunted physical and mental growth (in babies from mothers with the deficiency), cancer, depression, fatigue, difficulty breathing, change in mental status, weight gain, increased cold sensitivity, dry skin, thin hair, constipation, brittle nails, abnormal menstruation cycle
iron	dried thyme, spirulina, clams, mussels, oysters, liver, cashews, spinach, white beans, quinoa, squash/pumpkin seeds, cocoa powder	fatigue, developmental delay, cognitive impairment, anemia, hair loss, shortness of breath, dizziness, headache, pale skin, cold hands and feet, chest pain, cracked mouth corners
magnesium	leafy green veggies, rice bran, cocoa powder, cilantro/coriander, squash/pumpkin seeds, beans, brown rice, avocados, bananas, brazil nuts, mackerel, sunflower seeds, dried flax seeds, molasses, wheat germ	loss of appetite, tooth decay, fatigue, headache, migraine, blood clots, nausea, anxiety, panic attacks, asthma, bowel disease, urinary or bladder infection, heart disease, diabetes, depression, high blood pressure, low blood sugar, insomnia, kidney disease, liver disease, seizures, pre-menstrual symptoms, Reynaud's syndrome, numbness and tingling, personality changes, infertility, preeclampsia musculoskeletal conditions (e.g. cramps, , osteoporosis, fibromyalgia, back pain)

Table 27.2. (*continued*)

Mineral names	Healthy food sources	Result of deficiency
manganese	mussels, oysters, clams, cloves, saffron, rice bran, soy beans, hazelnuts, wheat germ, oat bran, cocoa powder, roasted pumpkin/squash seeds, flax seeds, sesame seeds, roasted sunflower seeds, chili powder	hypocholesterolemia, altered fat and carb metabolism, bone malformation, bone demineralization, stunted growth, skin rash, infertility, seizures, weakness, nausea and vomiting, dizziness, hearing loss, anemia, weak hair and nails, dermatitis
molybdenum	whole grains, legumes (e.g. beans, peas, lentils)	developmental delays, neurological changes, tachycardia, headache, night blindness, seizures
phosphorus	pumpkin seeds, mustard seed, wild salmon, scallops, brazil nuts, white beans, adzuki beans, chickpeas, cocoa powder, yellow beans	anorexia, anemia, muscle weakness, bone pain, impaired bone and teeth formation, rickets, stiff joints, fatigue, osteomalacia, loss of appetite, anxiety, irregular breathing, irritability, weight gain or loss, numbness
potassium	white beans, spinach, dried apricots, salmon, baked acorn squash, avocados, bananas	cardiac arrhythmias, muscle weakness, muscle cramps (mainly in toes, calves, backs of legs, and feet), confusion, extreme thirst, salt sensitivity, increased blood pressure, frequent urination, glucose intolerance, kidney stones

Table 27.2. (*continued*)

Mineral names	Healthy food sources	Result of deficiency
selenium	brazil nuts, cooked tuna, oysters, oat bran, crimini mushrooms, chia seeds, wheat germ, sesame seeds	keshan disease, skeletal muscle pain, fatigue, weakness, infertility, hair loss, fingernail discoloration, fatigue, poor concentration, miscarriage, hypothyroidism
sodium	sea salt, Himalayan salt, yeast extract, sun-dried tomatoes, saltwater crab (chances are you *don't* have a sodium deficiency, so move along please!)	brain swelling, loss of appetite, nausea, vomiting, headache, confusion, irritability, fatigue, hallucinations, muscle weakness, convulsions
sulfur	artichoke, arugula, broccoli, cabbage, cauliflower, leeks, brussels sprouts, onions, garlic, horseradish, avocado, kale, spinach, dill, steamed soy beans, sesame seeds, cashews, asparagus	itchy skin and scalp, eczema, acne, vomiting, digestion, diarrhea, migraines, atulence, hemorrhoids, painful nd irregular menstruation, sore roat, impotence, hay fever, joint in, toothache, nosebleeds, fever, bed wetting, breastfeeding problems
zinc	cooked oysters, spinach, toasted wheat germ, roasted pumpkin/squash seeds, sesame seeds, cashews, cocoa powder, mung beans, cooked white mushrooms	growth retardation, hair loss, diarrhea, anorexia, delayed sexual maturation, sexual impotence, lethargy, eye and skin lesions, cracked corners of the mouth, loss of appetite, delayed wound healing, weak immune system, impaired smell and taste

Holy shit! Look at all the ailments caused by nutrient deficiencies—and that's only a small selection of them! Hey, I have a question: why the fuck aren't we fixing people with nutrients?! I have another question: why the fuck aren't we fixing people with nutrients?! Same question, but it needs to be asked repeatedly and often. Do you know how much *cheaper* food is than medical care?! Health providers should be telling the pharmaceutical and supplement companies to "suck it," and then grow a garden and start treating their patients with *food*. All hospitals should have organic gardens, and the health providers should focus on pumping their patients full of powerful nutrients to allow for the best healing. Feeding tubes should be filled with powerful, organic superfood purees. I mean, c'mon—how the heck are patients supposed to heal while being fed shitty hospital food that inhibits their body from healing? Hey, I know! Let's keep them there as long as possible and rack up the bill!

Unfortunately—as I have previously discussed—there needs to be a lot of education thrown at our healthcare providers before the majority of them even *begin* to understand that nutrients can cure malnutrition problems—which we now know are at the root of most diseases. Here's where some good news comes in (about friggin' time, right?). Doctors are starting to take note, like the fabulous Dr. Robert Ostfeld, of the Bronx, New York. He started a Cardiac Wellness Program at Montefiore Hospital, which brings a "unique, nutrition-centered approach to the management of cardiovascular disease."[416] Simply put, they shove a shitload of whole plant foods into their patients (while having them sustain from all animal foods). These patients, who are being destroyed by heart disease, are seeing dramatic, life-changing results.

Even more exciting, Tulane University caught on to all of this "hippie-shit nutrition nonsense" and, in 2014, became the first university in the US to take a giant leap in the right direction. Their medical school opened a "teaching kitchen," so the doctors they spit out would actually be able to instruct their patients on how to use their pie-holes.[417] Righteous, eh?! Who knows what *kind* of nutrition they're teaching, but at least it's a giant leap in the right direction!

Okay, now don't hate me. Those micronutrient tables we just discussed? They simplify an exceptionally detailed, complicated relationship between nutrition and disease, which—if I'm going to be honest—is kind of bullshit. Here's why: the chances of you having only *one* vitamin or mineral deficiency are slim. If you are deficient in something (e.g. vitamin C), it's because you're not consuming enough foods that contain that nutrient (e.g. bell peppers, kale, broccoli, strawberries, oranges). Since those foods are full of many nutrients, than chances are you're also deficient in the *other* nutrients available in those foods. The tricky part is once you become deficient in more than one nutrient, the negative reactions within your body explode exponentially and create even more issues. With all of the nutrients out there, it is nearly impossible to predict the numerous reactions resulting from multiple nutrient deficiencies. What was the point of the chart then?! To piss you off, clearly. Or, it was there to show the possible result of a *simple* deficiency. Imagine if you accumulated *multiple* deficiencies. Suddenly your body breaks down in more ways that you can count, and the information becomes impossible to list on a chart.

SO WHAT'S THE FUCKING POINT OF THE CHART, THEN?! To educate you. If you make sure you're eating a wide variety of the foods listed by each vitamin in the chart, your chances of a nutrient deficiency significantly diminish. Just remember, this chart isn't exhaustive, and this journey is all about experimenting. If you get to a nutrient and don't like any of the foods listed next to it, get your research hat on and find other healthy options that tickle your pickle. Or, just fucking suck it up and eat the foods that are listed. The most important part is consuming a wide variety of foods to ensure you get all of your nutrients. You might not *love* everything you're initially eating, but you'll certainly love your new rockin' bod and superhero powers.

As you can see (unless you didn't actually skim through the chart), many powerful nutrients come from nuts, seeds, and herbs. Thus, one of the best habits to start forming is to flavor your foods with different fresh or dried herbs. Making nuts and seeds a regular meal additive or snack habit would also be fabulous. Personally, I keep jars of nuts (e.g. almonds, cashews, pistachios, pecans, walnuts, brazil), and seeds (e.g. pumpkin, sunflower, flax, chia, sesame, hemp) hanging out on my counter (or in my fridge), and regularly sprinkle them on, or incorporate them in my meals. They add excellent texture, and provide powerful nutrients I wouldn't have gotten elsewhere. Piss off, deficiencies!

Side note: if you want to get more specific with your nutrient intake, there are software programs that will estimate the nutrients you're getting from the foods you eat (the food logging website *www.cronometer.com* is one of them). You log your food, and the program spits out information on vitamins and minerals—which ones you may be lacking, and which ones you may be hoarding. If you choose to use a program like this, please realize that many of the target amounts might be set by the inaccurate RDAs, AIs, EARs, etc. that we mentioned earlier. Thus, use them with caution.

Before we forge on, I want to discuss vitamin D and vitamin B12 a bit further. "One of these things is not like the other . . ." Let's start with vitamin D. Big D is different from other vitamins as it functions more like a hormone, and we don't actually put it in our pie-holes (well, most of it anyway). I don't want you to get confused and think you're supposed to *eat* it, because over 90% of the vitamin D we get actually comes from the sun.[413] No, the sun doesn't shoot out little magical vitamin D microbes that scurry inside our bodies like some alien scene from a sci-fi movie. As cool as that would be, the ultraviolet (UV) light from the sun actually causes a reaction inside our bodies, which in turn allows us to produce our own vitamin D. Who knew our bodies were so friggin' rad!? I did! So, while companies seem to be stacking their man-made, vitamin D-infused products everywhere you look these days, they should *not* be the focus for your vitamin D intake. Instead, it's vital that you get your pasty ass outside and soak up some rays.

Eeeeeek! What about cancer?? Aren't UV rays demonic?! Hear me out. Unfortunately, we're told to avoid the sun's rays and lather ourselves in ridiculous amounts of sun block. Side note: I find it "hilarious," that most sun blocks—which are meant to protect you from skin cancer—have carcinogenic chemicals in them. Ha! Seriously. HA-HA!

Back to the lathering. Once we all look like albino zombies, we're then told to wear layers upon layers of clothes that shade us from the angry cancer monster in the sky. This becomes detrimental because if we hide from the sun we will develop a vitamin D deficiency, which will in turn shoot us to the bottom of the Nutrition Spectrum where diseases—like cancer—run rampant. Love me a good catch-22!

With vitamin D deficiency now considered a pandemic (in the US alone, 50% of the population is deficient, and in darker skinned individuals you'll see deficiencies in up to 82%), it has become more important than ever to make love to the sun's rays.[418] This leaves you in a bit of a pickle though, doesn't it? Expose yourself to the sun, increase your risk of skin cancer. Hide from the sun, get a vitamin D deficiency (which will increase your risk of cancer, heart disease, autoimmune diseases and a myriad of other problems).[413, 419-425] Time to find that sweet spot, eh?

Thus, while skin cancer is certainly a concern, when I say "get your lazy ass outside and soak up some sun," I'm not talking about lubing yourself up with Crisco and laying naked on a tin roof for days. I'm talking about getting some periodic *natural* sun exposure *without* sun block (which actually blocks the UV rays that start this magical process). I'm also talking about doing this *regularly*, so you can whip up your own vitamin D as needed.

This means you're outside for several minutes with a good amount of skin showing (arms, legs, and face will do folks—I don't want to be getting calls asking me to bail you out of jail for streaking through the park butt-naked chanting "come to me, Big D!"). It also means you have to be outside when the UV index is at a certain level (which takes into account the sun's strength based on latitude, time of day, and season)—and that magical UV number is generally three or greater. How long you need to stay outside varies greatly with the time of day, the season, the distance you are from the equator, and the darkness of your skin. I have a tool that may help you though. I was presented the information in table 27.3 during my nutrition studies.[426] It shows the estimated amount of time that you should spend outside in order to get adequate UVB rays to start pumping out vitamin D (based on your skin type and your local UV index).

Note: you can usually find your local UV index in any weather forecast (the part that most people ignore or skip over, because no one tells us what it actually means), or on environmental websites (check out the Environmental Protection Agency if you are in America). Also, for more accuracy, the recommended exposure times should be *doubled* if you are over fifty-five years of age.

Table 27.3. Exposure times (in minutes) for adequate vitamin D production

Skin Type	UV 0-2	UV 3-5	UV 6-7	UV 8-10	UV 11+
always burn, never tan	none	10-15	5-10	2-8	1-5
easily burn, rarely tan	none	15-20	10-15	5-8	2-8
occasionally burn, slowly tan	none	20-30	15-20	10-15	5-10
rarely burn, rapidly tan	none	30-40	20-30	15-20	10-15
never burn, always dark	none	40-60	30-40	20-30	15-20

Now, if it's winter, or you live far from the equator, you may be concerned that you can't actually see the sun for long periods of time (i.e. the sun isn't strong enough to do any good). Don't worry; your body actually stores vitamin D for situations like this. However, if you start to get bitchy mid-winter and need to take a vacation to a tropical paradise for "health" reasons, I say go for it.

I hate to be negative Nancy, but there's always a downside to everything. You see, even if you absorb copious amounts of sunshine, there are many reasons why your body might still struggle to properly utilize your stored vitamin D. You know what one of the main reasons is? Ingesting too much animal protein. I already mentioned that if you consume a diet based on animal foods, your body would enter an acidic state. This acidic environment greatly impacts the function of vitamin D in your body by shutting down the pathways involved in production.[427] One more point goes to the protein in plant foods (which don't have the same effect on vitamin D).

To summarize, whenever the sun is high in the sky in your neck of the woods (and the UV index is three or above), take advantage. You can't overdose on vitamin D from sun exposure, as our bodies don't allow over-production (rad, eh?). However, if you take vitamin D *supplements*, it is easy to overdose, and also extremely dangerous. Thus, if you're going to dabble in vitamin D supplementation, it should be done with extreme caution. And if you're going to dabble in animal-protein-hoarding, you may as well kiss your vitamin D goodbye.

Lastly, let's hit vitamin B_{12}. Similarly to vitamin D, B_{12} is "not like the others." *Unlike* vitamin D, you still have to consume B_{12}. And *unlike* most everything in this book, B_{12} doesn't come from plants. It also can't be produced by animals. What the? Where does this hidden necessity hide? Well, you see, B_{12} is actually produced by certain bacteria and archaea, which we need to consume to get our B_{12}. Most commonly, they reside in the guts of animals, and therefore vitamin B_{12} is available in most all animal foods (e.g. meat, seafood, dairy). There *are* some plant foods that contain a miniscule amount of B_{12}, but you will most likely come nowhere close to ingesting the amount your body requires by choosing those options.

This is where the plant-*based* diet comes into play. When people ask me where I get my vitamin B_{12} from, I simply say I eat enough foods with vitamin B_{12} in them. That doesn't mean that I'm not eating a plant-based diet. My diet is *based* on plants, and has other whole foods, such as wild fish and mollusks, scattered throughout it, ensuring I still obtain the nutrients my body needs.

If you are a vegan or even vegetarian, it's imperative you pay close attention here. The last thing you need is a vitamin B_{12} deficiency, and you're certainly not going to get enough B_{12} from fortified packaged foods or electric energy drinks that list a synthetic "vitamin B_{12}" on the ingredient label. If you refuse to eat meat or animal products in general (you have the right to make that choice), you must find a way to get B_{12}. You have a few options, and you're mainly looking at pills, powders, or injections. The choice is yours (head back a few pages to check out the side effects of a vitamin B_{12} deficiency if you need some motivation). If you're wondering where you stand on the B_{12} deficiency scale, go have someone jam a needle in your vein and analyze your blood.

Moral of the Story:

Malnutrition causes a million and one diseases and ailments. It's time we start looking to *nutrients* to cure mal*nutrition*. The best way to go about this is to consume a wide variety of whole, untainted foods.

Chapter 28

Probiotics, Flavonoids, and Carotenoids . . . Oh My!

I hate to add more complex terms to this learning experience, but not enough that I won't. #sorrynotsorry. Am I allowed to hashtag in a book? #fuckitijustdid

In addition to the fats, carbs, proteins, vitamins, and minerals we've discussed, there are several nutrient terms and smaller nutrients we haven't touched on. I feel it's important we discuss some of them, as you will most definitely find them ever-so-cleverly used on product labels, drawing you in and enticing you to take them home with you. Because, let's be honest—if you were looking for a certain product or food, you would most likely gravitate towards the option that boasted gut-enhancing probiotics and disease-fighting flavonoids and carotenoids, right? You may not be able to *define* those words, but hey, if they fight disease and give you a healthy gut, then shit—don't go home without them!

Before the marketing madness puts you on a leash and parades you around like a puppet, let's discuss how some of these nutrients and terms relate to nutrition, and whether or not they're even necessary. Time to throw that learning cap (cape?) on.

Supplements

Supplements are essentially anything added to your diet which help fulfill your nutritional needs by attempting to remedy any deficiencies (e.g. multivitamin, protein powder).

The only time you should take a supplement is when you are incapable of consuming your body's required nutrients from real food (or in the case of vitamin D, the sun). And even then, they should be used to get you to the *minimal* requirements—they should never be relied on to provide all of your nutrients. Real food should always be your first consideration. Remember, natural vitamins—found in the *whole* foods you should be consuming—never exist in isolation. Therefore, if a vitamin is offered in isolation (e.g. a whole bottle of vitamin C), than chances are it is man-made, and a bajillion times less effective than the natural stuff.[105, 428, 429]

I now give you permission to scoff at all the "fortified with 3,000% of your daily whatever" claims. Supplement companies are simply begging for your acceptance in the most pathetic of ways. They are there to sell products, and their claims have nothing to do with your nutrient needs or your health. And, since most people flock to vitamin claims faster than retirees can get to Florida, many people wind up with a toxicity of vitamins from over-consumption of supplements. Don't assume they're harmless—toxicities can be just as dangerous as deficiencies. For example, vitamins A, E, D, K, and beta carotene from supplements may *increase* mortality.[430] Ah, shit. And did you know that a regular 400mg daily calcium supplement will give you a 51% increased risk of prostate cancer.[156] Well, it will if you have a prostate. But you get my point. Many people take supplements because they figure "it can't hurt," when that's exactly what it may be doing.

Furthermore, if you thought FDA regulation was shady, you'll be thrilled to know that the FDA doesn't regulate supplements. In fact, *no one* actually regulates supplements. That's right—it is up to the "trustworthy" supplement companies to decide what ingredients are safe for their products. They can throw whatever they want in them, make whatever claims they want about them, and—wham, bam, thank you ma'am—send them straight to the shelves to be devoured. Are you eyeing your vitamin bottles and wondering what's in them yet? Or, better yet, wondering if you actually need them?

Superfoods

Superfoods are a mythical category of foods comprised of pure awesomeness. They're foods that have an enormous amount of powerful, health-promoting qualities, and are usually low in calories (fuck yeah!). Foods such as chard, arugula, turmeric, chia seeds, maca, cacao, spirulina, green tea, kale, watercress, hemp seed, flax seed, walnuts, goji berries, parsley, and papaya are all considered superfoods (and there are many more). You won't find a list of them anywhere though, as there isn't yet a way to classify them. They're kick-ass, however, because they help power your brain and immune system while fighting against infection as well as diseases and ailments like common colds, the flu, osteoporosis, heart disease, certain cancers, diabetes . . . and a million others. This is mainly because they "fill in" all of your deficiency issues with the assortment of nutrients they offer. Everyone should include superfoods in their diet,, so please add that to your "to do" list (noting that they're generally plant foods).

Phytonutrients

*Phyto*nutrients are brilliant little gems that *fight* against disease. Get it? Phyto—fight? Even though "phyto" technically means "plant," it's an easy way to remember what the heck that long word means: a fuckin' disease-fighter, that's what. Examples of foods high in phytonutrients are blackberries, walnuts, strawberries, artichokes, cranberries, raspberries, blueberries, cloves, prunes, and cabbage. Yes, phytonutrients are only found in plant foods (many of which could also be considered "superfoods"). Shocker.

Antioxidants

Listen up, because there's a big, stinky misconception about antioxidants. First off, you need to know that a process called "oxidation" is bad. Oxidation happens when little shits called "free radicals" are present in your body and lead to the destruction or death of your body's cells. To prevent this destructive oxidation, we require "anti"oxidants (molecules that fight against oxidation). You may have already put two and two together, but antioxidants therefore help maintain healthy cells and a healthy body . . . but, as always, there's a twist. Food additives like BHA and BHT (see the "Shit to Avoid Like the Plague" section) are technically "antioxidants" because they protect against the oxidizing, or spoiling of the food. Thus, please listen up: if you see "antioxidants" on a food label IT'S NOT A GOOD THING. Antioxidants occur *naturally* in foods—they shouldn't have to be added. If they are added, it's most likely not the good stuff, and signifies a highly-processed product looking to increase its shelf life. Examples of foods high in *real* antioxidants are: red beans, kidney beans, pinto beans, acai berries, blueberries, cranberries, blackberries, artichokes, prunes, turmeric, and pecans. Holy shit, there's another list of plant foods! Yes, plant foods have ridiculously higher levels of antioxidants than animal foods.[431] I love patterns.

Probiotics

Probiotics are tiny microorganisms (e.g. bacteria) that, when consumed, help us with our immunity, digestion, and metabolism. They live and thrive inside us. And, while consuming bacteria may sound weird or insane, the little suckers actually give us a "healthy gut" (as long as you consume *healthy* bacteria, and not the kind that will make you sick). Examples of foods high in probiotics (usually fermented foods) are: miso soup, kimchi, kombucha tea, pickles, sauerkraut, yogurt, kefir, and tempeh. Sea algae (e.g. spirulina, chlorella) also contain probiotics. You may not know what half of those foods are (heck my Microsoft Word spell check didn't even know what they were), but that's what the internet is for, so hop **to** it.

Are you cringing while thinking about eating bacteria? It will probably help you to know, that for you to function effectively, there should actually be more bacteria living in your body than human cells (there are around one hundred trillion of them living inside you if you're doing things right).[432] Stop squirming—the little guys keep us healthy, so imagine them as internal pets. Welcome them as part of the family, recognize their importance, and cross your fingers they will set up shop and thrive inside you.

Bacteria become even *more* important if you're taking (or have recently taken) antibiotics. *Anti*-biotics are precisely that, they are *anti*-bacteria, and are usually taken to kill off the invading bugs when someone has a bacterial infection. However, not only do antibiotics kill off the *bad* bacteria, but they also kill off the *good* bacteria, leaving you with a weakened immune system. This also creates oxidative stress, or oxidation (see "antioxidant" above), which opens the door for a myriad of health issues.[433] Next time you take *anti*biotics (you mostly likely won't if you get this nutrition shit down), be sure to follow up with a large dose of *pro*biotics to maintain your healthy gut. I'm sorry, I don't know why I'm telling you this. I'm sure your doctor lectured you about how important probiotics were last time they handed you an antibiotic prescription. Oh, they didn't? Well that's fuckin' strange.

Flavonoids

Flavonoids are a plant component with kick-ass antioxidant and anti-inflammatory healing properties. The following foods are bursting with these treasures: parsley, dill, thyme, kale, blueberries, cherries, cranberries, grapefruit, strawberries, peppers, tomatoes, eggplant, tea, wine, and dark chocolate.[434] I know what you're thinking. No smartass, this does not mean you can now go live on wine and chocolate. But hey, another point for the plants!

The FDA hasn't actually "recognized" flavonoids yet (they must be too busy approving harmful chemicals), and therefore, no one is allowed to make claims on them. Well, here goes my stubborn ass again: flavonoids have been shown to exhibit anti-allergic, anti-inflammatory, antioxidant, antimicrobial, antifungal, antiviral, anti-cancer, and anti-diarrheal properties.[435-446] Sounds AMAZING! Many of the most horrendous diseases known to man are initiated by inflammation or oxidation, so flavonoid-rich foods (which help prevent both) should be on the plate of every earthling. Get that wondrous stuff in your pie-hole, STAT!

Carotenoids

Carotenoids are the colorful pigments that give certain whole foods bright, vibrant hues (this doesn't include fluorescent packaged products). These pigments are important because they allow the body to make certain vitamins, and because they act as an antioxidant by preventing disease. People who consume a wide range of carotenoids avoid disease better than those who don't.[447-451] In other words, people who eat their (bright-colored) fruits, veggies, herbs, and spices are healthier than people who stay away from them. So many surprises.

The following foods are high in carotenoids: carrots, sweet potatoes, tomatoes, pumpkin, apricots, mango, papaya, cantaloupe, dark leafy greens, broccoli, turmeric, saffron, and cinnamon.

Pro tip: Use carotenoids to your advantage. Take your children to the store and tell them to pick out a "rainbow" of fresh foods (they have to find something naturally red, orange, yellow, etc. that they want to eat). Then take those kiddos home and they're more likely to eat those foods after having a hand in choosing them. Game on! Did I mention that carotenoids are only found in plant foods? PLANT FOODS!

According to everything you've just read, the key to fighting disease is highly powerful, immune-boosting, puts-hair-on-your-chest *plant* foods. By eating plant foods (preferably whole, organically grown versions), you will ingest all of the awesomely fabulous vitamins, minerals, phytonutrients, antioxidants, probiotics, flavonoids, and carotenoids that are rarely (sometimes never) available in animal or processed foods.

Do your best to avoid the hype of less-than-worthy synthetic vitamins, minerals, and supplements. Remember, they don't contain anything that can't be found—in a superior version—in real food.[105] If people selling and promoting these wonder-supplements tell you that "it is impossible for you to get all of your daily servings of fruits and veggies," and that "you *must* have their product because it's the *best* out there and the *best* way to ensure you meet your nutritional requirements," take a deep breath and say the following:

"It's pretty bold of you to tell me what I am, or am not, capable of eating. Also, did you know that the 'good' components of your product are actually available in *real* foods? Well they are, and I'm sure as shit going to try to get all my nutrients from *them* before I turn to your pill- or powder-in-a-can."

Then you pull a carrot out of your spandex superhero suit, give them a wink and a high-five, and fly into the sunset.

I have no issue getting all of my servings of fruits and vegetables; it's not hard at all, actually. I merely took a step back from the pressure of "faster and easier is better," ignored the hype of supplements and processed food products, and realized that I simply needed to start eating real, whole food. If you're struggling with this, the best way to kick start a natural nutrient-boost (which we'll discuss more in depth in the next chapter) is to incorporate a homemade juice or smoothie made from whole foods—perhaps *superfoods*—into your diet. You will then, without a doubt, catapult yourself ten steps closer to the amount, type, and variety of nutrients your body needs. And, of course, to the top of the Nutrition Spectrum. Hi-ho, Silver! AWAY!

Moral of the Story:

If you want to improve your health, eat *real* foods. Specifically, *plant* foods full of powerful nutrients that can't be found elsewhere. Don't waste your money by getting fake-ass nutrients out of a bottle. Ya hear?

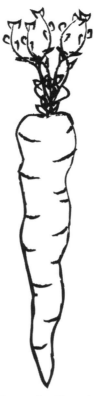

Holy shit, you're 3/4 of the way done!
By now you should be craving a carrot!
No? Well, go feed it to your fucking unicorn!

Chapter 29

Juices and Smoothies

What's a surefire way to get a kick-ass nutrient boost full of disease-fighting nutrients like antioxidants, phytonutrients, carotenoids, and flavonoids? Um, did you read the previous chapter? Start making your own juices or smoothies from *real* food! Think of drinking a juice or a smoothie as taking a much fresher, more powerful, and more natural version of a multi-vitamin or supplement. They can be consumed at home, on the road, by kids, by athletes, whomever. No one's going to die from a juice or smoothie (unless you dump something like glyphosate in them, which I don't recommend).

If you do it right, you'll get an organic, fresh boost of powerful nutrients that will save you from the void of nutrients in your body. Be sure to say "hello" to Captain America when you reach the top end of the Nutrition Spectrum, because you'll be headed there on the fast train. If this sounds pleasing to you, saddle up. If you're not interested in partaking, skip to the next chapter. The info is always here if you change your mind.

First and foremost, you need to decide whether you want to juice (which requires a juicer), or make smoothies (which requires a blender). Juicing involves removing the fiber and making a drink out of the water and nutrients of whole foods. On the other hand, a smoothie will contain *all* of the food, including the fiber. Both have benefits, and it generally comes down to preference.

Option 1: Juicing

The no-fiber option. Without the fiber, your digestive system won't have to work as hard to "break down" the nutrients, which in turn means that those nutrients are absorbed faster and at a higher quantity. Yay! The down side is that the fast absorption can give you a spike in blood sugar (take note, diabetics), and without the fiber you may still feel hungry after consuming one.

Option 2: Smoothies

The fiber option. With the fiber still there, the liquid is absorbed more slowly, which won't allow the spike in blood sugar you can get from a juice. Also, because the fiber is included, it will leave you feeling more "full" after consuming one. However, since the fiber *isn't* removed, the down side to making smoothies is that they can get *huge* fairly quickly (i.e. get ready to gulp down a gallon of goodness), whereas with juicing you can fit a lot more nutrients into less liquid since the fiber isn't taking up space.

Once you decide which one you want to tackle, you can start to piece together a fantastic, magical, superboost recipe (that *should* be called "Revive," "Defense," "Focus," or "Energy," in place of Coke's Vita-crap Water). Unfortunately, here's where most people go off the Richter and start chucking all of the super sweet foods they already eat and love (usually fruit) into a blender or juicer and feel they've built Rome in a day. Juicing or making smoothies is not about throwing a bunch of your favorite foods together—if they're your favorite foods, eat them in their whole form for fuck's sake. This is about finding a way to infuse new, powerful, superfoods into your body—ones you normally *wouldn't* touch— in order to fill the void of the nutrients.

This is where you may want to go back and reference the nutrient charts in chapter 27 to take a stab at what nutrients you may be lacking—either based on your ailments, or types of foods you don't regularly consume. You can also refer to the previous chapter and pick out some of the superfoods and flavonoid, carotenoid, and phytonutrient-dense foods. Start to piece together a recipe with a purpose (i.e. one that's full of foods you don't normally consume).

I get people asking me for my green smoothie recipe all of the time, and here's the thing: it's *my* recipe. And no, I'm not trying to patent the damn thing. It's simply based on *my* nutrient needs and the foods *I* already consume. It won't necessarily hurt you, but it's not necessarily going to help you either. It's important that you use your noggin to come up with a recipe that includes nutrients you might be lacking. Find importance and value in your new liquid "multi-vitamin."

But just so you can get an idea of what a smoothie may look like, I have included my recipe—not so you can copy the damn thing, but so you can perhaps determine some ingredient amounts. I generally choose to make smoothies over juices for various reasons: it's easier to clean a blender, it's easier to throw seeds and nuts in a smoothie, I prefer the thicker texture . . . the list goes on. That's *my* preference (but I also make juices on occasion).

This recipe makes three servings; one of them going to my son who downs them like they're going out of style, and has been doing so since he turned one. Also, we're pros at this, and our palates are quite used to these sort of tastes. If you're new to powerful nutrients, this will most likely taste like shart to you. Can't say I didn't warn ya.

Babich's Sweet-Ass Smoothie:

(Throw all in a blender)

- A few large leaves of curly kale (I frequently substitute any green leafy vegetable—like spinach, romaine lettuce, or chard—to increase my nutrient variety)
- 1 large carrot (or two small)
- 1/2 to 1 apple (amount depends on if my son gets his hands on the apple before I get it in the blender)
- A large handful of grapes (these bad boys are there so this drink doesn't taste like shit—leave them out if you can handle it, but they're a great way to sweeten your drink)
- 1/2 to 1 avocado or banana (I have only recently started using this as a "thickener" since we've been travelling and I don't have my kick-ass blender with me. The ho-hum one we purchased during our travels leaves the smoothie about as smooth as a gravel quarry)
- 1-2 tablespoons of maca powder
- 1-2 tablespoons of nutritional yeast
- 1-2 tablespoons of dried goji berries
- 1 teaspoon of spirulina powder
- A small handful of nuts (almonds, walnuts, brazil nuts, cashews, or pecans)
- A shitload of seeds (I usually put in a few tablespoons total of a variety of the following: flax seed, chia seed, sesame seed, hemp seed, sunflower seed, pumpkin seed)
- 1-2 cups of coconut water or filtered water (to get the desired consistency—don't forget this, or you'll feel like you're drinking cement)

That concoction will light my ass on fire and ensure that I'm getting all of my nutrients for the day (and if I drink it half-naked in the mid-day sun, my vitamin D gets taken care of as well). If we factor in all of the phytonutrients, carotenoids, antioxidants, and probiotics I packed into that thing, I could seriously give Captain

America a run for his money. Iron fortress immune system people. IRON FUCKING FORTRESS.

To make it incredibly easy on myself, I have all of the dried ingredients (e.g. nuts, seeds, yeast, berries) waiting patiently for me in plain sight (out of the sun) on my pantry shelves or in the fridge. This way I can easily scoop, scoop, scoop, scoop without much hassle. I suggest you do the same. The more often you see powerful ingredients, the more likely you are to use them (and not only in your juice or smoothie). If you hide them away in the depths of some cabinet, out of sight, out of mind. You don't hide your vitamin bottle, do you? You put it somewhere you can see it so you don't forget to take it, right? Well, throw out your vitamins and replace them with food. Keep that shit in sight.

Don't get hung up on the ingredients I use. Remember, I use them for a reason. You can add a billion other powerful foods like lemon, parsley, ginger, cucumber, celery, mango, or cranberries. Whatever you think your body needs a boost of, add it. See how it makes you feel. Experiment until you find something that works for you—meaning you can consume it without feeling like you're going to blow chunks. Who wants to drink something that tastes like shit?! I should ask everyone who drinks coffee and eats molasses. Seriously though, your juice or smoothie should taste good. If it doesn't taste good, work on adjusting your ingredients a bit, *without* completely compromising the nutrient content.

Initially, if your smoothie is too powerful for you to handle, try swapping out ingredients and slowly work your way back to the original recipe over time (i.e. use something less potent such as romaine lettuce rather than kale or spinach for the first few weeks). Or, simply nut up and drink the damn thing. Even if you're miserable for a few minutes of your day, the nutrients you get in those few minutes will give you energy for the rest of the day and will be worth it. My son has been downing "hulk juice" since he turned one, and no little kid is going to *choose* to gulp down something if it tastes like shit. Therefore, work on getting the ratio of ingredients just right so it still packs a punch when it comes to nutrients, yet tastes like "buttah" as my grandmother would say (not to be confused with "butter" which would be nasty).

Now to the actual drinking part. There are a couple of ways to consume a smoothie (or juice) that can make a huge difference. Plugging your nose and swigging it in one try-not-to-gag gulp is not one of them. First off, you want to make sure you drink it on an empty stomach so you are able to absorb as many of the nutrients as possible. This will help to avoid symptoms like heartburn, which can occur when eating it with, or right after, a meal. For this reason, I usually make our green smoothies as a mid-morning snack (a couple hours after breakfast, and about an hour before lunch).

Secondly, make sure you drink your smoothies (or juices) right after making them. They're not made to sit around or be stored for long periods (because they're *fresh* and not full of chemicals that help preserve them). If you must consume your smoothie or juice at a later time (i.e. you only have time to make it at breakfast, but want to drink it at work later) then look into getting a vacuum-sealed jar or mug that can remove the air, which will keep it from losing its potency. The longer it sits, the less powerful it will be, and the quicker it will become rancid. Tip it back immediately if you can.

Furthermore, did you know you're actually supposed to chew or swish your smoothies or juices? This is not my attempt to make you look like a jackass, promise. You may feel a bit ridiculous for doing so, but if we're talking about getting the full benefit, than this is how it's done. It's the same reason you're supposed to chew your food: the digestive enzymes in your mouth won't have the time to wake up and start the process of delivering the nutrients to your cells if those nutrients don't stay in your mouth for a bit. Without chewing or swishing, most of those wonderful nutrients will wind up going right through you. And wouldn't that be a shame (and a waste). So take a sip, swish it around your mouth a few times to wake up those digestive enzymes, and *then* throw it down the hatch like a badass.

Here's the down side to all of this: some people may argue that by drinking your nutrients you throw off the rate and efficacy of nutrient absorption, or that you wind up over-eating because you don't feel satiated after downing one. There is some truth to this. So let's be clear: I'm not promoting this as a meal replacement. I'm promoting it as an *extra* something to shove down your pie-hole to get nutrients in your system that otherwise haven't been finding their way there. Over time, if you can find ways to incorporate those nutrients in their whole form, *fantastic*. Until then, my opinion is that potential "less-than-optimal nutrient absorption" trumps completely absent nutrients any day. My advice then, is not to use smoothies or juices as a crutch, but to use them periodically, or specifically when you know your nutrient intake has been sucking hind-tit.

On a final note, the type of juicer or blender you get matters. I started with juicing, and I'll be totally honest—cleaning a juicer is about as fun as cleaning a diaper blow-out. I also felt horrible about wasting all of the "pulp" from the foods I was juicing (you can certainly use the pulp in recipes, but it wasn't happening for me, and I don't like to force anything). When I decided that I was going to make smoothies instead, I was fortunate enough to be able to buy a VitaMix blender system, and I wouldn't recommend anything else. They're expensive as fuck (compared with other blenders—not compared to a space shuttle), but I'm **pretty** sure we were made with two kidneys so we could sell one to pay for a VitaMix.

I have used several different blenders over the years, and nothing comes close to comparing. Other blenders left the smoothies chunky and gritty, and much less palatable than the smooth-as-silk smoothies I'd get from my VitaMix. We're talking professional quality, which makes consuming them a heck of a lot more enjoyable. Get a VitaMix if you can afford one, period (and they're actually much more than a blender—you can make soups, spreads, grind nuts and seeds, etc.) They're friggin' magic. If you're short on time or have the lazy gene, knowing that they're self-cleaning may help. No, I am not affiliated with VitaMix in any way (although the way I'm supporting you, VitaMix, a little sponsorship wouldn't hurt—wink, wink). Therefore, I have no reason to promote them other than the fact that their blenders are top-notch, kick-ass food machines.

If you decide to juice and want to buy a juicer instead, do your research on what brand and model you want to get (keeping in mind what the cleaning process may be like, because that will annoy the fuck out of you if it's hard to clean). Better yet, borrow a friend's juicer to make sure that you do, in fact, want to juice and not blend.

Moral of the Story:

If you want to knock malnutrition on its ass, get a head start and take care of your nutritional deficiencies by consuming a juice or smoothie packed with relevant, kick-ass ingredients.

Chapter 30

Poop on Cancer

The food you eat can be either the safest and most powerful form of medicine or the slowest form of poison.
—Ann Wigmore

Cancer is fucking horrible—I think we can all agree on that. And "we all know someone" affected by the disease, right? Heck, there's a good chance that *you've* had cancer, considering that every year diagnoses are being made in over fourteen million people worldwide. More specifically, in the US it is the leading cause of death in children, and diagnoses will be sent to every 1 in 2 men and every 1 in 3 women annually.[452-454] Fuck. Cancer.

The only problem, is that unlike obesity, heart disease, high blood pressure, etc. (which most people connect to poor lifestyle habits), most people don't associate cancer with diet. They think it's the "lightening" disease that strikes at random. Not so much. Here is the big red flag: you won't see the incidence of cancer in developing nations anywhere *near* that of developed nations.[455-458] The top cancer-go-getters are Australia/New Zealand, North America, and Europe. The folks with the lowest incidence hail from Africa, Central America, and South East/South Central Asia.[454] Why? For starters, they don't have the same shitty pie-hole habits, or the infestation of chemicals in their food system that you find in developed nations. The combination of "nutrients" (a term which I use lightly with our current food industry) that *developed* nations present to consumers leaves the deficiency disease door WIDE OPEN for cancer.

Most people in the developed world have heard the tagline "cancer doesn't discriminate." Pssshhh—*of course* cancer discriminates. If it didn't, we'd see an even spread of cancer across the globe (instead, there are these cancer "pockets"). Most cancers favor westernized malnutrition, chemical shit storms, and weak immune systems. If you're living in that type of environment (or you're a baby growing in one), then you, or your baby, are bound to have cells that say, "fuck this," and morph into cancerous cells. By now you should understand that the westernized food industry is one big fucking chemical *cyclone* that hurls people toward malnutrition faster than a prairie fire with a tail wind.

On a side note, most cancers are also *not* genetic, contrary to public belief. In actuality, only about 2-3% of cancers can be contributed to genes, which means that over 95% of cancers can be preventable if you can determine the cause of them.[459, 460] Well butter my butt and call me a biscuit! That's exciting! What's even *more* exciting is it's estimated that 40% of cancers are directly caused by a poor pie-hole usage. We could say *sayonara* to nearly *half* of cancer diagnoses if we learn to use our pie-holes correctly![461, 462] Past the 40% of cancers connected to nutrition, we're left with cancers caused by environmental factors—like pollutants, infections, and radiation— which are still preventable, but are outside of the scope of this guidebook.

Thus, while cancer infuriates me, I'm not actually mad at the actual cancer. I'm mad that over *95%* of cancers are preventable, and instead of focusing on *preventing* them, the focus is on "finding a cure." This means we're letting people *get* cancer first, and then trying to figure out how to help them—even though there's most likely a cure right under our noses. Do you see the problem with that? We're fighting a battle that most likely could have been prevented in the first place.

Unfortunately, the story usually goes like this: you get cancer, you go to your doctor, your doctor most likely doesn't have the nutrition background to know how to treat or prevent your cancer without poisoning you, and your cancer keeps returning because you don't actually change your habits or environment. It's a vicious cycle. We need to change our focus from treatment to *prevention*. However, education clearly needs to come first.

As I stated early on, our bodies have bitchin' immune systems. Well, they should anyway. A strong, properly fueled immune system can ward off cancer. You read that right; I'm not on crack, I promise. Hear me out. For instance, did you know that most people have pre-cancerous cells in their bodies? Yup. They have damaged cells that can go one of two ways: 1) their body either repairs or eliminates them, or 2) those cells grow into a tumor. If you have the internal environment and immune system you're supposed to, your body will go with option one, and you'll never know those little fuckers were ever there. However, if you have a *messed up* internal environment and a *weak* immune system, those damaged cells will divide and conquer. Hmmmm, I wonder what on earth might cause a messed up internal environment and weak immune system . . . WARNING, **PROFOUND** STATEMENT AHEAD: everything you put in your pie-hole will either fuel the cancer, or fight the cancer.

This is why people get confused when athletes get cancer. "I don't understand; he was so active!" Being active, does *not* make someone healthy. Remember when we talked about nutrition trumping exercise at the beginning of this guidebook? I didn't make that up. Who knows to what kind of shit that athlete has been around. Perhaps they drink a fuckload of Gatorade and Red Bull (which we now know are full of nasty shit). Perhaps they have poor nutrition in general. I know several athletes who do! Perhaps they're athletes who helped McDonald's be an Olympic sponsor at the last Olympics and really *did* eat the crap they promoted. Regardless, simply being an "athlete" (or being active in general) does not give you squeaky-clean, sparkling insides.

On the flipside, you'll see people who smoke all of their life and never get cancer. Why? Probability, that's why. If you dart across a busy intersection will you become road kill? Probably not. If you dart across a busy intersection a hundred times, will you *eventually* become road kill? Probably. Same goes for smoking. The more cigarettes you smoke, the more years you smoke them, the more second hand smoke you're around, etc. your probability of being a cancer statistic increases—it doesn't mean that everyone gets lung cancer because they smoke.

The folks that *don't* wind up with cancer simply beat the probability odds. Maybe they had a bitchin' immune system that kept cancer at bay. Or, perhaps they had a secret phytonutrient addiction. Who knows. There are infinite ways to fuel or fuck up your body (which would change your probability odds), so it's hard to say. What I *do* know is that cancer *does* discriminate, and if you provide it with an environment in which it can thrive, then it *probably* will.

Other than the "cancer doesn't discriminate" statement, you've also most likely seen someone roll their eyes at some point in your life, and sarcastically declare that "*everything* causes cancer." They're actually not that far off. I'd estimate that upwards of 90% of the "foods" and "beverages" in our food system today increase your probability of getting cancer if eaten regularly. This includes everything from restaurant foods, to processed foods drowning in chemicals, animal foods that may cause your protein intake to boil over, and non-organic plant foods that have been sprayed with chemicals. I'm assuming you didn't skip over the last section, which described the billions of types of food and beverage products that litter our food system. There are over *three thousand* chemicals directly added to the food that we eat, and it's becoming nearly impossible to hide from them.[161] Congratulations food manufacturers and agencies, you have undeniably made a genocidal food industry. Where's the Darwin award for *that*?!

One of the ways to obviously prevent cancer growth is to learn how to use your pie-hole. And one of the first steps you can take is to focus on the protein you're consuming—both the *amount* and the *type*. I mentioned previously that a diet high in protein—specifically animal protein—*will* promote cancer growth.[18-22, 126, 463] This means any diet primarily made up of foods like meat, seafood, eggs, dairy and protein supplements. It also means any diet lacking in fruits, vegetables, whole grains, legumes, herbs, nuts, and seeds (and the antioxidants, phytonutrients, carotenoids, etc. that come with them). Simply put, if you base your diet on animal foods and consume minimal plant foods, then you *will* be consuming a high-protein diet, and you will greatly increase your risk of cancer.

To support that, it might be good to mention that back in 1997, a review of *144* different nutrition studies showed that fruits and vegetables had a positive effect on all cancer rates.[464] In other words, people who ate the most fruits and veggies had the least cancer. There have been hundreds of similar studies published since then. On the other hand, there are only seventy . . . shit, no, wait—there are ZERO studies showing that animal foods have a protective effect on cancer. ZERO.

Speaking of animal foods, let's talk about casein: the main protein in cow's milk. It might shock you (or at this point, maybe it won't) that several well-known and renowned nutrition scientists have stated that they consider casein to be the most potent carcinogen known to man. You read that right. Damn you, cows! What kind of shit are you trying to pull?! I'm not saying that a cup of milk will kill you, but if you regularly consume foods that have casein in them (e.g. all dairy, most protein supplements, many processed foods), then your risk of cancer goes up.

Remember when we discussed the fact that high-protein diets have a correlation with cancer growth waaaaay back at the beginning of this mamajama? If not, don't worry—your memory will improve as your nutrition does. Anyway, I bet you won't believe it when I tell you that casein—A FUCKING PROTEIN IN COW'S MILK—was the protein used to demonstrate cancer growth in those high-protein diets.[126] Casein has shown to start and stop cancer growth—"like flipping a switch"—as it is added and removed from rat diets in the famous *China Study* (i.e. when the rats were fed casein their tumors grew, and when the casein was removed, their tumors stopped growing . . . they repeated this over and over with the same results).[126] Since most everyone in developed nations seems to consider both dairy and protein to be the bee's knees, you can see why we may have such a cancer crisis going on.

So, what the fuck do we do?! We poop on cancer! How do we poop on cancer? There is abundant evidence that a whole-food, plant-based diet can stop or even reverse cancer growth, so I'd start there.[126, 465] All you have to do is increase the organically grown, non-processed plant foods (full of the kick-ass, disease-fighting nutrients) into your diet, which will in turn reduce your intake of animal and processed foods. Adding a juice or smoothie will also help. If you're a processed food-whore, keep your eyes open for anything with caseinates, calcium caseinate, potassium caseinate, or sodium caseinate on the label, because they're all wonderful forms of casein that some jackass managed to whip up.

Just so this sticks in your head, I am not telling you to *eliminate* certain foods, I'm telling you that long-term, over-consumption of certain foods will drastically increase your risk of disease. I still eat meat and dairy on (very) rare occasions, but I eat *way* more plant foods. They have become the foundation of my diet, hopefully for obvious reasons.

Now here's the fun part (you may want to sit down for this); people are actually reversing and curing certain cancers on a regular basis—simply by manipulating their diets. Pump the breaks, *what*?! Yes, people have cured themselves of cancer (even advanced cancer!) by pumping so many disease-fighting plant nutrients (probiotics, flavonoids, and carotenoids . . . oh my!) into their bodies that their system takes hold of that cancer and tells it to fuck off, before drop kicking it out the door.

Why don't we hear about this? It could do with the fact that our doctors are the ones who help us with our cancer, and most of our doctors know jack shit about nutrition. Or, perhaps it's because when people *do* make positive, personal, individual lifestyle changes it's hard to publish scientific studies on them. Science is about control groups and study groups, and controlling as much of the environment as possible. You need a whole group of people doing the *exact same thing,* or the study will most likely be deemed useless and thrown out. Since many *different* people, with many *different* nutritional habits are getting many *different* types of cancer for many *different*, complicated reasons, it would be quite impossible to do a study controlled enough for scientific publication. What a bummer, eh? Any way you look at it, the fact that people ignore or scoff at natural cures is nuttier than a peanut party to me. It makes zero sense that we ignore such substantial evidence.

Hold up, what about chemotherapy and radiation? It's totally inspirational when you hear someone boast that they've "had cancer six times, and beaten it six times," right? Newsflash: if the cancer keeps coming back, they haven't beaten it. It's merely being suppressed while that person continues to poison themselves. If they still live in the same environment, and still eat the same foods, their cancer friend will permanently reside around the corner, and will make frequent visits. It's like detoxing or dieting: if you're going to do either, and then return to your original habits, what the hell do you think is going to happen? Answer: you're going to wind up detoxing and dieting at regular intervals for the rest of your life.

Same goes for cancer. If you have chemo treatments for the disease—which is most likely caused by something you're unintentionally doing, surrounding yourself with, or consuming—and then return to that same environment after your treatment, well, you can guess what I'm getting at. The story is going to end the same every time (unless you somehow beat the probability odds). You see, a 2015 study showed that colon cancer patients who chose the chemotherapy route (versus others who opted out) had a *worse* quality of life, were nearly *three* times more likely to have the cancer return within two years, and were *two* times more likely to die within two years.[466] Talk about pissing into the wind.

Why would you want to pump poison into yourself if you can just learn to eat? People are *curing* themselves (meaning the cancer *never* comes back), and it's because they're making permanent lifestyle changes. Do some searching to read about it for yourself. A good place to start is by looking up a place called The Gerson Institute, or by reading the books *The China Study* and *The Gerson Therapy*. Both offer a wealth of scientific, objective, and subjective evidence on how improvements in nutrition can reverse and cure cancer (and other "non-curable" diseases).[126, 467-473] Or just fucking Google "how I naturally cured my cancer," and I'm sure you'll come across more than enough stories and case studies depicting peoples' holistic journeys to bitchin' health. Don't believe them? Contact them and ask for proof—most of them will be thrilled to provide it.

Let's talk about The Gerson Institute for a bit. It's a pretty incredible place and has been around for almost a century. The folks there put all of their focus into providing natural illness treatments, mainly for cancer. There are currently only two treatment centers (one in Mexico, and one in Hungary) that practice the Gerson Therapy, and the results are *amazing*. We're talking about curing end-stage cancers—people who were told to prepare for the worst, and then took a final chance on a "silly" idea AND FUCKING SURVIVED!! Why aren't these miracle institutes on every street corner? Why haven't more people heard of this magical institute? For one, because they weren't even allowed to open doors in America. The therapy was considered too extreme and alternative (or was a fear for the pharmaceutical companies). Furthermore, the program didn't follow mainstream science and medicine and was therefore deemed unsafe. Unsafe to what? Eat fucking vegetables?! Oh, the frustration.

There was so much huffing and puffing about the fact that there weren't any scientific studies done on the therapy that it was considered nonsense. However, I encourage you to read all about what the Gerson Institute has accomplished. While you're at it, you can also read about the asshats who try to debunk this institution by saying there's no "scientific evidence" (i.e. published studies) to prove what they're doing is actually working.[468-473] Of course there isn't—because we're not lumping everyone into the same category and treating them with the same pill. Trust me, if scientific journals aren't shouting this theory from the rooftops it does not mean that it's not real. It simply means that there are other places to look for the evidence. Plenty of people have gone through the therapy and owe their life to it. Unfortunately, they don't have the same multi-billion dollar platform to share their message, and thus go unnoticed.

Thankfully, some people out there are using their connections to spread the word. Dr. David Brownstein, a board-certified, award-winning family physician from Bloomfield, Michigan once stated, "most cancer is caused by nutrient deficiencies." He's not the only one that believes this; more and more doctors are coming forward with their big boy and big girl panties on to discuss the truth about conventional care versus nutritional care. They are putting their reputation on the line, standing up for the truth, and we should praise them. Instead, they're often viewed as quacks, and are shunned.

Another brave soul putting his reputation on the line is John Kelly, a doctor from Dublin, Ireland. In 2014, he published a book entitled *Stop Feeding Your Cancer*. In the book, Dr. Kelly describes several of his patients' cases in great detail (most of whom had different types of cancers), and then declares that there is "convincing evidence . . . which shows that cancer can be stopped in its tracks and even reversed into a dormant state, allowing sufferers to regain good health and lead normal lives."[474] Dr. Kelly treats his patients with *nutrition*. This means sick people can beat cancer without spending hours in chemo chairs or getting poisoned by radiation. All they have is a grocery bill. There is one side effect though: feeling fucking awesome. Who's in?!

Dr. Brownstein and Dr. Kelly are two in a million though, and if most doctors had their knowledge, they'd be shoving powerful disease-fighting foods down their patients' throats. Alternatively, they'd be busing them off to treatment centers like the Gerson Institute instead of pumping them full of meds (which seem to have a lower success rate than the Gerson therapy).[469]

All of this is why I refuse to donate to organizations such as cancer societies. This view may sound harsh, but hear me out. Organizations such as the Cancer Society are interested in finding a *cure* for cancer. Sounds great, right? Not to me. Let me reiterate that this means people have to *get* cancer first. They have to *suffer* first. *Then* they get poisoned by chemo (literally poisoned, as some cancer drugs have been shown to *cause* cancer) while they sit patiently and wait for a cure.[475] Unlike these organizations, I'm much more interested in *preventing* cancer, you know, so no one has to suffer from the shit in the first place. Since I believe that cancer is largely a man-made disease, nearly all cancers are preventable, and almost half are caused by poor nutrition, it would make more sense to put money toward eradicating *malnutrition*. That way we can kill two (okay, thousands of) birds with one stone.

The bizarre part about all of this is that the American Institute for Cancer Research website states that "basing our diets on plant foods (like vegetables, fruits, whole grains and legumes such as beans), which contain fiber and other nutrients, can reduce our risk of cancer." Yet eating a plant-based diet seems to be the last thing you hear about when it comes to eradicating cancer. It seems to be all about giving money to "find a cure." SAVE YOUR MONEY AND BUY SOME GODDAMN VEGGIES. Let's kill that bitch *before* it invades our systems! For that reason, until organizations like the Cancer Society refocus their goal from "curing" to "preventing," they will get jack shit from me.

Even more aggravating, is the fact that organizations like the Cancer Society (as well as pharmaceutical companies) are not, in fact, winning the war on cancer (regardless of what they tell you).

This "war," has been going on for over forty years (even though President Nixon vowed to cure cancer within *five* years back in the '70s), and has had over $100 *billion* dollars pumped into it.[476] If *anyone, anywhere* tried to fight *any* other type of war for multiple decades without getting kick-ass results while draining *that* much money, people would go ape-shit. There would be a serious up rise and strike to stop the madness. Yet, that's not happening because the people in charge of the war on cancer are still convincing everyone that what they're doing is saintly.

In reality, they are fighting a static battle. Since 1950, the cancer death rate has only fallen about 5%.[476] That's simply the *death rate* though; not the number of people who have been diagnosed. My guess is that we're merely managing it better. Not so much winning going on there. I want to see fuckin' 70%, 80%, 90%, *100%* reductions in cancer. It's time to stop throwing our money away. It lays in *our* hands, and in the hands of the doctors who have their heads screwed on straight. Knock on wood you don't get cancer, but please know that if you do, it probably wasn't random, and you have options other than poisoning yourself.

Lastly, I could delve much deeper into the dangers of the chemicals in our environment and consumer products (e.g. laundry detergents, shampoos, household cleaners, feminine products, air fresheners, nicotine patches, nail polishes, deodorants, sun blocks, wall paints, carpet—all of which usually have synthetic chemicals and all of which we wind up inhaling or absorbing), but that is out of the scope of this guide. Once you figure out how to use your pie-hole, it may be in your best interest to open your eyes to the shit that's in *other* materials and objects around you.

Moral of the Story:
If you (or someone you know) has cancer, there's a pretty good
chance a change in diet can reverse or eliminate it. If you're the
lucky bastard that *doesn't* have cancer, it's up to you to make the
right nutrition decisions to prevent it.

Chapter 31

Other Shitty Diseases and the Common Thread

People who ate the most animal-based foods got the most chronic disease. . . .
People who ate the most plant-based foods were the healthiest and
tended to avoid chronic disease.
—Dr. T. Colin Campbell

I wouldn't be able to complete this guidebook without
discussing some other specific diseases and their relationships
to nutrition—specifically multiple sclerosis (MS). My mother was
diagnosed with MS around the time I was ten, even though she
had shown signs earlier in life (they didn't know what the heck
was attacking her back then). From primary school onwards, I
watched her slowly deteriorate. She suffered debilitating ailments
and began to struggle with basic tasks like eating, walking, and
bathing. She eventually had to walk with a cane, then use a wheel
chair, then a motorized scooter—until she left this world when I
was twenty. Watching the person I loved most in the world suffer
for a *decade* and then disappear before my eyes was the main fuel
for figuring this "how to be healthy" shit out.

I actually found myself more at peace when my mother passed.
The years prior were horrific, and I simply wanted the suffering to
end. No teenager should have to help bathe, feed, or toilet their

parent. No parent should have to have their teenager bathe, feed, or toilet them. The loss of independence was absolute torture for her, and witnessing it was incredibly upsetting to me. Thus, this section is dedicated to autoimmune diseases, which includes MS.

Let me start by telling you: knowing what I know now about multiple sclerosis, I would have gotten rid of her pills and pumped her full of as many different types of organic, whole plant foods as I could. That is, after I moved her straight to the equator (sunshine, vitamin D—you were paying attention, right?). You see, multiple sclerosis is much more prevalent the further you move from the equator.[477] However, the closer you get to the equator, and the more you boost vitamin D, there are considerably less cases of MS. Who knows what would have happened had we attempted that, but it certainly wouldn't have been worse than what did.

To rewind for a minute, I stated early on that I grew up mainly eating healthy, organically grown, local foods. So why would my mom end up with such a destructive disease? Well, for one, she probably acquired it *way* before my days (it's my understanding that she first showed signs of MS around the time she was twenty). She also grew up in New York, away from the equator, and on my grandmother's cooking—which I know wasn't the healthiest ("cottage cheese belongs on everything," by the way). Once my mom grew up, she started to eat healthier and change her habits (but even then her idea of healthy still included a bunch of meats and dairy). My guess is that my mother's body was on its way down the nutrition spectrum *way* before I came around. Therefore, who knows if my mother could have been saved by the time I was present. All I know is that if I can save someone now— perhaps someone's mom—then my job here is done.

So here goes: the following pages provide some information on select autoimmune diseases and how nutrition fits in. Before we begin though, let's examine what an autoimmune disease actually is. Diseases are classified as "autoimmune" if the body's immune system somehow gets confused, goes on autopilot, and starts attacking itself. This essentially leads to self-destruction. Systems break down, and sirens (i.e. symptoms) start going off.

There are forty some-odd autoimmune diseases out there, and, as a whole, they are diagnosed in around a quarter of a million people in the US each year, affecting about ten million people at any given time.[478] So yeah, this isn't a small problem. Some autoimmune diseases that you may have heard of are: MS, type 1 diabetes, rheumatoid arthritis, psoriasis, vitiligo, scleroderma, hyper- and hypothyroidism, and some people argue that Alzheimer's is on that list.[479]

Now, what if I were to tell you there's evidence that, by following a certain way of eating, there is a *significantly* decreased occurrence of all of those diseases? You'd probably say the same thing most people say when I tell them about this: "If that's true, why haven't I heard about it?" Hold on a sec—let me just pop that broken record on again. If someone presents to their doctor with signs of an autoimmune disease, we know it's going to be unlikely that they hear about the nutrition that can help them. Instead, they are more likely to be sent off to the pill factory. I have no idea how many pills my mother was on; I completely lost track. However, I *do* know exactly how many of the numerous doctors and specialists she saw over the years who recommended dietary changes. ZERO. In a *decade* (a DECADE!!) of regular visits to I-can't-even-count-how-many health professionals, not *one* of them talked to her about the shit she was putting in her pie-hole. Like tits on a tomcat, this system is fuckin' useless.

Thus, here I am to educate you. And let this be a lesson: If you haven't heard of a concept, idea, or plan, it doesn't mean it doesn't exist. If your doctor doesn't know about it, it doesn't mean it's bullshit (remember, it takes an average of seventeen years for a new idea or concept to circulate anyway). If it scares you to contemplate reaching for food rather than pills, it's okay—but it doesn't mean you shouldn't try. Especially when food doesn't come with a long list of side effects.

Let's start the educating by discussing how all of these autoimmune diseases differ from each other. As mentioned above, with autoimmune diseases the body gets confused and begins to attack itself. *Where* it attacks determines the type of autoimmune disease. If it attacks cells in the pancreas, you may wind up with type 1 diabetes. If it attacks the linings of the nerves, you may wind up with MS. If it attacks your joints, you may wind up with rheumatoid arthritis, etc. But wait—why on Earth would the body go all wacky and attack itself? In laymen's terms, our immune system is robotic. When foreign bodies (usually proteins) enter our body, our immune system creates little warriors (a.k.a. "antibodies") that fight against these protein invaders—usually without us ever knowing. Antibodies for the win!

Unfortunately, if those foreign protein invaders are similar to certain proteins that *we already have* in our bodies, this system doesn't go so well. The body mistakenly attacks *our* proteins as well as the nearly-identical foreign invaders, which results in a breakdown of one of our systems. Silly antibody warriors! So where do these similar foreign invader proteins come from? Answer: animals. Probably because, um, we're also animals?! What do all of these autoimmune diseases have in common? People who consume more animal foods than plant foods have an increased risk for autoimmune diseases.[126] Are high (animal) protein diets still sounding good to you?

Keeping with that concept, I'm about to explain one of the most alarming and substantial findings I have come across during my years of research analysis. Hold on to your hats, as this will be one of the most important topics on which to educate yourself.

We have already discussed casein, one of the proteins in cow's milk, and its relationship to cancer. Guess what? Casein is almost *identical* to the cells in our pancreas that produce insulin. When someone drinks cow's milk, their immune system creates an antibody for that foreign casein protein. Since the insulin-producing cells in the pancreas are so similar to the casein, that antibody also starts attacking *the pancreas* cells as well. Here's where shit hits the fan. Over time, that pancreas' luck may run out and it will no longer be able to produce insulin. That person is now stuck with type 1 diabetes. Well, crap.

Now, when is cow's milk usually "recommended"? At a young age; usually by the time a child is one (at the recommendation of the dairy industry, of course). This will "ensure that bones can grow big and strong!" Sometimes mothers choose not to breastfeed and start nursing their babies from a cow even earlier. Sometimes babies are fed infant formula, which is also usually loaded with the casein protein from cow's milk. When does someone usually get type 1 diabetes? Childhood.

There have been many, many, *many* studies that have shown the relationship between the protein in cow's milk and type 1 diabetes. One study in particular, that compared diabetic children to healthy children, showed that every single diabetic child had a high level of the antibody to casein, while every *healthy* child had lower antibody levels.[480] Basically, all of the children with diabetes had consumed more cow's milk. GASP.

Thus, children who drink more cow's milk are more likely to wind up with type 1 diabetes.[481-487] This has been known for *decades*, yet do you hear anything about it? Nope. The dairy industry is still up on a podium, still clinging to their golden calcium medal, and still has ties to the organizations that make dietary recommendations to us. Does this mean that everyone who drinks dairy milk will suddenly wind up with type 1 diabetes? Of course not. As I've reiterated many times, nutrition is a complex, multi-faceted game, and a lot of it comes down to probability. Many things will factor into whether or not someone winds up with *any* disease, so it's almost impossible to make blanket cause-and-effect statements. For example, you're not going to "get diabetes by drinking dairy milk," but yes, if you consume a bunch of it from an early age you will increase your risk of type 1 diabetes.

Side note: my child has never had cow's milk and is right as rain. Remember, you don't need certain *foods*; you need certain *nutrients* (I will say that as often as I'm able, so get used to it). I choose to stay the hell away from the casein in cow's milk. My son has always had organic almond milk, organic soy milk, and organic rice milk, and my son is thriving.

To infuriate you a bit more, casein isn't simply found in cow's milk these days. Since protein—specifically "complete," "high quality," animal protein—is highly sought out by misinformed consumers and considered the go-to nutrient, casein is extracted from milk and flung everywhere. You will find it in almost all supplements, protein bars, powders, and shakes; it's scattered far and wide throughout the processed food world. Diabetes for all! Ooooh, and cancer too!

Here's where the common thread comes into play. Throughout this guide it should have become obnoxiously apparent that it's imperative to eat lots of plant foods and get plenty of sunshine in order to get a wide variety of disease-fighting nutrients and to remedy any nutrient deficiencies. When you think about eating something packed with wonderful vitamins, do you picture a steak and cheese, or do you picture carrots and spinach? Even my most meat-eating clients tell me they realize "they don't eat enough veggies," and "they know that's where the good nutrients are." People *know* the good nutrients are mainly in plants, yet somehow they don't find the value in hunting them down.

All of this information connecting nutrition with autoimmune **disease** has been out for ages, yet we don't hear about it because it's "alternative," or, because people don't want to hear "medical" advice from anyone else than a doctor. They hear information like this from "hippies" like me, and label us "quacks" without even giving thought to the information being presented. Stop being swayed by the industries backing their own products and go read the fucking research (I have cited plenty). I dare you.

Speaking of research, the CDC once reported that US adults were only eating 27% and 33% of the necessary amounts of vegetables and fruits, respectively.[488] Well there's your fuckin' reason everyone is wandering around like malnourished zombies;

THEY *ARE* MALNOURISHED ZOMBIES. Want to know where the zombies are few and far between? Okinawa, Japan. They are legit longevity masters over there, and have been studied for decades because of their lower rates of disease and high life expectancy. Captain America has a summer home there.

Originally, the folks in Okinawa had diets based on whole grains and oodles of (non-processed, organic) soy and vegetables. Furthermore, Okinawa is the poorest area of Japan, so of course they had a hard time affording the "best" foods like meat, eggs, and dairy.[489] They drank water like mad, and spent much of their time outside building up vitamin D. They had one of the lowest rates of osteoporosis in the world, and, drum roll please—they didn't consume dairy! Shhh, don't tell the dairy industry! Heart disease and cancer were rare. What?! No, you don't say! In fact, about 97% of their lives were spent ailment-free.[490, 491] If what they did was wrong, then I don't want to be right.

Unfortunately, over the years the Okinawa residents' life expectancy has been declining, and disease has been on the rise. Thank goodness someone stepped in and did some more research to find out why, and I'm sure you've already guessed the results. Their nutrition habits were studied over a decade and suddenly they were found to be eating more meat and dairy, and less plant foods.[492] Suddenly heart disease, cancer, and diabetes were on the rise. Oh my gosh that's *crazy*; I didn't even see that coming! This shit is seriously taking me to frown town—somebody please tell those poor folks to cut themselves off from westernized diets and head back to their roots.

Side note: if you want to read more about communities like this, check out the book *The Blue Zones Solution*, by Dan Buettner.[493, 494] It details the lifestyles of five communities— Okinawa included— and why residents live longer and have the least disease in the world. Or, head over to Loma Linda, California, because that's one of the pockets. Funnily enough, all five "blue zones" eat mainly plants and little meat. Surprise!

This is—yet again—why I have chosen to base my nutrient intake around plants. I want a kick-ass immune system with the guts of a liger and the balls of a fighter pilot. *I* want to be a longevity master. Thus, I have put up an internal iron immunity fortress, so even if something external or environmental comes at me, I will samurai the shit out of it.

Again: the purpose of this guide is not to push my diet preferences on you. However, I have chosen my diet preferences based on a shitload of research, and I'm presenting that research to you. Eating a diet high in animal products (and processed food and beverage imitations) has been shown to increase your risk of disease, while eating a diet high in plant products can eliminate and prevent disease.[126, 463, 465, 495-500] Thus, even if you are a self-proclaimed "meat eater," it is imperative that you start choosing more plant foods if you give a rat's ass about longevity and your quality of life. Which plant foods? I don't give a shit—you chose!

Like everything else, "eating more plant foods" can be daunting and defined in many ways. I'm not talking about eating more french fries, highly processed veggie burgers, bottled vitamins, and veggie pizzas. I'm talking about using the knowledge you have gained thus far, and experimenting with whole, organically grown, un-fucked-with plant foods. Please head to Appendix B where several lists of nutrient-packed, disease-fighting plant foods await you. Aim to find several unfamiliar ones that you can start adding to your diet (and there are hundreds more). If you get through the list and cross them all off, please start the book over, and then try again.

Now here's the über cool thing about eating mainly plants (in case you didn't hear me mention it the initial fifteen times): their nutrient make-up will *automatically* be on par with the optimal percentages of fats, carbohydrates, and protein mentioned previously. You won't even have to think about it. NO MATH INVOLVED. Therefore, if you don't want to struggle with trying to get the right percentages of nutrients, eat mainly plant foods. Scatter some other shit in there if you absolutely feel you need to.

To tickle your pickle though, let's recall that, beyond not having to do math, eating a diet based mainly on whole (hopefully organically grown) plant foods will allow you to:

- boost your immune system;
- reduce your risk of disease;
- eat *more* food;
- lose *more* weight than a non-plant-based eater;
- lose weight *faster* than a non-plant-based eater;
- fit into your Captain America suit;
- live longer;
- look and feel younger;
- improve your quality of life;
- shoot happy rainbows from your face;
- substantially reduce healthcare costs; and
- help control world hunger and climate change.

I can't think of any reasons that trump those that would make me *not* want to eat a plant-based diet. Living longer, returning to a healthy weight, reducing your risk of disease, and feeling better should be reason enough for anyone to shift their diet towards plants.[501] [502, 503] Let me share a couple of relevant quotes with you that may help your decision. The first quote is from an article published in the journal *Preventive Cardiology* back in 2001:

> The single biggest step toward adopting this [disease fighting] strategy would be to have United States dietary guidelines support a plant-based diet. An expert committee purged of industrial and political influence is required to assure that science is the basis for dietary recommendations.[498]

Yup. The above quote essentially states that the corruption needs to go, and that people need to start focusing on the science that supports plant-based nutrition. That was said over a *decade* ago, and all I hear is fuckin' crickets chirping. The second quote comes more than a decade after the first one, and is from a 2013 Nutritional Update for American Physicians:

> Physicians should consider recommending a plant-based diet to all their patients, especially those with high blood pressure, diabetes, cardiovascular disease, or obesity.[495]

I can probably count on one hand how many physicians have read *either* of the above recommendations, *and* can define what a healthy plant-based diet is (enough to prescribe one to their patients). Even when someone like Dr. Kim A. Williams—the friggin' president-elect of the American College of Cardiology—touts that he recommends plant-based diets to his patients (after reversing his own cholesterol problems), many doctors *still* choose to turn a blind eye.[504]

Why is no one listening to these recommendations that have been made for over a decade? Unfortunately, it's because the recommendations have been muffled by the roaring sounds of filthy rich corporations, administrations, and industries that need to get more money in their pockets. The tables may be turning though. We are teetering on the brink of change and I want consumers worldwide to give their respective food system a major kick in the ass. Perhaps the "people in charge" will listen if we present them with another pyramid? Heck yes, they *love* pyramids! This is one I'd actually get behind . . . because I came up with it, and it's awesome. Duh.

Please note: the pyramid sections in the following diagram are not drawn to scale—ideally, the tip of the pyramid would be nearly non-existent and the base would take up 80%–90% of the pyramid. But, I wanted to provide pretty pictures, so roll with it. Also, we already discussed the better types of some of these foods. If you're going to eat fish, eat *wild* fish. If you're going to eat an apple, eat an *organic* apple. If you're going to eat processed cereal with food dyes and who-knows-what-else, then march your ass right back to page one.

Regardless of what you choose to eat, forget about all of the other food "groups" that have been used over the years (meat, dairy, fruits, vegetables, etc.) and simply focus on where your foods are coming from: mainly eat foods from plants.

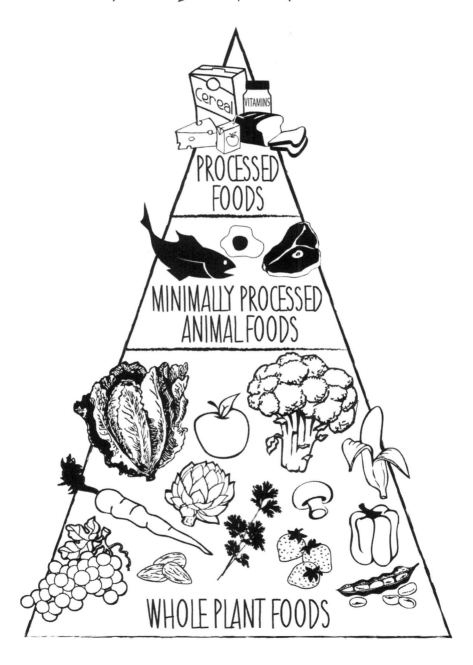

Moral of the Story:

Disease sucks. There's overwhelming evidence that a diet high in animal foods and processed foods can increase your risk of disease, while a diet high in plant foods can help inhibit and cure disease. Therefore, in order to promote health, healing, and longevity, cram plant foods in your pie-hole.

SECTION V

Suits on! Shields up!
Balls to the Wall!

Chapter 32

Connect Your Brain
to Your Mouth

Here's where the panic starts to set in. I have dished out a *mammoth* amount of information, and now it's up to you to put it to use. "SHIT, WHERE DO I START?!" Panic, panic, panic . . . breathe. We have this whole section to talk about making changes and implementing this information into your life.

The first step is to turn the brain on. Initially, this may take some work (especially if your brain is being fueled by less-than-optimal crap), but the idea is to actually *think* about what you're putting in your pie-hole every time you go to shove something in it. *Think* about what you've already eaten that day, and what types of foods you may be lacking. *Think* about new, powerful, plant foods that you can start incorporating in your diet on a regular basis. *Think* about how many whole plant foods, versus animal and processed foods, you're eating. *Think* about the fact that you only need a certain amount of energy and how you're going to make every calorie count. *Think* about regularly spending time in the sun. *Think* about other, non-food products (e.g. cough drops, toothpaste, pills) that you ingest and the ingredients that may be in them. *Think* about making foods from scratch, rather than buying something pre-made or processed (if someone else can make it, so can *you*). *Think* about new recipes that excite you *and* nourish your body. *Think* about hydrating yourself with natural liquids and eliminating the unnecessary junk liquids. Okay, thinking about all of that at once might get a little overwhelming, but you get my point. Think, think, *think*. Don't SHOVE, SHOVE, SHOVE. Check out (or even photocopy) Appendix E if you need help with thinking.

Over time, the whole thinking thing will get easier and will morph into an automatic response (*whew*). I know this because it's second nature to me and I'm not some sort of nutrition wizard. Here's how my day usually goes: My breakfast usually consists of homemade, nut-and-seed-packed, oat-based muesli with organic almond milk and berries. Sometimes I have lemon water prior to that if I feel like it (that's an actual chunk of lemon squeezed into a glass of water, for clarification). Then I might have a peppermint tea after breakfast to stimulate my senses. My mid-morning snack sometimes consists of a green smoothie crammed with veggies and superfoods. My lunch usually consists of a plant-based, homemade soup, salad, or sandwich, and a side of fruit. My afternoon snack usually consists of a piece of fruit or a handful of nuts (or both). Dinner consists of one of the healthy plant-based recipes I've concocted over the years. I usually end the day with a nice warm chai tea, and possibly a piece of organic dark chocolate. I drink filtered water out of my nifty stainless steel water bottle all day, and I make sure to get outside to soak up some UV rays (I usually eat lunch outside).

I'm also a grazer (because when you eat whole plant foods, you can graze all you want), thus I always have healthy snacks scattered around my house that I can nibble on (like humus and carrots, grapes, and cashews). By the end of every day I'm left feeling kick-ass because I *know* I've filled myself up with a variety of powerful nutrients that will make my body thrive. None of this is a chore for me, it's simply life. I have grown to enjoy the fuel I choose to consume, but even if I didn't, it wouldn't matter. I have detached from the "eating is a hobby" notion. This means I'm not trying to please myself with food. It means that, instead, I'm trying to *nurture* my body. Sure, I choose foods that I enjoy, but at the end of the day when I know that I've pie-holed a bunch of powerful nutrients, *that's* what makes me happy. I wouldn't be lying if I told you that every time I cook I think , "how can I make this meal so nutritionally fierce that rainbows shoot from my fucking stomach?!"Then I usually throw a few more nutritionally-dense, whole, plant foods in the mix and give myself a roaring high-five for one-upping the original meal. There's no reason why you can't do the same. It is, after all, a choice—which, of course, requires *thought*.

Another goal of mine (and hopefully soon to be yours) is to try new recipes and "cycle" foods often. No one wants to become bored with eating, and we already know that variety is key. Thus, it is important not to get stuck eating the same foods (even if they're "healthy"), and choose foods that are in season (which means they regularly change), and are therefore the freshest, most nutritious, and cheapest. It's also important to always continue to expand your recipe repertoire. If you have kids, search for fun ways to include them. For instance, I often have my son join in the food prep process. I also find fun ways to present his food to him, like shaping his food into a face or a car. Or, when it comes to his green smoothie "hulk juice," he enjoys adding ingredients to the blender and pushing the buttons. He shouts with joy as the blender goes to work. Then we pound our chests, make hulk grunts, and shout "HULK SMASH!" right before we down them. Why not? You only live once, folks.

There was a time that I counted calories and looked up nutrients, and it may have taken me a while to get where I am, but my family eats with *purpose*. As soon as you start to eat with a purpose, *and* do so with foods that you enjoy, you will get in the groove and start loving life. You will learn to enjoy your choices because you will understand what it means to feel like Captain America. You will understand what it means to not need caffeine to stay awake all day. You will understand what it means to not get the flu shot, and then not get the flu. You will understand what it means to look five, ten, perhaps twenty years younger than you do right now (unless you're five . . . but if you are, I'd like to congratulate you on your reading skills). Simply put, you will understand what optimal health is, and what it feels like to truly thrive. Over the next several chapters I will give you the tools you need to start building your own nutrition plan. It's about fuckin' time, right?!

Moral of the Story:
Use your brain not only to assemble a nutrition routine that is full of kick-ass nutrients, but one that is also mentally and physically satisfying.

Chapter 33

10 Simple Steps to Using Your Pie-Hole Correctly

When you change your diet, you change your entire physiology and you can heal.
—Charlotte Gerson

Does that chapter title make you laugh so hard you shart your pants? There's no friggin' *way* we're contorting everything in this guide into "10 Simple Steps." You should know better, and you should also now be able to understand why, when someone with a "western" diet ask me to put together a simple food plan for them, my brain short-circuits. There is *nothing* simple about avoiding malnutrition if you consider what our food system has become.

The best thing we can do is discuss where to start, as it's been a wild, wild ride, and we've attacked a ridiculous amount of information. To start, the morals listed at the end of all chapters are conveniently listed in Appendix A if you need a refresher. Or, read the whole book again. Read it twenty times. Do whatever it takes to get to a place where you feel like you actually know what to do with that pie-hole of yours.

Everyone will have a different path (hence why there's no set formula or menu plan for this). I have worked with people who are so ridiculously ready to make changes, that they throw their old habits out the window cold turkey and become born-again, plant-based nutrition warriors in a month. I have met others who need to take baby steps that last years, and that's okay as well. Some people eternally log their food because it holds them accountable, and some people never do it. Whatever tickles your pickle, do it. Mmmm, pickles. Ever made your own?

As you start making changes (did you ever go pick up that fucking glass of water?), please realize that *all* changes—whether they be big, small, one-off, or continuous—are a step in the right direction. Not just for us as individuals, but for consumers as a whole. Together we can eradicate malnutrition and the shitty diseases that come with it. That may sound corny and heroic, but I fucking mean it (and I'm wearing a superhero suit, so I'm allowed to spout heroic nonsense). Spandex suits on, shields up, and balls to the walls, people!

First thing's first: is your brain really connected to your mouth (in other words, are you ready to eat with purpose)? Seriously if it isn't, this will all be for nothing and you'll be right up shit creek as soon as you put this book down. You *need* to consider every step and action you take. You *need* to understand what you're shoving down your throat: what it is, where it came from, what it contains. No more eating for a hobby; no more robotic movements or decisions based on emotion.

You're about to step into the world of finding, cooking, and eating your own food. After all, that is the point of all of this. If you don't learn, we're not solving the greater problem. And without learning, you're just going to run out, spend hours hunting down delicious, healthy foods, and then get home and have no idea what the fuck to do with them. Let's start by doing a little happy dance first though. We are finally learning how to fucking eat! Seriously—get up and shake what your mama gave ya, because . . . "we're gonna have a good time tonight. Let's celebrate, it's all right."

(*Cue Celebration by Kool & The Gang.*)

Don't pretend you didn't just start singing.

Step one: *don't* do some silly detox or cleanse. Both are completely unnecessary and there's no time to waste. You don't need to eat lemons for a week to "reset" your body. The body is perfectly capable of detoxing on its own (we have a liver and kidneys for a reason), and as soon as you start shoving good shit down your pie-hole, the detoxing will begin.

The next step is optional (who am I kidding—all of this is fucking optional), and is to figure out approximately how much you need to eat. If you skipped over the math in chapter 9, you may want to head back and get 'er done. Or, maybe you don't. If you know you're someone who is going to take baby steps, I recommend tracking calories because that will at least keep your portions in control while you're making the long journey. If you're taking the fast or cold-turkey track, and head straight for the plant-based diet, you can scrap the "figuring out how much to eat" all together. Because remember, the *amount* of food you eat becomes insignificant if you're solely eating plant foods.

Side note: if *you* change (lose or gain weight, have a baby, etc.), the *amount* you eat will also have to change. Recognize this. The key to this journey will be learning to adapt and to not get stuck into one set number or system.

Once you determine approximately how *much* you're supposed to eat—whether you choose to log, or just go off how you feel— the next thing I usually recommend is to break your day down and pick apart each meal. Let's say you've gone the logging route (if you haven't, just bear with me for a second), and figured out that you need to be eating around 2,000 calories per day. If we distribute those nutrients over the day throughout your meals, it might look something like this (which looks a lot like my day):

7:00 a.m.—Breakfast (400 calories)
10:00 a.m.—Mid-morning Snack (200 calories)
12:30 p.m.—Lunch (500 calories)
3:00 p.m.—Afternoon Snack (200 calories)
6:00 p.m.—Dinner (550 calories)
8:00 p.m.—Evening Snack (150 calories)

This doesn't mean you must eat six meals a day; some people feel better eating three or four meals per day. Experiment with a few different meal frequencies and find out what feels best for you. When my son goes through growth spurts he eats about fifty meals per day, and I'm not about to try to stand between him and his fork. He naturally knows what he needs, and I let him have it (and he gorges on vegetables, so really, who cares?). Most of us have fucked up our food radar system though, and have reprogrammed our brains to make it seem okay to eat whenever and whatever we feel like, rather than what we really need, when we need it. Learn to listen to your body and get a feel for what's actually needed.

Back to breaking apart your day. I usually have people start with breakfast because a lot of people skip it, and need to add it in. That's right, if you're a breakfast-skipper, this shit's specifically for you. Cut the bullshit; you need breakfast.

(Cue Mission Impossible theme song.)

Man! We really *are* having a party here! Your first mission, should you choose to accept it, will be to first find a healthy—hopefully organic—whole-plant-food-based-breakfast *that you enjoy*. If you're following the calorie route, you'll want that kickass breaky to ring in around 400 calories, per the example. You're probably saying, "well what the heck makes up a 400-calorie breakfast?!" We'll get there, I promise! Here's where *type* and *variety* come into play. We must choose wisely.

How do you choose a good breakfast? Um, you search! You ask friends! You buy a cookbook! You find someone who has figured their shit out, and ask them to share a recipe! You avoid pre-made items that come in a box and have an excess of chemicals. You aim for health-promoting plants. Recipes aren't going to magically pop up in your kitchen, so yes, you'll initially have to do some work and hunt them down. If you're doing an internet search, try to use words like "whole-food," "plant-based," or "healthy." Remember though, most people have pretty skewed definitions of "healthy." Don't go eating a whole sugar-filled banana pie for breakfast simply because it's called *"healthy* banana pie."

Once you find a recipe that you think you may enjoy, look at the ingredients and use your judgment. If they're mainly all whole, healthy foods, *great!* If all but one of the ingredients is fair game, see if you can eliminate or substitute the bad one. If most of the ingredients are from an animal or are processed shit, try again. Then you go buy the best versions of the recipe ingredients you can find (e.g. raw, untainted, organic) and have a go. For now, I'll get you started with my kick-ass muesli.

Babich's Bitchin' Muesli:

9-10 cups rolled oats	1/2 cup pumpkin seeds
3 cups raisins or any dried fruit	1/2 cup sunflower seeds
1 1/2 cups slivered almonds	1/4 cup chia seeds
1 cup toasted wheat germ	1/4 cup flax seed
1 cup wheat bran	1/4 cup cinnamon

Instructions: Mix all of those beautiful, kick-ass plant ingredients together. Place 1/2 to 1 cup of muesli (per serving) into a pot, depending on your size and activity level. Cover with the non-dairy milk of your choice, and slowly heat. Dance while you wait. Feel free to top with berries or a chopped banana if you want to make this extra orgasmic. Don't you dare add sugar.

The portion I pie-hole has about 500 calories (approximately a generous cup). I determined this by totaling up the calorie amounts of each ingredient above, and then dividing by twenty (because it makes about twenty cups).

Side note: I don't magically know all of the calorie amounts of foods. I *do* know many of them though, and that's because I've done this long enough. If you're not skilled in calories, chances are you may need a calorie calculator to assist you with figuring this shit out. Head on over to *www.calorieking.com*, where you can search for most foods—even toxic food—and it will give you the corresponding calorie amount.

Back to the grind. I just figured out that I eat around a 500-calorie breakfast. Unfortunately, for the 2,000-calorie day example we're using, I should have only eaten 400 calories for breakfast. Crap! Fail! I may as well go drown myself in some donuts! Hell no, the game isn't over yet. I still have several options, so I'm not about to get my panties in a bunch. The first option is that I can eat less muesli (not going to happen, I love my muesli). Alternatively, I can rearrange some of my calories for the day (i.e. instead of having a 200-calorie mid-morning snack, I have a 100-calorie mid-morning snack and keep the extra 100 calories for my big breakfast). Nah, too complicated. Perhaps I simply eat the 500-calorie breakfast, wind up with 2,100 calories for the day, and not give a shit about the extra calories because I'm downing 100% plants! Bingo. And from now on, I don't need to calculate my breakfast; I just eat (until I want to experiment with another recipe).

This gets easier and easier every time you search out a new recipe. Eventually you'll become a master and construct your own recipes. You'll automatically know how much to eat without busting out the calculator. In time, you will ideally have several breakfast options you can cycle through, and all will be well in the world. Have I mentioned my breakfast smoothie option yet? When I'm short on time I just chuck a banana, a cup of almond milk, a tablespoon of chia seeds, a sprinkle of cinnamon, and a tablespoon of cacao powder (not *cocoa* powder—there's a big difference) into a blender and then suck down the magical, "chocolate" smoothie as I fly out the door. D-friggin'-lish.

Can you guess the next step? After you get your breakfast sorted, you'll go on to do the same thing with lunch, then dinner, and then snacks. You may even learn how to make healthy desserts (fuck yeah, you will)! I recommend not moving on to another meal until you've made a habit with the first one though—unless you enjoy feeling panicky and overwhelmed. Remember, it's important to not rush this. This is a journey and it's important you do it right. With each step you'll need to create a habit, and habits take time. Start slow—I can't say that enough. Learn one recipe, for one meal, and *then* move on.

As you move along, remember to focus on the *types* of foods you're choosing. Always seek out recipes that use whole foods, not a bunch of processed food products. For instance, choose whole tomatoes over canned, diced tomatoes. If you *do* ever find a processed food product staring you in the face, remember to head straight for the ingredient list, as that is the most important part. If there are ingredients you can't pronounce, or that bring back memories of the "Shit to Avoid like the Plague" section of this book, put it back and find a way to use a whole-food as a substitute. Also, now that you've read about controversial foods like soy, fish, dairy, eggs, and GMOs, you can make an educated decision on whether or not you want to decrease your consumption of them, or eat them period.

Always aim for *variety*—specifically organically grown, whole, fresh, in-season foods—and try not to mutilate them when you cook or use them. Reflect on what you've already eaten, and more importantly, foods that have nutrients you may be lacking. Don't hesitate to add a green smoothie or juice periodically to help boost your nutrient intake, which will, in turn, help to eliminate any nutrient deficiencies.

Get your family, roommates, *whomever*, involved, because if someone sees value in what you're doing or helps prepare a meal, they're more likely to eat it—even kids. This should be a household effort, not a single effort. Everyone should be on board, and everyone should care about getting healthy. If they don't care, it means that they haven't discovered the significance of nutrition yet, so help them find it. If you merely try to force them to eat new foods, they won't see the value, they *will* be miserable, and they *will* create an uprising against you. They will start informing their friends about how you have gone off the deep end and are trying to get them to eat "crazy" foods like nuts and seeds. Everyone must be on the same page. I can't stress that enough.

Being open to learning about (and learning to enjoy) new foods is extremely important as well. If you're not used to eating whole, untainted foods, everything may initially taste like dry tree bark to you. It's not the food though—it's the fact that your taste buds are so out of whack that you literally can't taste the food. It's not going to taste like fried, fatty, sugary goodness, because it's not fried, fatty, sugary goodness. Your taste buds *will* come around, so give it time. Please don't eat a meal, decide it's horrible, bitch about how much this sucks, and then completely throw in the towel. Muffle those temper tantrums and realize that this is a life journey, you won't hit the nail on the head every time, and you will have to build new habits. It's not a temporary diet or fix. This shit takes time and effort, remember?

You will eventually be amazed at how much taste buds can change. Every now and then my husband and I go out for a meal that is, shall I say, "less than healthy." Why? Obviously because we feel like suffering and punishing ourselves. Or, because we're not perfect and we get cravings sometimes (even though I don't eat certain foods on a regular basis, it doesn't mean I don't think they taste wonderful). Each occasion leaves both of us insisting that "the food wasn't good" (as in "it tasted like shit and we'll never order *that* again"). In reality, the food tastes exactly like it's supposed to (and like it always has), it's just that our taste buds have gotten so used to "clean" food, that the not-so-healthy food we stupidly chose to eat tastes like fucking poison (yet before we ate a clean diet, it tasted like heaven). Then, after we don't come close to enjoying our less-than-healthy meal, we usually wind up with the runs and bloating for a day or two. Masochists, I say!

My point is that you have to give your taste buds time. Find foods that you *think* you may enjoy and test them out for a while. Let your taste buds crawl out of the shit-swamp they've been drowning in; let them detox from the sugar, salt, and chemicals. If you *still* can't stand something after giving it a good go, *then* give yourself permission to move on to something else.

Above all, always listen to your body. In other words, choose foods that don't make you feel like ass. If you happen to eat something and soon feel like you're ten months pregnant or feel like your insides are trying to jump out of your throat, make sure you take note and don't make the same mistake twice. It doesn't mean you can't eat that meal again, it simply means there may be an *ingredient* in that meal that doesn't agree with your body. Keep a journal if you need to, so that you can discover trends. It's a trial and error process, and you *will* find foods that make you feel awesome if you keep putting one foot in front of the other.

Use your brain, have fun experimenting, and try to eat as clean as possible (meaning decrease your consumption of chemical-packed, nutrient-void, processed foods). Remember: it only gets easier. The more you learn about food, the sooner you will be a kitchen master, creating and experimenting with new foods on a regular basis. It all starts with learning one new recipe. Eventually, you will have replaced all of your meals with healthier options or versions. Maybe it takes a month, maybe it takes a year. Let it take as long as it needs to take.

The next concept you need to understand, is that there's a big difference between consistency and perfection. If you try to follow every single piece of information in this guide, you will surpass even me. While most people assume my family and I eat "perfectly," we, instead, eat *consistently*. Meaning, we don't have big ups and downs in our diet. We mainly cook all of our meals at home from whole plant foods, and a very small percentage of the time we do "something else." Trying to be perfect is the number one way to fail (and end up in the mental ward). Nobody is perfect, and there will be some things you won't want to "give"

on. It becomes all about how far up that Nutrition Spectrum
you're willing to climb. Are you comfortable only wearing
Captain America socks, or do you want to don the whole fucking
outfit—shield and all?

If you're not comfortable with the thought of up-scaling all of
your meals, consider changing something else. Here are some
ideas on other places to start:

- focus on the *amount* you're eating, and more specifically,
  your portion size (if you're not ready to change the *types* of
  food you eat)
- analyze the *types* of foods you eat (animal versus plant) and
  see where you may be comfortable making changes
- eliminate or reduce foods that come in boxes and packages
- chew less gum (or eliminate it completely)
- reduce or eliminate beverages that may not be needed
- investigate water filters
- eat out less, cook more at home
- eat slower, chew more
- ditch the vitamins and miracle pills
- give your pantry a make-over so you have wholesome foods
  readily available to you (like grains, nuts, and seeds)
- weed out your fridge and pantry, and ditch the fake food
- aim to increase the *variety* of foods you eat by experimenting
  with new foods (refer to Appendix B)
- figure out how to make a power-packed juice or smoothie
- experiment with a new, organically grown, whole foods
- start an herb or vegetable garden, or plant some fruit trees
- venture out to your local farmer's market
- *talk* to vendors at your local farmer's market
- research local restaurants to see if any of them support your
  new eating habits
- stop supporting large companies that have no regard for
  consumer health—even if they have organic spin off brands
- research a topic that may be confusing or interesting to you

- resist charring meat on your grill
- make your own almond milk
- discuss your journey with other like-minded people
- start eating to fuel yourself, instead of for pleasure
- focus on getting your pee clear and your poop submarine-y
- dress up like Captain America, fly around your neighborhood, and shout nutrition knowledge from the rooftops

There are endless possibilities on where to start, and there's no cookie-cutter formula or path to take. Just start with whatever feels best to you. Rome wasn't built in a day, and neither was our horrible food system. It has been on a downward spiral for decades, so I don't expect anyone to pop out of it in a day and be magically healthy. You should, however, notice immediate (*immediate*!) changes like having more energy, weight loss, or skin that clears up. You may find that you sleep better and your memory improves. The significant ailments will take more time (i.e. you're not going to kick your cancer in a day), but your body *will* try to take care of them and eliminate them as it becomes well-nourished and capable of fighting disease. Be patient.

Knowing that, ask yourself how long you've been overweight, underweight, or unhealthy. Then, ask yourself how long you've been trying to improve your health *without* seeing results (yo-yoing up and down doesn't count). If it's more than a week, you've been headed down the wrong road. If it's more than a *year*, well shit, pull your head out of your ass and try something new.

Let's talk more about not striving for perfection. There's a group of foods and beverages that I like to call "sparingly foods." These are foods that I would consider to "not be perfectly healthy, but periodically desired." Basically, foods that I would throw a temper tantrum over if I could never have them again. These foods differ from the "everything in moderation" concept because they're only eaten once in a blue moon, rather than regularly in moderation. They also differ from "cheat" foods because you should never label something a "cheat" unless you automatically want to feel like shit for consuming it. It's not about "cheating." If you love something, you should be able to enjoy it *sparingly.* This means infrequently enough that perhaps you can't recall the last time you had it. Unless you're craving something like crystal meth—that's not the kind of shit I'm condoning.

For instance, take chocolate. I'm a self-proclaimed chocoholic. I love chocolate and there's no way I'd *ever* eliminate it from my diet. However, my body obviously doesn't *need* chocolate (like it doesn't *need* broccoli or apples). Yes, chocolate may have some good components (especially certified organic, dark chocolate), but like I said previously, if something has a few good components it doesn't mean it's the best option for you (or that it doesn't also have a bunch of hidden shit in it).

So, I eat chocolate. How often? I can't say. I have it **when** I want it—but I'm at a point where I truly want to eat healthy and crave nutrients my body actually *needs.* Therefore, I don't seek chocolate all the time. When I do, I grab some chocolate . . . just not enough that it sends me into a panic-stricken depression for "falling off the wagon" or for "cheating." I also choose the *best* chocolate I can find: the certified organic, all-natural, dark chocolate—which happens to contain about five times the amount of iron than beef does, in case you were wondering. Yes, that is me justifying my chocolate addiction. Shut up and let me indulge. Lastly, I also try to buy locally-made products to support local businesses, rather than supporting the big-ass companies that are creating much of this cluster fuck in the first place.

There are some other non-chocolate cravings I get periodically, and I make an educated decision on whether or not I should have whatever I'm craving based on the last time I ate something on my "sparingly" list. It's funny; if I decide to fulfill that craving (for example, buffalo wings, which I had an addiction to during my teenage years), I usually wind up feeling physically sick afterward, and that craving gets suppressed for another year. Eating one "bad" thing that infrequently is not going to kill me—

especially when the rest of my diet is kickass. It's not going to physically help me either though. Moral of the story: as long as you can find the sweet spot between kicking your cravings and flinging yourself overboard, you've won the battle.

Staying in control gets easier. The healthier you eat, the less you'll want to sabotage yourself. Shitty foods will start to taste more and more disgusting. Your body will actually start to crave healthier foods, and you will want the "sparingly" foods less. The unhealthy foods you used to gorge on will suddenly leave you feeling ill after only a few bites. This happens because your body has detoxified itself—and without having to survive on lemons, green tea, and dandelion root for a week. It automatically flushes out all of the "bad," and makes room for the "good." You put more "bad" in it, and it shouts, "WHAT THE FUCK ARE YOU DOING?! I THOUGHT WE WERE DONE WITH THIS SHIT!!" Don't believe me? There's only one way to find out.

Side note: I have to let you in on a little secret. My family has thrown out a lot of food that has been gifted to us over the years. I don't care if it's the holidays or what; I'm not willing to sabotage myself for the sake of the gift-giver. I'm also not willing to re-gift something that has a bunch of shit in it so someone else ingests that crap. I'm therefore sorry to say that if you have given me or my family delicious processed treats, candies, or baked goods over the past several years, they have most likely ended up in the trash (okay, perhaps after one bite). This is not a reflection of your cooking skills or lack of generosity; this is our decision to put health before anything else. Don't be afraid to do the same.

In the end, the truth of the matter is that even if you only take *one* thing from this guidebook, you will be healthier. How much healthier you get depends on how many steps you're willing to take. Shuffle on up that Nutrition Spectrum. Heck, crawl if you need to. Remember that every little improvement you make is an improvement. Any little change you make will be a step towards optimal health and a step away from imminent ailments and disease. Always keep that in mind. String a bunch of little changes together, and VOILA! Suddenly you'll find a lycra superhero suit plastered to your ass!

Try not to get hung up on where you're going to end up though, because—trust me—you have no idea where that will be. Even if you *think* you know right now, your goals and desires will change as you change. Focus on the present moment and make one small change at a time. How far you go will be determined by how you feel when you get there. It won't be determined now, so don't freak out about foods "you can't live without," when you haven't even gotten there yet. If there *is* something you're currently freaking out about, leave it and start with something else. Down the road, when you've progressed to a point where you're comfortable, you can make the decision to stop, or to go further. Don't go farther than you're comfortable going, because you won't stay there. Once you've made a bunch of changes and you think you're done, come find me so I can give you a high-five.

Moral of the Story:

Learning how to use your pie-hole is never going to be as simple as "10 Simple Steps," so stop trying to make it such. Find the parts of your nutrition habits you're willing to change first, and begin the extensive journey. Focus on one small change at a time. String a bunch of small changes together. Be consistent. Be *perfectly* consistent. But don't you dare try to be perfect.

Chapter 34

Where the Fuck
Do I Find Real Food?

To plant a garden is to believe in tomorrow.
—Audrey Hepburn

If you don't know where to search for real food, then I imagine you've been snoozing at the wheel. Farmer's markets. Community Supported Agriculture programs. Natural Grocers. Your own friggin' garden. Okay, *possibly* a conventional grocery store. But seriously, have you ever seen Captain America in a grocery store?! Of course not. He's got his shit figured out, and probably has a garden the size of Texas. However, since most people flock to grocery stores, I'll play nice and cover the topic—as long as you promise to walk outside afterwards and start turning up some soil for your new garden.

When it comes to buying processed food in a grocery store, one of the first things many people look for is the nutrition label. Therefore, we should become nutrition label masters, right? Wrong. I'm going to make this simple for you: most of the foods you should be buying won't *have* nutrition labels. Why? As my good friend Jamie Oliver put it (kidding, we've never met—but hey, Jamie, let's do lunch!), "Real food doesn't have ingredients, real food *is* ingredients." Get it? Real food is *whole* food that doesn't come with an ingredient label. Whole, friggin' food.

Sure, real food can *become* an ingredient, but it shouldn't be full of them. Therefore, I'm not even going to discuss reading nutrition labels, which unfortunately seems to be the focus of the US government at the moment (or at least making them "easier for the public to understand").[505] Because—and I'm going to be Captain Obvious here—the more we focus on getting people to read nutrition labels, the more processed, chemical-filled foods they're going to reach for. So yeah, that seems like the dumbest plan ever.

All I'm going to say is this: if you must purchase something that comes in a package, can, jar, or box, look at the nutrition label (which will most likely be in fine print to make the bad news difficult to decipher). Skip right over the actual nutrient info—the fats, carbs, protein, sugar, etc.—because there's something of greater importance: the list of *ingredients*. If you can, without a doubt, say that every ingredient on that list is healthy and won't fuck you up in some way, then that product is fair game. Most "fair game" products (and there *are* some, but they will most likely be found in health food isles or stores), will have a short list of ingredients—perhaps five at max—and will all be recognizable foods. Foods like "apple" or "cinnamon," and not "vitamin E," "hydrolyzed proteins," or "antioxidants" (which may sound healthy but aren't actually real foods). If you pick up a product and you don't know if all of the ingredients are healthy, put the product back. Simple. This is the point in the game where you start to realize how much crap is hiding in food.

I'm now going to take you on a wild ride through a conventional grocery store so you can navigate the shit out of it. Hold on to your hats. Commence "Mission: find *real* food." The helpful part is most grocery stores are laid out pretty much the same. Around the outside are the whole foods (or minimally processed foods) like the produce, deli, seafood, and frozen foods. On the inside of the store you have the crap isle, the shit isle, the chemical isle, and the kill-you isle. Near the cashiers, you have a bunch of completely unnecessary and enticing items that will stare you in the hunger-laden face. Basically, you should generally try to buy from the outside isles of the store. Anything on the inside isles can generally be made from whole foods originating from the outside isles. Mind. Blown.

Let's start in the produce section. Here you'll find a wide variety of foods like fruits, vegetables, and fresh herbs. You also may find some pre-packaged versions of those items (e.g. cut up pineapple). Let me give you some hints: First of all, you're perfectly capable of cutting your own damn pineapple. Secondly, whatever you're buying is going to be (and taste) the freshest if it hasn't been fucked with. Thus, try to buy whole, un-cut, un-tampered food if you can. Learn how to cut a fucking pineapple!!

There are three different versions of produce we're going to touch upon:

1. Genetically modified organisms, or GMOs (red light!)
2. Conventionally grown foods (yellow light!)
3. Organically grown foods (green light!)

We already know that GMOs are extremely controversial, are laced with chemicals, and are horrible for the environment. Steering clear of them to err on the side of caution, *and* to show that you don't vote for chemical companies invading our food system, seems like common sense to me—but I'll leave that decision up to you.

Conventionally grown produce items are not genetically modified, but are generally contaminated with chemicals like herbicides, pesticides, and fertilizers. They may also contain systemic chemicals (chemicals that are injected directly into the plant, and therefore exist in all parts of the plant). We haven't discussed systemic chemicals yet, mainly because I didn't want to completely overload you with shitty information. But basically, even if you wash your non-organic foods, they're probably still laced with systemic chemicals. Bummer.

Organically grown food—or simply, "food"—is grown naturally from organic seed, and is chemical-free. Simple as that. Obviously organic foods are the best option for health, but how can you tell which is which, and what if you can't afford to buy all-organic foods? You keep reading, that's what you do!

Telling which is which is generally simple: most of the certified organic foods are labeled as such (since they're the ones who have to dish out the extra money to prove that their product is real and untainted). There also may be an "organic" section that showcases all of the organic foods together.

When in doubt, referring to the price look-up code (PLU) number may help. Most fruits and veggies have stickers on them that clearly show a four or five digit PLU number (unless it's a bag of grapes or something, which, in that case, the number will be printed on the bag). Those stickers aren't there purely to piss us off folks—they're there for a reason (and it's not just to leave a sticky, chemical residue on your produce). If the number is four digits, it's conventionally grown. For example, the number 4318 signifies a conventionally-grown cantaloupe. If there's a fifth digit, that will signify that it's *not* conventionally grown, and instead is either organically grown or genetically modified. If the PLU on the cantaloupe has an "8" in front of it (e.g. "84318"), it would mean the cantaloupe was genetically modified. If that number were to have a "9" on the front of it (e.g. "94318"), cha-ching! It's organically grown![506] To recap:

- a 5-digit code starting with an "8" signifies a genetically modified, chemical-laden produce (red light!)
- a 4-digit code signifies a conventionally grown, *non*-GMO, chemical-laden produce (yellow light!)
- a 5-digit code starting with a "9" signifies organically grown (green light!)
- a 6-digit code means someone fucked up their stickers

Buuuuut, once again there's a catch. These numbers are completely optional, and I'll let you guess how many of the GMO companies want to label their products as so. As of today, I have never seen a five-digit PLU starting with an "8." However, the conventional foods that have the 4-digit codes, or the organically grown foods that have a "9" on the front of the 4-digit codes, should be fairly reliable, and are frequently used.

Now we get into the price issue. I'm not even going to discuss the price of GMOs because I don't believe they're worth my time. As far as the other two categories go, organically grown foods are generally slightly more expensive than their conventionally-grown equivalents. Therefore, if you must pick and choose which foods to buy organic and on which foods to take a risk, here are some hints. First, meet "the dirty dozen."[387]

apples	grapes	snap peas
celery	nectarines	spinach
cherry tomatoes	peaches	strawberries
cucumbers	potatoes	sweet bell peppers

These foods are known to deliver a dazzling chemical blast (more so than other produce), and you are therefore going to want to buy them in *organic* versions when at all possible. When I say "chemical blast," I'm referring to the chemicals that are sprayed around them or injected into them, which includes carcinogens, neurotoxins, hormone disruptors, and developmental and reproductive toxins. Don't take this dirty dozen lightly. Two foods that didn't make that list, but still get coated in chemicals are hot peppers and leafy greens (e.g. kale, collards, spinach, swiss chard, mustard greens). Thus, grab organic versions of those as well.

Now meet "the clean fifteen."[387] This would be a list of non-organic produce items that are generally *less* coated in chemicals (but still not completely clean, of course):

asparagus	eggplant	papayas
avocados	grapefruit	pineapples
cabbage	kiwi	sweet corn
cantaloupe	mangoes	sweet peas (frozen)
cauliflower	onions	sweet potatoes

If you can't afford to buy all organic, the foods on the clean fifteen list are safer to buy in conventional form, as they contain far less chemicals than other produce tested.

Of course, there are many other types of produce that are not listed on the "dirty dozen" or "clean fifteen" lists. They fall somewhere in the "questionable zone" and you'll have to make the decision on what form to buy them in. If you can't buy organically grown produce, wash the heck out of the conventional versions you buy (even the clean fifteen). The scrub-down may not take care of the systemic chemicals *inside* the food, but at least you'll wash off some of the ones on the outside. Just be wary of what you choose to wash with, because there's no point to wash off harsh chemicals with more harsh chemicals. A sixty-second wash under simple tap water will be your best option.[507]

Now, unless you want to only eat produce for the rest of your days, we must venture further into this chemical plant—I mean *grocery store*. If your grocer has bulk bins (which are usually somewhere near the produce), hit those up next. Bulk bins are a great place to buy dried foods like nuts, seeds, whole grains, and legumes. You don't pay for the packaging, and you can buy them in raw form (but if they're not labeled as "organic," you're living on the edge my friend). This is a great way to stock up on some "staple" items for your pantry. I buy several foods in bulk (e.g. dried beans, nuts, seeds), and have them stored in glass jars out of the sunlight—patiently waiting to be thrown into a recipe. It makes it simple to make something like muesli in an emergency breakfast situation. Be cautious though, as some companies may add chemicals to their bulk bin products to make them last longer. All ingredients should be listed on the bin though, so as an example, if you're looking at a bin of black beans, the only item listed should be "black beans."

Next stop: meat and seafood counter. If you're a meat or seafood eater, it's time to locate the grass-fed, pasture-raised, wild versions of whatever you're buying. Try to avoid buying factory farmed, caged anything (it might not be labeled as such though, so you'll have to ask). Again, if they don't know if something is wild or grass-fed, move along. They should know what they're selling—and if they don't, it's a ginormous red flag. Just remember to keep tabs on your intake of animal products if you have any concern for long-term health. When my family chooses to have animal products (usually wild-caught seafood—we're in New Zealand for fuck's sake), it's usually a small part of the dish, not the *main* part of the dish.

Past the meat and seafood, usually tucked along the back corner of the store, is the frozen section. This can be hit or miss, and one of the most common questions I get asked is: "Which is better: frozen or canned?" My answer is always "local, organically grown, and fresh," which, of course, pisses people off. Seriously though, if you can't find it fresh from a local farm it's because it's not in season and it's been shipped in from some other corner of the planet. Those foods that *are* shipped in (and possibly frozen first) are usually conventionally grown and sprayed or waxed to go the distance. In fact, the average distance your food travels before you consume it is 1,500 miles.[508] That's like living Boston, and getting a burger delivered from Miami. Gross.

If you *must* buy canned or frozen, I'm going to tell you the same thing I previously have: look at the ingredients. If you can pick up a can of corn and compare it to frozen corn, and one has chemicals and one doesn't, buy the one that doesn't. Simple. One is usually packaged in a can, and one is usually packaged in plastic. We already know that chemicals seep out of cans into their products, so if it were me, I'd go the frozen route (as long as that frozen thing isn't packed with chemicals). *Organic*, frozen foods can be a great option for something like fruits or veggies (because they were picked fresh, frozen with nutrients locked in, and then shipped to you without any chemicals added). We add organic, frozen berries to our homemade muesli quite often when they're out of season, because that's generally the best option at that time.

Moving along. Sometimes you may need to venture into one of the middle isles to grab something like tea, honey, spices etc. If that's the case, buckle up—it's going to be a wild ride. Now you're entering the land of highly-processed, packaged, can-survive-on-a-shelf-for-a-year "food" and "beverage" products. Put your blinders on and stay the course.

If you happen to come across something irresistible that comes in a package, find the list of ingredients on the nutrition label immediately and put it through the test. Do you know what all of the ingredients are? If the answer is "no," put it back. If the answer is "yes," and you can undeniably say that those ingredients are health promoting, then congratulations you have found a one-in-a-million product. GRAB IT AND RUN.

Whatever you do, do *not* go off what the front of the package says. We already saw "100% fruit juice" that had other crap in it, and we know that companies will do and say anything to entice you to buy their product. Pretty, healthy-looking packages mean jack shit. Don't fall for it.

Pressing on. We've thankfully foraged through most the store unscathed . . . but unfortunately, as soon as you go to pay for your items, you're put to the test and punched in the conscience by the chocolate, gum, and who-knows-what-other-shit hanging out by the cash register. Punch that shit right back, let them know who's boss, and get the fuck outta dodge (but please pay for your healthy food first). You made it! Whew!

Now, here's something a lot of people don't take into consideration when they begin to transition to eating whole, fresh foods: *frequency* of shopping. Remember, fresh foods are exactly that—they're *fresh*. Most of them will not last on your shelf for months because they haven't been tampered with, and therefore don't have chemical additives that keep them from decomposing (except for some of the dried, bulk items which can last quite a while if stored correctly). Hell, many of your fresh foods won't last a *week* (especially if they're organically grown). Thus, you *will* be shopping more. If you think about it though, your cumulative time at the store is probably about the same (or less if you learn to fly past all of the enticing, harmful shit). Therefore, rather than going once per week and spending an hour stocking up for the next seven days, you may instead shoot by the grocery store or farmers market several times per week and spend five to ten minutes grabbing some food for the next day or two. I buy food daily, and I'm in the store for five minutes tops (except on the days I hit up the farmer's market). It's part of my daily routine, and it might just become part of yours as well. If you live out in the wilderness, and there isn't a store within a stone's throw, then you will obviously have to come up with the next best option. Hint: huge-ass garden.

Take some time to get acquainted with the parts of your store or market you may have previously ignored. It's all part of the journey, so get your compass and explore. Allow yourself to become familiar with new foods that used to go unnoticed. Don't be embarrassed. *Learn.* Talk to store employees (some of them may not have a clue, so find the ones that do). Please don't go out and buy a bunch of random food yet—that is not using your brain. You'll want to have a plan of what you're going to do with the food first (i.e. a breakfast recipe) before you go and waste your money.

If you venture out to a local farmer's market or use a Community Supported Agriculture program always talk to the growers or providers about their products. Ask them if they grow the food they're selling, and whether or not they spray them with chemicals. Unfortunately, some farmer's markets don't require all food to be certified organic, and some vendors are actually selling food they've purchased from another store and then marked-up. Trickery everywhere!

If you can't get to a farmer's market or join a Community Supported Agriculture program, and it's not feasible for you to plant a garden (are you *sure*?), find a local health food shop that sells wholesome foods, and won't have as much of the "junk" mixed in to make your head spin. Everything may seem foreign to you in there, but don't let that deter you. People who work in health food stores generally know more about health foods (duh), so don't hold back on the questions. If all of that is a no-go (but seriously, try your best), then a conventional grocery store will have to do—and thank goodness you now know how to navigate one. Grab the list of ingredients for your new, healthy recipe, throw on your smart-pants and shitty-food blinders, and do your best to avoid the massive, festering sea of deception classically known as "advertising."

Moral of the Story:
Wherever the fuck you decide to hunt down your edibles, the majority of them should come *without* nutrition labels, and preferably be whole, organically grown, in-season foods.

Chapter 35

I Have Real Food! Now How the Fuck Do I Cook It?

Congrats! You made it out of your grocery store, garden, or market alive. Head to the medic before proceeding if you need to tend to any battle wounds. Make haste though because this train is on the move and the next stop is coming up fast: cooking and preparing food.

I mentioned this earlier, and the fact of the matter is that not all cooking methods are created equal. Food preparation is a science, and an extremely important one at that. Cooking a carrot in a microwave, versus baking a carrot in the oven, versus frying a carrot in oil, versus eating canned carrots, versus eating a carrot raw, will all dish up different nutrients once that carrot gets shoved down your pie-hole.[509, 510] This is a *huge* concept to get under your belt. What a shame it would be to change your nutrition for the better, only to cook the shit out of your food so you're left malnourished again.

The US Department of Agriculture has an awesome report on "nutrient retention." It explains how foods change, based on the methods you use to cook them.[511] For instance, if a nutrient in a certain food—let's say the vitamin C in a orange bell pepper—has been given a factor of 100 for a specific method of cooking, it means that 100% of the vitamin C in that pepper will be retained during that particular cooking process. If something has a nutrient factor of 45, it means only 45% of that nutrient will be retained with that cooking method. Basically, just because you're eating healthy foods, it doesn't necessarily mean you're getting adequate nutrients from them. How you cook (or don't cook) matters.

As an example, take sweet potatoes—you could bake or boil them (and for this example, we will leave the skin on). If you bake a sweet potato, you will retain 100% of the calcium, iron, magnesium, phosphorus, potassium, sodium, zinc, and copper. If you boil that same sweet potato, you will lose 5%–10% of all of those nutrients. That's not a huge loss, but if you enjoy both cooking methods, you now know to bake so you can get the most out of your damn sweet potato. Since we're dabbling in science and math in this guidebook, why not throw in a little spelling as well?! You'll notice that I did not include an "e" on the end of the singular word "potato." Why? BECAUSE IT DOESN'T FUCKING HAVE ONE. Every time someone contacts me regarding something with "potatoe" in it, a little piece of me dies. Please stop.

Back to the important stuff. What you do to your food determines which nutrients you ultimately end up with. As an example, I have heard many people bark about how liver is incredibly high in iron (which must mean we need it) before smearing processed liver pâté on a chemical-filled cracker. Well guess what? If that liver was simmered, it has already lost 40% of the iron in it. You may as well go eat your shoe! Not to mention you will also lose 55% of the potassium, sodium, B_3, and B_6. Essentially, you're left with a nutrient-depleted mound of foul-smelling organ. It's time to learn about appropriate cooking methods so you're not eating nutrient-depleted foods.

What are the best cooking methods? Well, that's not easy to say, because every food reacts differently to each method, and every vitamin and mineral acts differently within each food. BUT, in general, the less you cook or process a food, the more nutrients it will retain. If you cook a food in liquid, or if a food loses liquid while cooking, nutrients will leach out into the liquid. If you want those nutrients, you must consume the liquid as well (easy for something like a soup, not so easy for the greasy liquid dripping off your roasted chicken).

Ideally, you also want to incorporate numerous raw foods into your diet to get their powerful hit of nutrients. I'm not talking about clambering around ripping the heads off of live chickens for a snack—I'm talking about eating raw *plant* foods like herbs, nuts, seeds, vegetables, legumes, and fruits (you know, the ones with all of the kick-ass disease-fighting nutrients mentioned earlier).

All of these recommendations are based on the assumption that you're using fresh foods to begin with. The longer a food sits on a shelf or in the sun, or the farther a food is being shipped, the more nutrients it will lose before it even gets to your kitchen. Therefore, buy fresh, and then *lightly* cook your foods (if at all), incorporating any liquids into your meals when you can. As for raw foods, try to hit them when they're *ripe*, as this is when their nutrients will benefit you most (i.e. wait until the green banana has brown spots).

If you're going to try to prepare your foods ahead of time (cutting up your foods and storing them in the fridge, for example), try to minimize the time between cutting and eating. The second you cut, peel, or prep a food, it will begin to lose nutrients (and flavor). However, you also have to weigh your options. If the only way you can eat nutritious foods is to prep them on a Sunday and store them in your fridge for the week, then losing a bit of those awesome nutrients is going to beat running out for fast food daily because you don't have time to get your ass in the kitchen during the week. Prep ahead of time only if you need to.

An ideal scenario would be that you grow your own food, or buy fresh, local food. You would eat those foods within a few days from being harvested, and you would prepare them just prior to the meal. You would do your best to find a cooking method that won't send every nutrient in your meal packing, and you would eat that meal shortly after preparing it. Let's not kid ourselves though—this world is far from perfect. Find a balance and the best methods that work for you.

Before we discuss different cooking methods, please know that regardless of the method you choose, it's not necessary to drown your food in oil. Like anything else, oil isn't needed. For starters, we learned about how oils can make your omega-6 levels explode, sending you to inflammationville. The more oil you consume, the more inflammation you're likely to have, the more disease you may experience. Furthermore, when oil heats up high enough it can release free radicals (which you will wind up eating, and can damage your system). The amount of free radicals the oil releases depends on how old the oil is, the temperature it is heated to, and the type of fat the oil harbors (saturated versus mono or poly unsaturated, which we have not discussed, so don't think you're losing your memory).

Free radicals are *not* something you want an abundance of in your system. Thus, if you cook with oils, not only does low heat trump high heat, but less oil (or no oil) trumps more oil. If you "must" use oil, here are a couple of hints: coconut oil is less likely to produce free radicals than most other oils, and won't go rancid for a good year or so. Canola oil, on the other hand, goes rancid quickly, is likely to produce high amounts of free radicals, and is one of the most genetically modified commodities out there. I would recommend avoiding canola oil at all costs. Really though, you don't actually need to cook with oil (seriously, you don't—food is perfectly capable of cooking without it). You *may,* however, need to personally lube up with oil in order to initially slither into your spandex superhero suit, so I wouldn't dispose of it just yet.

Boiling/Simmering

Unless you plan on consuming the liquid you're boiling your food in, I don't suggest using this method. Many of the wonderful nutrients from your food will leak out into the water and end up being poured down your drain instead of poured down your throat. Save the boiling method for dishes like stews and soups.

Frying/Stir Frying

While I perceive this method to be a bit better than boiling, it really depends on if you use oil, what oil you use, how much oil you use, and the level of heat at which you cook. Soaking your veggies in canola oil and turning that bad boy to high, versus simply lining the pan with some organic coconut oil (or just water) and heating on a low heat (OH MY GOD IT WILL TAKE FIVE MINUTES LONGER TO COOK THOUGH!!) will have completely different effects on your food. If you're going to use oil, use it sparingly when stir frying, and try adding water to the dish if you are concerned about it drying out or sticking to your pan. Any way you look at it though, your food will retain more nutrients than if you boiled it.

Oven: Baking/Roasting/Broiling

Similar to frying, the outcome of these methods depend on if you use oil and how much you use. Baking something without oil will yield a different nutrient-packed food than roasting something submerged in oil. If your taste buds are used to heavily oiled foods, it may take some time to learn to eat them in their whole form (and actually enjoy the taste of the food, rather than the oil). And if we're talking about retaining nutrients, it's a good idea to bake foods in their whole form, and then cut them prior to *eating* rather than prior to cooking.

Steaming

I would consider this one of the better methods of cooking. As long as you don't steam the shit out of whatever you're about to cook, you can retain a lot of the nutrients in your food this way. However, you must steam *minimally* so your food retains its shape and structure (and fiber). If you hold up a steamed piece of asparagus it should hold its shape; it shouldn't look like it's auditioning for an erectile dysfunction commercial. In addition, although it may seem natural to chop whatever you're steaming into lots of little pieces *before* steaming them, this will cause the most nutrient loss. Keep the food whole, or in the largest pieces you're able, and then cut them *after* the food is steamed, just prior to being pie-holed.

Grilling

If you decide to grill, there are a few points that might interest you. First off, depending on the heat of your grill, nutrients are often well maintained while grilling (as long as you leave the food intact before doing so; the more you cut the food prior to throwing it on the barbie, the more nutrients it will release). Secondly, grilling usually involves high heat, and unfortunately when you're specifically grilling meat ("what else do you fucking put on a grill?!") you should be extra cautious. The reason is that when meat is cooked at high temperatures—especially as it begins to "char"—it will start to produce cancer-causing compounds.

Again, this is something that is well-known, but generally not public knowledge. Some of these carcinogenic compounds are called "heterocyclic amines," in case your fingers are feeling Google-happy. Those little bitches are mean as fuck and will rip you apart if you ingest them regularly. A 2014 study recommended that people should avoid "grilled, fried, and broiled meats to reduce the risk of cancers of the colon, rectum, breast, prostate, kidney, and pancreas."[156] Basically, the more charred or high-heat-cooked meat you eat (and not only by grilling), the more likely you are to be knocking on cancer's door. To avoid this, if you are grilling meat, it is imperative you do so gradually on minimal heat to avoid any "charring" or "blackening."[512-515] Just make sure you don't down twelve more beers in the extra time it takes to brown your steak.

Microwaving

Ahhh yes, the controversial magic cooking box. The one we so quickly throw our inedible food into because it miraculously makes it edible by heating it up faster than we can say "what the fuck is this magic box doing to my food?" The answer, my friends, is that a microwave oven heats food by exposing it to a good dose of electromagnetic radiation, which probably sounds scarier than it actually is. Electromagnetic radiation waves are actually quite similar to radio waves, but move back and forth a bit quicker.

Microwaving actually has some great benefits (why else would they be in almost every kitchen in the developed world?). First off, they're quick. We all know that "quicker is better" when it comes to food. No one wants to starve to death in their kitchen while waiting for a pot of water to boil or for an oven to heat. Problem solved! Zap that sucker in the magic box! Past being lightning-quick, microwaves also allow foods to retain nutrients better than other cooking methods, because the time at which the foods are cooking are considerably decreased (in general, the longer something cooks, the more nutrients it loses).[516-518] Lastly, microwaves are safer while in use, meaning you're not going to burn yourself on a microwave like you would on a stovetop or oven.

Therefore, to the microwave's credit, it has solved several "issues" when it comes to cooking. However, regardless of those wonderful cooking improvements, it's always important to look at the big picture: microwaves leak radiation. How much radiation? Not much. Probably about the same amount that comes from your TV or computer screen, for what that's worth. For this reason though, many people believe microwaves can cause cancer.

It seems, based on the information I have read and gathered, that the main fears regarding microwaves stem from one (yes, *one*) study published back in 1992. It was published in the Swiss publication *Journal Franz Weber* (which I can't actually find in English) by a Dr Hans Hertel and a Dr Bernard Blanc, of the Swiss Federal Institute of Technology and the University Institute for

Biochemistry. This study apparently pointed to microwaves having the ability to "change" our blood in a way that would be similar to how cancer would change our blood. There has been much controversy over this one little study, as well as several lawsuits surrounding it.[519] There is *much* more evidence surrounding the cancer-causing compounds produced by grilling meat at high heat, yet no one seems to be scared of grilling, and everyone and their mother seems to fear the microwave (with little evidence pointing to it being harmful).

Who knows what we're supposed to believe, or how much water that little study mentioned above actually holds. For me—even though there really isn't substantiated evidence against microwaves—I still don't like to use them. Mainly because they cook unevenly and leave my food mushy and foul-tasting. I'd use a *convection* oven (which simply blows hot air over your food) over a microwave oven any day. That's a decision I made based on my personal feelings about microwaves. You can draw your own conclusions. If you do decide to use a microwave, please make sure you use containers that won't leech carcinogenic compounds into your food.[520] Reach for glass, parchment paper, or even paper towels before you reach for plastic or Styrofoam containers. Metal is, of course, completely frowned upon.

Raw (Not Cooked)

As mentioned earlier, it is crucial to incorporate raw foods into all diets. Raw foods will retain all of their nutrients as long as they haven't been shipped in from afar, and haven't been sitting in the hot sun for a decade.

To clarify though, a food is technically still considered "raw" if it is cooked in heat no hotter than 118°F (48°C). This is understood to be the maximum temperature that will maintain the enzymes in the food (which help with nutrient absorption and digestion). Thus, heat 'em up if you'd like, but keep that temp low. People who maintain raw food diets use food dehydrators to help with slightly "cooking" their food. The dehydrator will slowly and mildly heat the food by blowing hot air over it. A dehydrator may be something to consider if you want to go gung-ho with this nutrition stuff.

In the big scheme of things, if you're eating whole foods, period, you're doing fantastic—so don't stress about whether you eat raw or slightly un-raw foods. Mix it up and do whatever puts a bunch of whole, healthy foods down your throat.

Moral of the Story:
Eat some raw plant foods. Past that, try to cook minimally with little to no oil on low heat, and consume any resulting liquids along with your meal.

Chapter 36

I Cooked My Food! Now How the Fuck Do I Eat It?

Picture a ferocious lion snarling and snorting as it viciously rips into a zebra carcass, devouring every last bit of it as quickly as possible, thinking the world is ending and this is its last meal. *That*, my friends, is how my husband eats, and that, my friends, is a surefire way to waste precious nutrients. I wish I could embed a video here for your viewing pleasure, but unfortunately hubby has not released the rights. For fuck's sake, if you're going to take the time to buy the best foods and cook your precious foods properly, you may as well get the most out of them. I mean shit, don't you want to taste your food?!

Here's some more brain-power for you: Digestion (which includes the process of delivering beloved nutrients to various parts of your body) actually begins directly behind your pie-hole, in your mouth. For the same reason we discussed the need to "chew" your green juice or smoothie, you also need to spend time chewing whatever other foods you shove in your mouth. If you swallow your food whole, or only partially chewed, the digestive enzymes (which start the process of prepping those kick-ass nutrients for absorption) will not be able to get to work on breaking them down. This is crucial, as nutrients won't be able to squeeze through the tiny nutrient shuttle-system into your bloodstream if you skip this step.[521]

Instead, those larger particles you've decided to inhale will sit in your gut and will most likely cause constipation, bloating, gas, pain, and cramping. Not to mention you've skipped the nutrient-absorption part. If you just take the time to friggin' *chew* your food, the smaller enzyme-enhanced particles will be absorbed into your bloodstream and will provide you with abundant energy. In other words, you won't waste a shitload of nutrients. So let's see: you can opt to feel lethargic, bloated, and heavy, *or* you can opt to take the time to actually chew your food, savor the taste, and at the same time optimize your energy. Can someone please teach my husband to chew his food? He wonders why he has no energy when he "eats so well."

If one of your goals is weight loss, you'll be thrilled to know that if you spend more time chewing, you will actually control your portion size a bit more. In other words, you'll eat less than you would if you were playing the role of the lion. *But,* regardless of how fast or slow you eat, putting the amount of food you actually *need* on your plate (and not going back for seconds and thirds) is the best way to assure that you don't over eat. If you pile a heap of edible brilliance on your plate and attempt to "stop when you're full," you will most likely fuck up. It takes about twenty minutes for your body to signal you that it has had enough, and by then you would have completely over-eaten.[522]

Pro tips: First, try to avoid associating your portion size with the size of your plate (i.e. eat what you *need*, not how much food your plate will hold). Also, if you want to slow down your eating, try using your non-dominant hand to hold your shovel—I mean your *fork*—or even try using chopsticks (if you don't know how to use chopsticks, you'll *really* slow down that shoveling). You can also count how many times you chew. Try at least five to ten chews per bite (depending on how hard or soft your food is). Even if something is soft (e.g. organic coconut yogurt), you still need to "chew" it to wake up those digestive enzymes. Or, get up and dance the Macarena between each bite. That'll certainly slow you down (as well as everyone else at the table, as they'll be wondering what the fuck you're doing). Whatever works for you, do it.

Let's also talk beverages. First and foremost, if you're properly hydrated, you should never feel thirsty or feel the *need* to drink water (or anything else) during a meal. Secondly, gulping down large amounts of fluids *with* your food may actually reduce your body's ability to absorb the nutrients you're eating.[523, 524] Therefore, 'sip' wisely. If you want to gulp, do so *in between* meals or during the new kick-ass workouts you suddenly have the energy for.

Finally, this may be stating the obvious, but the only way you're going to *eat* healthy foods, is if you *have* healthy foods available. Therefore, you must plan ahead. Keep healthy staple foods at home, plan your meals ahead of time, make sure you have time to prep and cook them, and bring foods with you wherever you go. That way you won't get stuck in a drive thru when you're out of your comfort bubble.

Moral of the Story:
Take the time **to** chew your food, you gluttonous vacuum!
(That may or may not be a direct message for my husband.)

Chapter 37

Eating Out 101

Fact: people who cook at home are healthier than people who eat out.[525-527] This is, of course, because the majority of establishments that make or sell foods and beverages process them to oblivion and then hide a bunch of shit in them in order to help "sell" their product. This includes fast food joints, cafes, diners, restaurants, taverns, food trucks, etc. (either they add the shit themselves, or they use pre-made condiments and products that have already been tainted by other companies). If you make your own food, from untainted foods, in the comfort of your own home, you can avoid this madness. This doesn't mean you never eat out again (put the panic away); it means you eat at home more than you venture out, and when you *do* venture out, you learn how to pick the best options and have control when wolfing them down.

When you eat out, it's crucial to choose an establishment that supports your new habits. If you allow yourself to enter the danger zone of a less-than-worthy food joint, you're guaranteed to get spit out a little less healthy than when you walked in. Don't do that to yourself. Hunt down a healthy place. This usually means they source local, organically grown ingredients. It also means the servers and cooks can actually *tell* you about those ingredients—like where they came from, and how fresh they are. What it *doesn't* mean is a dollar menu and drive-thru-boasting shithouse. If you're dining where the servers and cooks only know about super-sizing your meal and giving you extra ketchup packets, you have not found the right place. Keep hunting.

Please, please, *please* (for the love of god, PLEASE), don't assume places are "safe" or "healthy" because they're advertized as so or have a trendy, healthy-sounding name (you should be able to smell a marketing scheme from a mile away by now). For example, take Subway sandwiches, which everyone seems to assume is the "healthy," go-to fast-food joint—mainly because that's how they promote themselves, and their cheeky slogan, "eat fresh" helps. Unfortunately, there are enough chemicals hiding in their "food" to build a periodic table.

Do me a favor. Next time you're in Subway, ask them who makes their bread dough and where they get their "fresh" ingredients from. Watch them stumble over their words. Ask them what's so "fresh" about thiamine mononitrate, silicon dioxide, disodium phosphate, sodium propinate, sodium nitrite, caramel color, yellow 5, sodium benzoate, calcium disodium EDTA, dimethylpolysiloxane, or tert-Butylhydroquinone—all of which are all hanging out in their breads, veggies, meats, cheeses and condiments. At least in the US, they are.[528] Or, simply ask them if their "natural flavors" come from beaver ass—what a *fantastic* conversation starter that would be! Subway throws so much shit in their food it's mind-boggling. Even the "fresh" veggies have been doused with chemicals "to maintain freshness." A bit of a hypocritical statement there, if you ask me.

Moral of the story: don't flock to places you *assume* are healthy, as Subway is not the only one pulling the wool over your eyes. Research and discover food joints that *are* healthy. If you're too timid to talk to an employee face-to-face, call first and fire away with however many questions it takes for you to feel satisfied you've found your answer. If they're willing to take the time to answer, you've most likely found a winner.

Then, after you believe you've found a safe place to eat, it's time to find the best meal option. If you've truly found a healthy establishment, all meals should be fair go. However, since those places are about as common as a nipple ring on a Barbie doll, you'll most likely still have to be wary of your menu options. Your best bet is to try to aim for meals where you can actually *see* all of the original foods (i.e. whole foods that are all identifiable). Meaning, if something has a sauce smothering it, how do you know the sauce isn't being held together by "natural" ingredients like donkey shart and whale jizz? Answer: you *don't*. If you ask your server, and they don't know either, then RED FLAG. Sauces are a fantastic place for restaurants to hide addictive additives and unhealthy ingredients that suck you in and keep you coming back for more. Beware the special sauce. Aim for meals that use spices or simple liquids like fresh-squeezed lemon juice to flavor them instead. Also beware all processed foods like breads, pastas, tortillas, etc. as you have no idea what they were made with (unless they come bearing an ingredient list).

You won't know what's hiding in your food unless you ask. Thankfully, the people who showed you your seat and took your order actually talk! They're there for a reason. If you want to be 100% certain you're not eating crap, you simply need to ask. However, you probably want to word it nicely—asking if they've "put any shit in this" will probably get you a blank stare and an attitude. And perhaps some spit in your food. Instead, ask questions like:

- "Do you source local ingredients?"
- "Are your meals made from organically grown foods?"
- "Is everything made fresh?"
- "Do you make your (bread, pasta, etc.) from scratch?"
- "Do you use additives like MSG?"
- "Will you piss in my food if I continue to ask questions?"

If you are in a healthy establishment, they should be able to answer these questions without hesitation. If you get that look— the one that says, "why the fuck are you asking so many questions, just order some goddamn food so I can get my tip"— you know you're not in the right place. Hand them this book (which I'm sure you will carry with you everywhere), and then make beeping sounds as you slowly back your ass out the door.

When in doubt, order the salad. I'm joking. Ordering a salad because it's the "healthy" option when it's a dreary 5,000-calorie heap of wilted lettuce covered in bacon, ranch dressing, five eggs and a cheeseburger, is so 1995. Salads have the ability to be the *worst* option—especially if you use the restaurant's salad dressing, which is most likely filled to the brim with chemical junk. Instead, if you can get a salad that's labeled as "organic," and loaded with ingredients like veggies, nuts, seeds, or fruit, with a simple dressing like apple cider vinegar or fresh squeezed lemon, you'll be closer to the jackpot.

If you're afraid of sauces after I just revealed that they're a great hiding spot for crap, you should feel the same about salad dressings. Thus, don't hesitate to bring your own version of either. If you have a healthy version at home (perhaps *you* made it, wink, wink), and you *know* your restaurant meal won't be complete without it, throw some in your purse or man-bag and bring it with you. Why the fuck not—it's your *health* with which we're dealing. If anyone gives you a hard time, simply tell them it's your liquid vitamins (because all real foods have vitamins, tee hee hee).

Now, on to calories. Isn't it *great* that restaurants are now slapping calorie amounts on their menu items? Since everyone *clearly* knows all about calories, this must be a good concept, right? Not so much. You see, 700 calories of an organically grown, plant-based, whole-food meal *not* covered in special sauce is a quadrillion times a better choice than the 300 calories of a nutrient-void, chemical-filled, highly-processed meal. That 300-calorie meal, when eaten over time, will most likely gift you a list of life-long ailments. Meals should be chosen based on the *nutrients* they provide, not their calorie amount.

If you're worried about calories because you're trying to lose weight, order the 700-calorie, healthy, whole-food meal that will fuel your success, and only eat half of it. Whatever you do, do not base your meal decisions on the calorie number next to them. If you're completely on the whole-food, plant-based food train, feel free to ignore calories completely.

Last point: eating out comes with a lot of trust. You need to *trust* that employees will give you the right information (and not simply say whatever they need to entice you to buy their food). You need to *trust* that if they say their food is organically grown, that it is, in fact, organically grown. If it isn't, you need to then *trust* that they've done their due diligence and washed the chemically-doused conventional ingredients well enough that you're not eating a chemical explosion. Finally, you need to *trust* that they're not going to piss in your food if you annoy them with too many questions.

Hopefully, in the next decade—if things go my way—there will be healthy, organic, whole-food, plant-based establishments that use local, fresh ingredients popping up on every corner. And when you sit down to eat at one of them, you will automatically know that anything you order on the menu is health-promoting, and fair game. Wouldn't *that* be nice?

Moral of the Story:

Eating out is manageable if you know where to go, and what to look for on a menu. First step: start searching your area for restaurants, cafes, diners, or other eateries that may cater to your brilliant, new, healthy eating habits.

Chapter 38

The Fruit of Our Loins

Let's raise children who won't have to recover from their childhoods.
—Pam Leo

In the same respect that I can remember what it was like to be asked if you wanted to sit in the "smoking," or "non smoking" section when dining out, I'd love the next several generations to be able to reminisce and ask questions like, "do you remember when foods were infused with toxic chemicals and caused debilitating diseases?" Or, "do you remember when consumables were so processed you couldn't even determine from which real foods they originated?"

A great deal needs to happen before either of those questions becomes a reality. We need to educate ourselves, and opt out en masse. We need to break this malnutrition-death cycle by giving a giant middle finger to all of the companies and organizations that have shoved our health to the back burner. We need to bring back *food*—actual real food—so our future generations can survive.

I get incredibly upset when I see unhealthy, malnourished kids—either overweight or underweight—who are falling behind their potential. Like, I-want-to-fucking-strangle-someone upset. Kids are none-the-wiser, which means someone else has essentially put them in that position—either in utero or after birth.

419

No one is doing this on purpose—I'm mean, who would purposely want to fuck up a kid? But the truth is, most caregivers don't know what to put in little, growing pie-holes (or in their own pie hole when they're pregnant).

Because of this, kids around the world are getting fatter and becoming more and more riddled with ailments and disease— even "adult" diseases like type 2 diabetes. Heck, one in *five* kids in America is now suffering from high cholesterol (which means they're at risk for heart disease and stroke).[529] Consequently, kids are starting to be pumped full of drugs to "manage" their health issues (because who wants to invest time into changing a child's habits?!). I blame the same people and organizations that I did at the beginning of this guide, whose greed and guidelines have led to the presentation of beautifully advertised, child-targeted, poisonous food. Without proper guidance, it has become the norm to reward our children with sugar, and shove toxic shit down their precious throats: "You sat through a hair cut! Well done! Here's an artificially-colored, sugar-filed lollypop!" Enough is fucking enough.

Jennifer Silverberg—the brains behind the "Eat Yourself Well" website—puts it bluntly and beautifully: "[I hope] that one day it will be as socially unacceptable to give a child a lab-created-sugar-and-chemically-filled-junk-food as it is today to hand them a cigarette."[530] A-FUCKING-MEN. Do you see any difference between cigarettes and many of the foods targeted at kids these days? At this point you shouldn't—they're both toxic and both cause addiction and disease. Unfortunately, parents are tricked into thinking otherwise. Thus, if you're not comfortable handing a cigarette to your child, you shouldn't be comfortable handing 80% of "foods" and "beverages" to your child.

Thankfully, a 2014 study on childhood obesity (which spanned ten to fifteen years) found that obesity rates in some developed countries are actually starting to plateau. The *bad* news is they're simply starting to plateau, when in reality, they should be taking a death-defying nose-dive toward optimal health. Thus, we still have intense work ahead of us, especially since childhood obesity is still rising in *developing* countries.[531] Hopefully you Greeks are reading, since your country now tops the charts for childhood obesity (with 44% of boys and 38% of girls being overweight or obese—which is sickening). In case you're curious, the other countries that round off the top ten rankings for child obesity are: Italy, New Zealand, Slovenia, The United States, Mexico, Spain, Canada, South Korea, and Israel.[532] Regardless if your country is in the top ten or not, we all need to get our shit together. This has become a global crisis.

I mentioned a woman by the name of Robyn O'Brien during our discussion on genetically modified foods. She is a mother, author, public speaker, and founder of the AllergyKids Foundation, which is based on the following principle:

> The AllergyKids Foundation consists of a team of leading medical advisors, nutritionists, industry consultants and concerned corporate and everyday citizens in the hopes that together, we can inspire change in our food system and protect the 1 in 3 American children that now has autism, ADHD, allergies and asthma from the chemicals in the US food supply.[533]

The foundation has therefore studied and researched how foods are, and have been, affecting our children over the past several decades, and has come up with some staggering statistics. In the last twenty years, the rates at which certain childhood ailments are increasing are as follows:

- 300% increase in asthma
- 400% increase in allergies
- 400% increase in ADHD
- 1,500%–6,000% increase in autism spectrum disorders[240]

I absolutely *refuse* to believe it's simply a coincidence that we add a bunch of shit to our food supply, give that shit to our children, and get these results. And these statistics don't even include all of the heart diseases, cancers, auto immune diseases, etc. that are also ripping kids apart. If we continue to poison our future, we won't have one.

Therefore, we have a couple of choices. First off, *having* children is generally a choice. If you don't want a child, keep your vag closed or your dick in your pants. If you *do* choose to breed, the next choice becomes whether or not you choose to provide your offspring with kick-ass fuel, or make them a statistic. When I say "statistic," I mean providing them with shitty, artificial, highly processed "foods" and "beverages" that will set them up for years of frustration and health **problems** from not knowing how to use their pie-hole. Let's face it, it's not *a child's* job to know how to use their pie-hole; it's *yours*. Don't turn them into a statistic.

The decision to fuel children properly should start early, as "after 24 months [of age] children become reluctant to try new things and start to reject foods."[534] Basically, a child's first two years are crucial. A 2014 study done at the University of Leeds in the UK showed just how shapeable babies' palates are.[535] "Shockingly," it seems that if you regularly offer certain foods— even healthy foods—to a child before the age of two, those tastes will become "fixed" and set the tone for their adult food preferences.[536] Well duh, that's why the majority of people are walking around sick and miserable—because they were fed formulas and artificial crap instead of (human) breast milk and real food from a young age.

The above mentioned study also axed down the myth that children have to have healthy foods smothered in unhealthy sauces in order to like them. Therefore, no disguising, no trickery; simply present them with real food. The more you hide and disguise healthy foods, the more they're going to think something is wrong with those foods, and the less they're going to want to try them.

Unfortunately, I feel like most parents are concerned with "making their child happy" by "giving them what they want" over anything else. You know what? Babies and kids want *food*. They don't know what McDonald's is unless *you* present that shit to them. A parent should be asking, "what am I going to fuel my child with so they get the best nutrients possible and grow and develop to their full potential?" Sadly, if you do the opposite—and provide your child with crappy nutrients—you are unquestionably stunting their physical and mental growth. This will not—I repeat, will *not*—make them happy in the long run. They will be weaker, both physically and scholastically. How friggin' unfair to them; from the beginning some kids quite frankly never stand a chance.

I've heard parents respond with statements like, "well my daughter is smart," or "my son is strong," and you know what, that could very well be true . . . to some extent. But, if they're "strong" or "smart" being fueled by shitty nutrients, imagine what they *could* be like if they were fueled by *awesome* nutrients. The truth is, you will never know a child's full potential unless they are fueled as intended, and are *able* to reach their full potential. It's like the example I used early on—how many of my clients are amazed at how *great* they feel after making changes. They realized that even though they originally thought they felt amazing, in reality they had no idea what "amazing" felt like. For fuck's sake, *please* let your kids know what "amazing," and "smart," and "strong" *really* feel like. That way they'll be able to look after you when you're 115 years old and can no longer pull your own parachute cord.

If you're reading this book, chances are you've, at some point, struggled with nutrition. If *you* know how hard it is, why on earth would you want to pass that difficulty on to your children? If we all step back and take a second to realize that we're potentially setting our children up for disaster, we can then stop packing them full of the highly processed crap that shouldn't be considered "food" or "beverages" in the first place. This way, no one has to deal with trying to figure out how to fucking *eat* later in life (which would obviously mean my book sales would take a nose dive—but I sincerely wouldn't give a shit if it meant that kids weren't being poisoned).

What does this mean? This means you don't take children through the drive-thru of a fast food shithole purely because *you're* tired or "don't have time" to get something healthy for them. You don't let them eat crap simply because it's disguised in some cute little kiddie package and specifically boasts that it's "made for kids." Spend a dollar and shove a carrot and an apple in their hand—that stuff will fill them up and provide them with more nutrients than any processed shit would. And, while *you* may not find those foods exciting, you will no doubt find excitement in the fact that your child is building habits around consuming real foods—and enjoying them.

If you *do* choose to give them shit, then you need to recognize that you're giving them shit and be okay knowing that you could be making life harder for them. This destructive way of fueling your child not only increases their risk of disease, but it opens the floodgates on them. Their palate is only just developing, and this is a crucial time for them. Once they've tasted the chemicals that are made to suck people in and are addictive in nature, there's no going back. It makes *your* job that much harder.

My favorite example, which I hear all of the time is, "what am I supposed to do? My child comes home and devours a whole bag of chips" (or a whole pint of ice cream, a liter of soda, etc.). Well, pardon my French, but what fucking creature crawled into your pantry or fridge and put that shit there in the first place?! *You* did. You cannot get mad at your children for eating the food you have purchased and placed within their reach. Don't buy the shit, and they won't eat the shit.

As we have learned, sometimes the "shit" is unfortunately disguised or presented as being "okay" though, and this is where you need to keep those smart pants handy. For instance, take Flintstones vitamins. They have to be good, right? I'm pretty sure nine out of ten pediatricians recommend them, and most parents scramble to get them in their child's pie-hole, because of the assumption there's "*no way* they can possibly get all of their nutrients naturally these days!" GROAN. Here's some lovely (I mean *horrifying*) information for you. Check out the list of shit you are putting in your child when you give them Flintstones Complete Multivitamins.[537]

calcium carbonate	calcium pantothenate
dextrose monohydrate	cupric oxide
sugar	blue 2
microcrystalline cellulose	red 40
maltodextrin	yellow 6
sorbitol	folic acid
sodium ascorbate	magnesium stearate
ferrous fumarate	niacinamide
natural and artificial flavors	potassium iodide
hydrogenated soybean oil	pyridoxine hydrochloride
pregelatinized starch	riboflavin
gelatin	silicon dioxide
vitamin E acetate	thiamine mononitrate
stearic acid	vitamin a acetate
corn starch	vitamin B_{12}
aspartame	vitamin D_3(cholecalciferol)
beta-carotene	zinc oxide
biotin	

That shit ain't just vitamins, Barney Rubble! Food dyes, aspartame, nitrates, maybe some beaver ass—basically everything that was in the "Shit to Avoid like the Plague" chapter of this book. Let me break it down for you: this is a ticking time-bomb of hazardous, cancer-causing, genetically modified, chemical concoction that targets millions of *children*.[538, 539] Yes, "the norm" has become to shove highly processed and highly marketed crap into our kids—when perfectly good vitamins and minerals are already surrounding us. For fuck's sake, whose brilliant idea was this? Whomever they are, I wish them endless years of festering ass warts. If you have any children's vitamins laying around your house (heck, *any* vitamins for that matter), I suggest ditching them ASAP and exploring this concept: give your children real food, with real fucking vitamins! THIS IS ME SHOUTING BECAUSE I'M FURIOUS (not at *you*, at the companies targeting our children).

So here's the deal: if, for a second, you think you're depriving your child by keeping all of the shitty foods and beverages out of their reach (or better yet, out of the house completely), please realize that you *are*, in fact, depriving your child—but not how you'd imagine. You are depriving them of years of disease, struggle, and frustration stemming from poor nutrition. If we're going to deprive our children, let us *please* deprive them of that.

What should parents do? Let me start by saying that if you already have kids with poor nutrition, this is going to be much harder for you, as you now have to break habits, and there will most definitely be tears (but put your big boy or girl panties on and consider the long-term goal here). If you're starting to *contemplate* having children, this will be a bit easier for you.

Let's break this down and go step-by-step. First and foremost, you figure out how to use your own pie-hole (see book entitled *How to Use Your Pie-hole*, by Jennifer M. Babich). Once that's done, you give your child(ren) the greatest gift you could ever give: physical and mental health via correct pie-hole usage.

I'm going to use myself as an example here. What I did with my son was choose to give him the gift of health. In spite of what most people believe, the gift of health doesn't begin when a child is born. Step one begins from the minute you decide you want to procreate, and when you start asking yourself these questions:

- Is my body capable of procreating in an optimal manner?
- Is my partner's body capable?
- Do I live near chemical-sprayed food crops (i.e. do I want my child to have a 60% increased risk of autism)?
- Have I (or my partner) taken oral contraceptives that have stopped the natural process allowing procreation to occur?
- Is the penis that will be involved functioning well enough to get the job done, or does it looked like a limp asparagus?
- Is the semen in that penis healthy and capable of fertilizing an egg? Or, has it been effected by pesticide residue from non-organic food, leaving a significantly low sperm count?

Most people forget that it takes two to tango, meaning the health of the man is just as important as the health of the woman. You put a fucked-up sperm into a healthy egg, you're still going to have fucked-up results. A healthy sperm and a healthy egg are imperative if you want to build a healthy child—and they both come from two people who know how to use their pie-holes. Thus, please get *your* shit straight before you put the D in the V and attempt to create life.

Moving along. Prior to getting pregnant, you women know it's "imperative" you take your folic acid (a.k.a. vitamin B9) to reduce the likelihood of miscarriage and birth defects, right? Well, were you aware that it's just as important for men to have the correct amount of vitamin B9 as woman? And that men who are deficient in vitamin B9 can cause similar birth defects in their future child?[540] On the flip side, for all of you moms who are jamming folic acid down your throat like you're smuggling diamonds, were you also aware that folate (the *natural* version of folic acid) exists in food? I'm not even joking! The vitamin "folate" naturally exists! In *real* food. Future moms and dads should start pumping their bodies full of folate-rich foods (e.g. spinach, broccoli, asparagus, avocado, mango, beans, and sunflower seeds), and screw the synthetic "folic acid" pills.

Next step: humping. Unfortunately, there are so many reasons why a couple may not be able to conceive. Many of them stem from throwing the wrong shit through your pie hole, which— believe it or not— includes oral contraceptives. I can't tell you how many people I know (too many), that had to wait friggin' dog's years for their body to start functioning normally again after years of taking birth control. It took some women *years* to get their cycles back (please revisit the dangers of oral contraception listed in chapter 22). That's far from normal, and frankly, if you've ever tried to make a baby before, it can be quite exhausting. I can't imagine *years* of trying and wondering why the fuck a baby isn't knocking on my vagina's door.

Eventually we arrive at pregnancy. Congrats! If you're the knocked-up woman, do you know what time it is? It's time to throw every fucking excuse as to why you have to eat shitty foods just because you're craving them out the window. You are now growing a child inside of you. A fucking *child*! Seriously, ponder that for a moment. Women are capable of growing *human beings* when given the proper seed. That's mind-blowing, and requires an immense amount of time and energy. That being said, everything a pregnant woman eats fuels the growth of that fetus. Do you want to grow your future child with toxic, chemical-laden, nutrient-depleted crap? *Or,* do you want to grow your child with organically grown, whole, powerful nutrients? Which do you suppose will grow the healthiest, smartest child with the most potential? You have a choice, and I'm guessing you love your child more than you love a bucket of ice cream. Well, I'm hoping.

On a side note, if you've ever pushed a baby through a vagina before, you know there's a direct correlation with the size of the baby and how much you want to commit murder. If you eat healthy during pregnancy, you have the power to control the size of your baby (to some extent, as genes are also involved here). If you want to spew forth a diabetic, ginormo-baby, eat sugar-filled, chemical-laden shit, and eat lots of it! If you want to deliver a healthy-sized child that eases through your vaginal canal like a sailboat down the Seine (hey, one can dream), then don't. There is a direct correlation between fetal growth and woman's nutrition, so binge wisely. You also may (or at this point, may not) be surprised to know that there's a correlation between the amount of animal protein a mother eats and her child's weight later on in life. A child born to a mother who consumes higher amounts of animal protein is shown to be two to three times more likely to be overweight than a child born to a plant-food-hoarding mother.[541] A "normal," "healthy-sized" baby comes from a mother who has her shit together nutritionally, and who doesn't overdose on animal foods.[542]

When my husband and I conceived (which we had no problems with because we were super-powered and healthy as Larry (who *is* Larry, by the way??), it was game on for me. Step one done, now onto step two: pregnancy. I didn't even think about cravings. I got to work making sure I was building the most incredible, powerful human being inside of me. I wanted my child to fly out of my vagina wearing a cape! Most people get this step backwards though. They think, "Sweeeeeeet, I'm preggo! I can lounge around, eat pickles and mac and cheese for days, and throw everything health-related out the window because look at me: I'm knocked up, and shit, I deserve it!"

This is indisputably *the* most important time for a woman to be spot on with her nutrition. I hate to say it, but we are bringing children into this world who have already fallen behind their potential. A poor diet during pregnancy *can* result in long-term, permanent, physical and mental health issues for your child.[543-547] Here's a scary fact for you: a mother with high cholesterol can literally give her fetus heart disease.[548] That's right: babies are being born with heart disease. All because mama decided that her tub-per-day of ice cream was a justified craving.

It's not simply foods and beverages that you need be concerned with. There are "other" things that people shove down their pie-hole with little thought, simply because they're assumed safe. You read about some of them in the "Shit to Avoid like the Plague" section. Something we mentioned but didn't discuss in depth was over-the counter meds like ibuprofen (e.g. Advil, Midol, Motrin, Nurofen) and acetaminophen (e.g. Panadol, Paracetemol, Tylenol). You know, for all of the pregnancy pains that women go through. That pain has to be muffled somehow, right?

Check this out: Both ibuprofen and acetaminophen were considered "safe" during pregnancy at one point. Then the tables turned. First ibuprofen was deemed harmful (as well as other similar drugs like naproxen and diclofenac), and apparently increased the risk of miscarriage.[549] Women were therefore strongly advised to take acetaminophen during pregnancy instead. Great! Problem solved; the women are pain free, and the pharmaceutical companies are still raking in the dough. Then *acetaminophen* was linked to ADHD, and *ibuprofen* was suddenly deemed safe again.[550, 551] Fool me once pharmaceutical bastards, and then FUCK YOU. The healthier you are, the better you will be able to handle your pregnancy, and the less you'll feel like crap. Either way, don't pop pills—Freddy the fetus can't handle the shit.

Then—just past mid-pregnancy—you'll have to give your doctor a big kick in the cooter when they prescribe the glucose tolerance test for you. Here's why: 1) that shit they're about to pour down your throat is NOT purely glucose, and 2) glucose is simply sugar. You may as well go drink some sugar water and skip the "other" ingredients, listed here:

dextrose	brominated soybean oil
citric acid	yellow 6
natural flavoring	sodium hexametaphosphate
modified food starch	BHA
glycerol ester of wood rosin	sodium benzoate

Does that entice your taste buds? Heck it's marketed as being "certified kosher," with a "great taste," and it also comes in an amazing "plastic shatterproof bottle"![552] Great taste my ass. If you've ever tried this brew before, you'll know it tastes like sweaty gym crotch. This is probably why the bottle is shatterproof—because the women who feel they've just been poisoned usually hurl the shit at the closest nurse. The ingredients for the concoction above were from an "orange" flavor, by the way. Check out how much "orange" is listed there. Then check out how many of those "shit to avoid like the plague" ingredients you're poisoning your growing child with. Please, please, please ask your doctor or midwife for an alternative test. If they tell you there are no other options, beeline it to another doctor who understands your concern and provides you with a better option.

After many months of (hopefully) eating healthy, a woman pops out a child. Congrats! Here we go to step three: now it's time to keep that child's physical and mental growth on the fast-track to full potential—which is hugely influenced by what you put in their pie-hole. Children aren't born craving candy bars and gummy bears. They will only crave those types of foods if they're given to them. They would also crave broccoli and apples if given the chance. I shit you not.

From day one, I gave my child the nutrients his body *needed* (which then became the nutrients he *wanted*, because that's all he knew). I breastfed for thirteen months (and would have gone longer if I wasn't spending two months travelling and moving cross-country). You know why? Because my breast milk was specifically designed for my child. Furthermore, my breast milk altered its healing and growth benefits based on what my baby needed. You think formula can do that? Formula was *not* what he needed (nor was the breast milk of any other animal, as we have discovered), and has also proven to have less optimal results than breastfeeding.[553-559]

Some may argue that the differences between breast and formula fed babies are minimal, and to them I ask two questions: 1) "do you work for the dairy or baby formula industries?" And, 2) "do you want your babies to be healthy and smart, or healthi*est* and smart*est*?" To be fair, it's up to the mother, but I don't understand wanting to inhibit your child in any way. Again, you won't know the true potential of your child unless you give them the fuel they are designed to have. If you are able to breastfeed, make it happen. If you're fueling yourself probably, you shouldn't have any problem lactating. I spouted milk like a geyser, and could have probably fed my whole neighborhood.

If, for whatever reason, you're *unable* to breastfeed, do you know what the next best option is? BREAST MILK FROM ANOTHER HUMAN. If you just cringed, I'm going to smack you. If you have no problem drinking breast milk from a swollen, infected cow nipple, you shouldn't have any problem drinking milk from another human. There are programs out there that sell clean breast milk. Seek and ye shall find.

Remember, we discovered back in the "Other Shitty Diseases" chapter that there is most likely a connection between cow's milk consumption and type 1 diabetes. Many studies have compared breastfed babies with babies who were given dairy milk at a young age. Many of them point to the possibility that children who drink cow's milk from a young age (or who aren't breastfed for the majority of their first year), are more likely to wind up with type 1 diabetes.[480-487] If you're someone who has lived with type 1 diabetes, I'm sure you'll agree that you'd be willing to do whatever it takes to keep the disease from your child. Breastfeed, dammit—from *your* breast, not another mammal's.

Side note: for those of you non-parents out there, instead of getting angry at a woman for boobing her child in public, give that woman a high-five and a salute for doing what's right for her child (but perhaps wait until she's done). A breastfeeding mother should be considered a kick-ass, healthy individual, and should be allowed to provide her child with healthy nutrients wherever and whenever that milk extractor needs it.

Moving along. When my son was six months old we added some solid foods to his diet (he already had most of his teeth then—they came in like a stampede of cattle around four months). These solids consisted of organically grown, whole foods like avocado, peaches, sweet potato, and spinach that I would puree. They did not come out of a container, had not been sprayed with shit, and therefore did not include any other unwanted ingredients. We already learned that non-organic, pre-made baby foods contain harmful chemicals, so stay the fuck away.[393]

Fast forward to today, and my son will be three soon (or seven by the time I finish writing this damn thing). His current favorite foods (which he regularly requests on his own accord) are:

cashews	broccoli	strawberries
walnuts	cauliflower	blueberries
almonds	mushrooms	raspberries
prunes	bananas	olives
seaweed	apples	beans
peas	kiwi	quinoa
carrots	mangoes	corn
cucumber	avocados	coconut kefir
hummus	tomatoes	green smoothies

Those are mainly all whole, unpackaged, unprocessed (and usually organically grown) foods. He loves all of them and gets super excited when he sees them on his plate. When I ask him what he wants for a meal, he always rambles off whole foods— he's never once told me that he wants pizza or any other "meal" (other than our green smoothies, which are made from a bunch of whole, powerful foods). It's so friggin' easy to "cook" for him—I can simply throw an avocado, some beets, some nuts, a carrot, a plum, and some beans on a plate, and he's *stoked*.

He's also obsessed with the garden, and thinks all foods come from one. He regularly wants to go out and pick foods to eat. We sit in the grass, open up some peapods together, and share some peas. It's an amazing feeling watching your child enjoy healthy foods, knowing that you are leading them down a fantastic path toward health, wellness, and prosperity.

Because of his food habits, we often have people stare at him like he's some sort of circus act. Ladies and Gentleman, the kid who eats real food! People often make statements like, "wow, I wish my child would eat that!" My response is always, "they're not the ones who choose their food." You'd be surprised what your child may eat (especially if they feel it's *their* choice, and you're not forcing them to eat something). During a recent preschool dinner gathering, several kids crowded around my son's meal and asked for carrot and cucumber sticks. Their parents (who were still holding the McDonald's they had brought for their children), were shocked that their child would actually ask to eat veggies. His school actually wound up taking photos of him eating his lunch soon thereafter and hung them on the wall so everyone could see what a healthy lunch looked like. Even though we often are, we shouldn't be the odd ones out.

Side note: please don't force your children to eat more than they want. They naturally know how much they should be eating. If you force them to eat more, you will merely give them undesired over-eating habits. Ever have one of those? Yeah, they suck and are not advisable Let your child(ren)'s natural eating instincts take over. Realize that sometimes they'll want more (during growth spurts), and sometimes they may want less (in between growth spurts, or when they're under the weather). If they look and act healthy, they are. Don't freak out if they don't finish the mound of food in front of them. Instead, take note and learn about portion control from them.

It's up to you how much you want to control your child's nutrition habits. Within the past couple of years, there have been times when my son has been exposed to what I would consider disease-promoting foods. These times usually come during the holidays or someone's birthday. Our decision is usually to bring our own food. It seems so simple, I know. And I've never encountered anyone who is offended by these actions (or at least they don't tell me to my face). To be honest, I wouldn't care if they *were* offended. Everyone should respect your desire to fuel yourself properly. They might not understand it (they most definitely won't understand it), and may discuss how "weird" and "extreme" you are behind your back, but hey, that comes from their lack of pie-hole knowledge, so not your problem. Just hope that one day they'll take the time to learn like you have.

I even send my son to daycare with food for the time he's there, because I don't want him eating the "healthy," "approved" (highly processed and chemical-filled) snacks they serve to the kids. Simple. My son is happy with this choice. He regularly tells me about the cookies the other kids eat, and then lights up when he tells me that he got a *banana* and *orange* instead! He feels special, and asks me if cookies come from a garden—because where else would they come from? He also loves to try new foods that he sees mommy and daddy eat. He's far from a picky eater, unless it comes to highly-processed food, because it looks foreign and strange to him. This means that our children are capable of eating healthy *and* surviving! Mind blowing!

Does this mean we "deprive" him of a birthday cake for his birthday? Of course not. We either find healthy ways to make cake with ingredients that aren't going to tear his insides apart, or we buy local from someone we know uses all-natural ingredients and let him indulge once a year. We most certainly do not buy packaged, processed cake mixes—they are full of shit, and it's completely simple to make your own cake using healthier ingredients.

Feeding my son real foods has become easy, because that's all he wants. I don't want to have to pry Jell-O and chicken nuggets out of his hands—and I won't have to, because he would never pick them up anyway. In fact, he has the same nutrition habits as my husband and I: on top of the processed crap we don't consume, he also doesn't eat meat or dairy (oh, the looks I get). "*What*?! How is he growing so big and strong?!" Remember, no one *needs* meat or dairy. Our preference is to not have them, and I make sure he gets all of the nutrients his little body needs. When he gets older, he can make his own decisions. For now, he is a living example of how this works. He has always hovered around the ninety-fifth percentile for height, he made it through his first two years without getting sick (most parents would call that a miracle), and frequently receives comments about how "great his skin is." And, if you missed it the first twenty times I said it: he has enough energy to power a small city.

Here's a funny story: Throughout my son's second year, during a series of his monthly well-being checkups, I had the same nurse repeatedly ask me when I was starting him on whole milk. She'd say it with the inclination as if it were *imperative* that every child in the world should be sucking at a cow's teat. Every time she'd ask, I'd tell her that he was never going to have whole milk as long as he was under my roof. She would look confused, would jot down some notes, and leave. The same thing would happen at the next visit. And the next. Eventually, I told her that it was quite frustrating that she was asking me the same question over and over, and also that I was always going to continue to give her the same answer: he was never going to have cow's milk. This time, when she looked confused, I asked her why he needed cow's milk. Her non-educated answer, of course, was, "for the calcium, for his bones." "Great!" I said. "He has organic almond milk daily, which has *more* calcium than dairy milk does. He also eats spinach and broccoli like they're going out of style . . . but you didn't ask me if I was finding a way to get him *calcium*." She looked even more confused. And beaten. And embarrassed.

It wasn't my intention to embarrass her, but I did want to make a point. I definitely made it, because she soon left and came back with the doctor, who ordered blood tests for my son. Doctor "hasn't-got-nutrition-knowledge" was suddenly worried about my son's nutrition, and thus worried that he may be anemic (i.e. have low iron levels) since he didn't eat meat. I explained that the kid eats a daily truckload of leafy greens, beans, nuts, and seeds, and they looked bewildered as to what that had to do with him potentially being anemic (those foods are high in iron). I let them do the blood tests for shits and giggles, as well as for personal reassurance. A week later, I received a call with the results—and they were horrible. For fuck's sake, I'm joking! To quote the nurse directly, "the blood work came back absolutely perfect." Yay! I'm not a fuck-up!

Do your homework folks. Understand that you have options when it comes to fueling your child. Unfortunately, your pediatrician—as well as his or her nurses—most likely don't know the best options for nutrition if they have the standard medical training. But don't be afraid to pry them for information to see if they do! For instance, it was New Year's Day 2014, when our family got struck down with norovirus. Happy New Year to us! My son was the first to get it, and to be on the safe side we brought him to the doc to make sure it wasn't something more serious. We were weary because this was only the second time since birth that he had ever thrown up (he never even *spit up* as a baby). To reminisce for a second, the first time was directly into my husband's mouth. Talk about shit you don't want to put in your pie-hole!

Anyway, the doctor confirmed that it was a "nasty tummy virus" and recommended we keep his "sugars" and "electrolytes" high. Then he recommended Pedialyte. "What's that?" I asked (knowing fair well what it was—I'm a little shit, I know). After looking startled (had no one else ever asked that question before?), he replied, "it's specifically formulated for children" with this cutting inflection in his voice. Well, that didn't answer my question, so I continued, "really, what's in it?" He replied, "exactly what your child needs." Except this time he threw a look at me that shouted, "how dare you question me! I'm a doctor, BITCH!" Time to slowly back away from the medical professional who doesn't know jack shit about what he's prescribing.

I didn't want to embarrass him anymore, as he either clearly didn't know how to explain what Pedialyte was, or was completely shocked that any parent in their right mind would be concerned about what they were putting in their child's mouth— especially when it was "specifically formulated for children." He was also clearly agitated with me, so I asked to see a bottle. Right on the front of the electric-pink-liquid-filled-bottle it stated: "Artificial Bubble Gum Flavour." YAY! Exactly what a child would *love*! How convenient; I'll take a case! Wait, seriously? NO THANK YOU. I'm simply going to keep my child naturally hydrated and properly fueled with the natural REAL liquids I have at home. I do not need any "specifically formulated" chemical solution that a pharmaceutical company pays my doctor to sell to me. In case you were wondering, my son *survived*! He got over it in only two days—about four days shorter than the average person who had the virus. Miracles happening everywhere!

Okay, enough with story time, let's get back on track. With your help, your lovely child will begin to develop physically and mentally from the nutrients you provide them with, and you will start to wonder if they're hitting all of their "milestones" a child "should hit." My son flourished and thrived, hitting milestones sometimes a *year* ahead of schedule (and when you're only two, that's a huge deal). In other words, I was reassured that he was being fueled properly.

Once a child hits school, it's a conveyor belt of learning. If they can't keep up, they will fall right off the belt (let's hope those bones are strong). There are numerous studies on the effects of poor nutrition on developing children. Not only can poor nutrition lead to diminished *physical* growth, but it can also lead to altered mental states like attention disorders and cognitive problems (which could all be grouped under "**malnutrition**" if you think about it!).[553, 560-563] If you feed crappy food to your child, you are, without a doubt, making it more difficult for them to learn and maintain good behavior. They may fall behind, get frustrated, and act out all because you're shoving the wrong shit down their pie-hole. Then, of course, they get carted off to the doctor, who slaps some term on them like "ADHD," prescribes them some pills, and voila! Problem solved!

Not quite. Not only is your child functioning at partial-capacity, but their little system is now getting pumped full of chemicals merely masking the problem, and in the same breath experiencing some pretty nasty side effects. What the heck are we doing to our poor little babies?! All they need is *food*. Proper pie-hole usage will allow their brains to function properly, and will give them clarity in everything they're trying to absorb. Their worn out teachers will actually have grounded, focused children in their classrooms, rather than chemical-filled crazy monsters who are scaling walls, throwing tantrums, and eating scissors.

The last step comes when—whether you want it to happen or not—your child reaches adulthood. It will get to a point where they'll have to make nutrition decisions on their own (when they leave for college, when they're at friends' houses, etc.). Only *then* will you see if you've provided them with the habits they need to survive and thrive, and not crash and burn at the bottom of the Nutrition Spectrum. Like I mentioned earlier, when I arrived at college I was suddenly surrounded by a bunch of shitty, chemical-filled, highly-processed foods. I tried them because I was curious. I also tried them because there was a food joint on campus—that we dubbed "the crack shack"—which would conveniently deliver greasy food straight to my door whenever I asked for it. It was like a five-star resort to me, and I was going to take advantage of the service if it was the last thing I did! Regrettably, I finally opened up my eyes and realized that campus food was killing me.

Due to my upbringing, I was thankfully able to make the educated decision to return to my nutritious food habits. Moral of the story: if you fuel your children properly, they *can* grow up to be smarter than smart, and *can* make smarter than smart decisions. Give them the best chance at survival.

* * *

"I already have children—is there hope?!" Nope. No hope— you're completely fucked. Your kids will most definitely wind up in juvie after their less-than-optimally-fueled brain told them it was okay to dress like a ninja and reenact *Gone in 60 Seconds*.

Of course there's hope! If you're a parent who already has kids, and you're already past the conception, pregnancy, and initial growth part, a challenge awaits. Don't stress about what you did or didn't do while you were trying to conceive, or while you were pregnant—that's over and done with and can't be changed. Move on and look forward. Focus on what you *can* change (e.g. the not-so-good habits your child(ren) may have acquired). Remember, you must try to avoid thinking about depriving them of certain foods they want, and instead think about depriving them of toxic chemicals and imminent disease. Buck up and do this. Whatever stage they're in, whatever habits they have, start NOW. If they're old enough to understand, tell them *why* you're making changes, and get them eating the same foods you are. Have fun with food, let them help cook, make foods colorful and in fun shapes; whatever it takes.

To the folks that make three different meals every night because your partner eats something different than you, and your child refuses to eat, let's say, vegetables: you're insane. In case you've forgotten, if *you're* cooking, then *you're* in charge. Make *one* nutritious meal that will fuel everyone, and call it a day. If your partner throws a tantrum, then they truly don't understand why you're making changes. Talk to them again, and get them on the same page. If your child throws a tantrum, it's not as easy because they most likely won't listen when you try to explain the importance of proper nutrition. It doesn't matter—you're still in charge. Be firm and try your best to make things fun. If they refuse to eat a meal, fine. Don't force it—they need to make the decision on their own if they don't' want to feel like they're being forced into something. They're not going to starve to death. They'll eventually give in and will have to choose to eat whatever is available to them. Let them know that these are the foods they'll be eating now, and the foods that will make them stronger and superheroesque. They need to know that a healthy diet won't kill them. In fact, it will help *not* kill them.

Before we move on, I realize that at the beginning of this guide I stated that no two people can eat the same way, and now I'm telling you to get your family to all eat the same foods. I'm not a complete moron, I promise. When I say you should cook *one* meal, it should encompass everyone's nutrient needs. And thank goodness your children are genetically similar to you, live in the same climate, and have the same foods available! I have found that most families can find one way of eating that works for the whole family, and makes everyone thrive.

In the rare case that one person physically feels miserable from the way you eat, well they'll have to figure out their own nutrition habits. For example, let's say someone is having trouble eating cucumbers. You can either eliminate cucumbers from everyone's diet, OR, you decide to make two meals; one that has cucumbers, and one that doesn't. If it were me, I'd simply want to make one cucumber-free meal and call it a day.

On top of that, let's not forget about portion control. Everyone's portions should be directly related to their age, gender, size and activity level. For example, you shouldn't evenly divide your meal between yourself, your three-hundred-pound husband who plays rugby twelve times per week, and your seventy-five-pound daughter who spends the whole week scrapbooking. Use your brain, and size portions appropriately.

Moral of the Story:

Children won't know what a donut is unless you present them with a donut. They also won't know what broccoli is, unless you present them with broccoli. If you want healthy, optimally-fueled kids, stay away from the fucking donut.

Chapter 39

Dumbass Debunking

Here's the truth: the majority of people in developed nations eat shit and are malnourished. Therefore, if you clean up your nutrition and wiggle your way up the Nutrition Spectrum to the "no disease" zone, you will officially be in the minority (eek!). People will judge you and consider you strange and extreme for being concerned about food additives, getting a water filter, buying from farmer's markets, and making your own food from scratch. It will happen. Many of those people will also say some pretty absurd and unreasonable things to you, mainly due to ignorance (by no fault of their own, as we have learned).

How do I know this? Because I've been the minority for a long time and have fielded some of the strangest questions or statements you could imagine. The most common question I field is: "so what do you eat? Grass?" Yup, now get out of my way so I can drop to all fours and graze, bitches! Hopefully I find a nice, buttery dandelion for dessert. Then, when I try to explain that all I, in fact, do is eat real food, they get even more confused and say, "like what?"

"Real food."

"Yeah, but like what?"

"Food that hasn't been fucked with."

"What do you mean?"

"Real food."

The Abbot and Costello conversation doesn't continue much further, because at this point we're both frustrated we're not getting anywhere. But hey, I know a good book that should explain my eating habits.

To help prepare you for the nutty statements and questions that may come your way, I have compiled some common examples (and appropriate responses) to ease your pain. Enjoy.

> **Question/statement**: "I have never met a healthy vegan or vegetarian." (Insinuating that if you don't consume meat, dairy, or eggs, you won't be healthy.)
>
> **Answer/rebuttal**: "They must not exist then! I have never met a healthy Argentinean either. Actually, I have never met an Argentinean, period. Argentineans must not exist!"

> **Question/statement**: "You must have to take supplements if you eat like that, right?"
>
> **Answer/rebuttal**: "I'm the one eating real food here. As in real food, with plenty of real nutrients. I'm less likely to need supplements than anyone else, and supplement pushers know to stay the hell away from me."

> **Question/statement**: "What do you *eat*?!" (If you're like me and eat a plant-based diet with rare appearances from meat, dairy, and eggs.)
>
> **Answer/rebuttal**: "Fucking FOOD. What the hell do *you* eat?!"

> **Question/statement**: "You can't possibly get all of your servings of fruits and veggies!" (Most supplement businesses will shout this at anyone within ear shot.)
>
> **Answer/rebuttal**: "See this hole here? (Point to mouth.) This is my pie-hole, and this is where I shall shove all of my servings of fruits and veggies."

Question/statement: "That's a little extreme, don't cha think?" (Referring to someone's "alternative"—a.k.a. *healthy*—eating habits.)

Answer/rebuttal: "Extreme? What about eating chemicals from a box that has sat on a shelf for a year, travelled half way across the country, and was pieced together from different nutrient-depleted ingredients from different corners of the world. *That* would seem extreme to me. Or wait, were you referring to this Captain America suit I'm wearing? Yeah, I guess that's a little extreme."

Question/statement: "I can't afford to eat healthy."
Answer/rebuttal: "Sure you can. Don't buy expensive food."

Question/statement: "I want to do a detox so I can get healthy."
Answer/rebuttal: "If your body is holding onto toxins, you don't need a detox, you need a new liver."

Question/Statement: "You'll have weak bones if you don't drink your [cow's] milk!"
Answer/Rebuttal: "Do you work for the dairy industry? Also, I'm not a cow, so I'd prefer not to nurse from one."

Question/Statement: "Where do you get your protein?" (Insinuating that protein only comes from "meat," and thus implies if someone doesn't eat meat, or only eats a little meat, they must be protein deficient.)
Answer/Rebuttal: "Would you ask a buffalo, panda, elephant, rhino, hippo, or gorilla that question? No? Well you should, because they eat less meat than I do." (Those animals are huge, strong-as-hell beasts, and also all herbivores— meaning their diets are comprised of 100% plant foods.)

Question/Statement: "But we've been eating (insert food here) for years!" (Insinuating that length in time something is consumed correlates with its safety, and therefore must be good for us)

Answer/Rebuttal: "You know what else we've been doing for even *longer* than eating (insert food here)? Murdering each other and using each other as slaves. Those things must be fair game too, then. Hey, want to be my slave?" (Say yes, or I'll murder you.)

Question/Statement: "It's okay that I ate at McDonald's, because I got the salad!"

Answer/Rebuttal: "False! Not only are you eating a month-old salad that's been leaking nutrients since it began its trip around the world and is probably sprayed with shit, shit, and more shit, but YOU ARE STILL FUCKING SUPPORTING A COMPANY THAT DOESN'T GIVE A SHIT ABOUT CONSUMER HEALTH. Stop buying from the problem. Don't support them in any way, even if you *think* one thing they make might be healthy. Chances are it's not, and your support to them is making them pump out more and more shitty products, making the greater problem worse. Sorry, my brain doesn't know how to handle statements like that."

Question/Statement: "Eating healthy means my food will taste like crap."

Answer/Rebuttal: "So, you've tasted crap? Oh, and by the way, *you're* going to be the one making your food. If tastes like crap, it's your own fucking fault."

Moral of the Story:

Once you sort your shit out, have fun fielding nutrition questions. After nutrition, laughter may just be the best medicine.

Chapter 40

Food Fight!!

The wonderful thing about food is you get three votes a day.
Every one of them has the potential to change the world.
—Michael Pollan

We have the right to know what we're consuming. Period. Anyone who disagrees with this is hiding something. We also have the right not to be dicked around by food companies who put harmful shit in consumables, and then market them as the latest-and-greatest. We also have the right to choose what foods we purchase, and where we purchase them from. Therefore, *we*, as consumers, have the ability to change the food industry. In the book *The Omnivore's Dilemma*, Michael Pollan puts it perfectly by stating: "But that's the challenge—to change the system more than it changes you." Let's fucking *change* this backward, disease-promoting food system!!

I want to start a food fight (WHO'S WITH ME?!). It's time to take back our food system, and gain control of what we're putting in our pie-holes. It's time for a food system that actually nourishes us and heals us. When I say "food fight," I, of course, mean taking a stand and boycotting the companies and organizations that don't deserve our time, attention, or dollars. Don't get me wrong, I would certainly *love* to hurl some meat loaf and custard at the FDA, medical schools, and food companies that have shown zero interest in our health. However, in reality, this is about everyone coming together, educating ourselves, and taking action that will lead to a better system.

Food and beverage products survive because people buy them. Plain and simple. Don't buy them, and they shrivel up and die (take that, bitches). Therefore, if we do this right, the shitty foods will die off and whole, organically grown, real foods will become "the norm" again. We will see disease of all forms dwindle or even cease to exist. Let's get this straight—we don't need laws to stop certain foods, beverages, or additives from being produced. And we certainly shouldn't hold our breath waiting for companies to change their ways. We simply need to STOP BUYING THEIR PRODUCTS AND SNUFF THEM OUT. We cut to the chase, go straight to the root of the problem, and without saying a word, tell them to fuck off.

The only way this is going to happen is if the consumer outsmarts the companies and organizations behind the madness. We must educate and raise awareness so we can all learn to see through all of their ridiculously misleading products and slogans (even if they're blaring from the "Health TV" at your doctor's office), and stop being so quick to jump on board the trendy nutrition crazes.

Which foods should we boycott? Pretty much anything with a marketing team behind it. Basically, anything making claims with a tag line, advertisement, or commercial. The foods you should be eating shouldn't *have* to make claims about having less sugar, less fat, or more protein. Healthy foods are generally untainted and untouched, and usually come tag-line free. Tag-lines, claims, and slogans should be viewed as marketing strategies, and huge red flags.

The food fight must begin now, before we're royally fucked and too sick to take action. We cannot let money-hungry companies manipulate and mind-fuck us. We must support the people who are growing, producing, and selling *real* food. Or, better yet, we must grow our own foods in our own gardens. By doing so, we can create a healthier society that functions better, has a heightened quality of life, creates smarter, more focused children, wastes less money on disease treatment, and has more money to spend on nutrition education. Essentially, we begin to thrive as a whole. Spread the word and get to it. It is up to us.

Fooood Fiiiiiiighttt!!

Moral of the Story:
Educate yourself and then vote like hell with your pie-hole.
Start a fucking FOOD FIGHT.

Chapter 41

Do Your Research, Dammit!

See this guidebook you're holding? Take a good look at it. It's merely the tip of the tip of the *tip* of the iceberg when it comes to nutrition knowledge (and even then you may need to read it several times to fully grasp the information it holds). It would take a lifetime to write about the whole, forever-evolving iceberg. Furthermore, just like nutrition is a multi-facetted expedition, so is health. And, just because you learn to use your pie-hole correctly, it doesn't mean you're in the clear. Your stress levels, your sleep patterns, what you put *on* your body, and your environmental factors are all contributing components when it comes to one's overall health. *But*, the closer you are to Captain America status on the Nutrition Spectrum, the more bitchin' of an immune system you will have, and the more likely you are to ward off anything that comes at you (except maybe Captain America himself).

As stated at the beginning of this guide, the scope of this book was to discuss nutrition-related ways to grab your health by the balls and tell it to buck up. Yet, I still stand firm when I say, "don't let people dictate what you put in your pie-hole." This includes me. I would rather you *doubt* my words than simply hop on my back and ride me to the future. Go out and research the fuck out of whatever changes you're considering. Just make sure you find reputable sources that don't work for the industry they're backing or researching—which will take research in itself.

Before you begin, I urge you to throw out your current beliefs. Start with a clean slate and build new beliefs as you go. Every story has two sides, and there are always people arguing both. You'll have to decide which side makes more sense to you. After years of research, I presented what I believed to make the most sense. You may hop on another train—and that's *okay*. At least you would have used your brain, learned about your body and health, and made *educated* decisions based off your findings. To assist you, I recommend reading, watching, and listening to people who have your well-being in their best interest.

Here are some places to start gaining knowledge. The more you read, see, listen, watch, and learn, the better. Now go forth and conquer, young food warrior! Up, up, and away!

Books to Read

- *Breaking the Food Seduction* by Neal Barnard
- *Cooked* by Michael Pollan
- *Diet for a New America* by John Robbins
- *Disease-Proof Your Child: Feeding Kids Right* by Joel Fuhrman
- *Eat, Drink, Vote* by Marion Nestle
- *Eating on the Wild Side* by Jo Robinson
- *Eat-Taste-Heal* by Thomas Yarema, Daniel Rhoda, and Johnny Brannigan
- *Food Politics* by Marion Nestle
- *Food Rules* by Michael Pollan
- *Forks Over Knives* by T. Colin Campbell, Caldwell B. Esselstyn, Jr., and Gene Stone
- *Healthy at 100* by John Robbins
- *How not to Die* by Michael Gregor
- *In Defense of Food* by Michael Pollan
- *My Beef with Meat* by Rip Esselstyn
- *Power Foods for the Brain* by Neal Barnard
- *Prevent and Reverse Heart Disease* by Caldwell B. Esselstyn, Jr.
- *The Art of Simple Food* by Alice Waters

- *The Cancer Survivor's Guide: Foods that Help You Fight Back* by Jennifer K. Reilly and Neal Barnard
- *The China Study* by T. Colin Campbell
- *The End of Dieting: How to Live for Life* by Joel Fuhrman
- *The Food Revolution* by John Robbins
- *The Forks Over Knives Plan* by Alona Pulde and Matthew Lederman
- *The Gerson Therapy* by Charlotte Gerson and Morton Walker
- *The Low-Carb Fraud* by T. Colin Campbell
- *The McDougall Program: Twelve Days to Dynamic Health* by John McDougall
- *The Okinawa Program* by Bradley J. Wilcox, D. Craig Wilcox, and Makoto Suzuki
- *The Omnivore's Dilemma* by Michael Pollan
- *The Plant-Based Journey* by Lani Muelrath
- *The Pleasure Trap* by Doug Lisle
- *The Starch Solution* by John McDougall
- *The Unhealthy Truth* by Robyn O'Brien
- *What to Eat* by Marion Nestle
- *Whole: Rethinking the Science of Nutrition* by T. Colin Campbell

Movies and Documentaries to Watch
- *Cowspiracy* (2014)
- *Crazy Sexy Cancer* (2007)
- *Cut Poison Burn* (2010)
- *Dirt! The Movie* (2009)
- *Dying to Have Known* (2006)
- *Earthlings* (2005)
- *Fat, Sick, and Nearly Dead* (2010)
- *Fat, Sick, and Nearly Dead 2* (2014)
- *Fed Up!* (2014)
- *Food Inc.* (2008)
- *Food Matters* (2008)
- *Forks Over Knives* (2011)
- *Frankensteer* (2005)

- *Fresh the Movie* (2009)
- *Heal Yourself, Heal the World* (2013)
- *Hungry For Change* (2012)
- *In Defense of Food* (2015)
- *King Corn* (2007)
- *One Man, One Cow, One **Planet*** (2007)
- *Open Sesame: The Story of Seeds* (2014)
- *PlantPure Nation* (2015)
- *Processed People* (2009)
- *Rethinking Cancer* (2009)
- *Second Opinion* (2014)
- *Simply Raw, Reversing Diabetes in 30 Days* (2009)
- *Super Size Me* (2004)
- *That Sugar Film* (2014)
- *The Beautiful Truth* (2008)
- *The Food Cure* (2015)
- *The Gerson Miracle* (2004)
- *The Human Experiment* (2015)
- *Vanishing of the Bees* (2009)

Applications to Use

- Buycott
- Calorie King
- Clean Plates
- Cronometer
- Farmstand
- Forks Over Knives
- Food Scores
- Fooducate
- GoodGuide
- HealthyOut
- Ingredient 1
- Non-GMO Project Shopping Guide
- Shopwell
- True Foods

Websites to Visit

- Calorie King (to look up calorie amounts of different foods and beverages): *www.calorieking.com*
- Center for Food Safety (to learn about food safety regulations, news, current events, etc.): *www.centerforfoodsafety.org*
- Cronometer (to log your food and get a detailed breakdown on the nutrients you may, or may not be, getting): *www.cronometer.com*
- eCornell Plant-Based Nutrition Certificate (to obtain more education about plant-based eating): *http://www.ecornell.com/certificates/plant-based-nutrition/certificate-in-plant-based-nutrition/*
- Environmental Working Group (a database that scores food based on the shit that's on it and how it's processed): *http://www.ewg.org/foodscores*
- Forks Over Knives (plant-based recipes!): *http://www.forksoverknives.com/recipes/*
- Fox News . . . just kidding! I wanted to see if you were still reading. Fox News: "where *not* to get your nutrition information."
- My Whole Food Life (recipes galore!): *http://mywholefoodlife.com/recipes/*
- Nutrient Database (to look up nutrient data in foods): *https://ndb.nal.usda.gov/ndb/search*
- Physicians Committee for Responsible Medicine: Food for Life Program (to learn and become certified to teach disease prevention and survival through nutrition): *http://www.pcrm.org/health/diets/ffl/training*
- Pub Med (for you science-y folks who want to read copious amounts of raw data on studies that have been done): *www.ncbi.nlm.nih.gov/pubmed*
- Non-GMO Project (to keep up to date on all of the latest GMO news and facts): *www.nongmoproject.org*
- Nutrition Data (to learn about what foods contain what nutrients): *www.nutritiondata.self.com*

- Nutrition in Medicine (offers FREE online courses on dozens of nutrition-related topics): *www.nutritioninmedicine.org*
- Plant-Based Doctor Database (to find a plant-based doctor near you): *www.plantbaseddoctors.org*
- Plant-Based Katie Mae (recipes!): *http://www.plantbasedkatie.com/project/recipes*
- Raw Food Recipes (more recipes!): *http://rawfoodrecipes.com/recipe-categories/*
- Sweet Potato Soul (even *more* recipes): *http://sweetpotatosoul.com/recipes*
- T. Colin Campbell Center for Nutrition Studies (plant-based recipes for days!): *http://nutritionstudies.org/recipes/*
- VitaMix (to check out the wonderful blender systems that will make you want to blend shit for days. Then you'll want to head over to *www.kidney.org/* to find out how to donate a kidney to pay for one): *www.vitamix.com/Home*
- What's on my food (to learn about what else you're buying when you don't buy organically grown foods): *www.whatsonmyfood.com*

Moral of the Story:
Knowledge isn't going to hurdle itself into your head.
Get out there, put in some long hours, and educate yourself. Be wise and nutritionize.

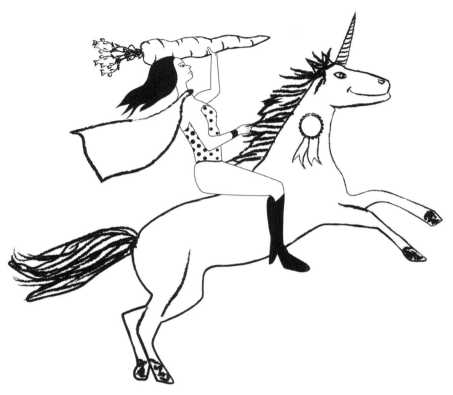

You ROCKSTAR—you fucking made it!
Now ride off into the sunset, you superhero!

Appendix A

The Morals of this Long-Ass Story

Introduction: Chances are you're confused as fuck about what you should be putting in your pie-hole. This guide will help you find the specific nutrients *you* need in order to achieve optimal health, eliminate disease, and return to your natural weight. Fist pumps all around.

SECTION I

Chapter 1: Following someone else's diet plan will get you nowhere. It's imperative to learn about *your* body and what nutrients it needs. If you have no aliments to speak of, and you can pull a tractor with your eyelids, you've nailed it.

Chapter 2: You don't need to be a professional, and you don't need a professional's help to fucking figure out how to EAT. You just need to know how to read (or be read to). Hey! I know a good book!

Chapter 3: Nutrition trumps exercise. End of story.

Chapter 4: Being "skinny" or "buff" does *not* mean you're "healthy." Malnourishment comes in many forms, and if you have any ailments of any kind, chances are you're malnourished. Nutrients, and not chemicals, should be used to heal malnourishment. Duh.

Chapter 5: Everything you consume becomes your fuel. Don't shove shit down your pie-hole and then act surprised when you feel or look like Turd McShitty. Grab your cape and haul your ass up that Nutrition Spectrum.

Chapter 6: Our food and healthcare systems are completely fucked up and have left people more confused than a fart in a fan factory. It seems as though *you* may have to take it upon yourself to fuel that brain up and pull yourself out.

Chapter 7: We're spending a buttload of money intervening and treating diseases, rather than focusing on preventing them from ever happening in the first place. That makes sense how?

SECTION II

Chapter 8: Nutrition is fucking COM-PLEX. But, you can't let that deter you. The Nutrition Triad concept—which will help factor in the amount, type, and variety of what you're shoving down your pie-hole—will let you discover how to adequately fuel yourself *and* fit into your Captain America suit.

Chapter 9: Your body requires a specific amount of fuel. That amount can change daily, and is impossible to pinpoint. However, for those of you who have absolutely no fucking clue how much food you're supposed to be eating, initially learning about calories can help you understand them and provide you with a range to shoot for.

Chapter 10: Finding the right amount of fuel is important, and will eventually become second nature. If you hate calorie counting and want to enjoy larger portions, focus on whole, plant foods.

Chapter 11: Drink more water, dammit.

SECTION III

Chapter 12: The *types* of nutrients you consume are far more significant than the *amount* you consume, or any diet label you feel like giving yourself. Choose the *healthiest* nutrients, and you'll prevent a ginormous crotch-hole from forming in your pants.

Chapter 13: Whole foods are the key to health. Find the ones that turn you into a plate-humper, and then shove them into the depths of your pie-hole as often as you're able.

Chapter 14: You heard the doc: your body will perceive most processed foods as sugar, and will drag you into a net of ailments, syndromes, and diseases. Most of the medical system is built on false assumptions that pills will solve those issues, when they most likely won't. Quit wasting your time going to the doctor for your lifestyle problems, and learn how to heal your body yourself.

Chapter 15: Food is made up of numerous types of nutrients, and can also be categorized into animal foods, plant foods, and processed foods. If you give two shits about your long-term health, you'll learn which types of foods to avoid, you'll head straight for the whole foods, and you'll chow down on the best, most untainted nutrients.

Chapter 16: A third of your calories should come from fats, so stop trying to hide from them. Instead, rip into the non-processed, whole foods that have healthy fats.

Chapter 17: Fear not the whole, high-carb foods. After all, half of your diet should come from them. Instead, fear the artificial and highly processed, nutrient-void, full-of-additives carbs that have been produced by none other than our very own food system.

Chapter 18: Don't be a protein pirate. Pull protein off its high horse and put it on the same horse as fats and carbohydrates.

Chapter 19: Have I mentioned that you should drink a bunch of water?

Chapter 20: To achieve optimal health, it's important to make sure everything you consume comes together to hit the recommended nutrient percentages. If you don't have ESP, I would recommend using a food logging site to assist you.

Chapter 21: Consumer products are littered with toxic chemicals—whether they're processed foods, restaurant foods, or whole foods that have been sprayed. If you don't want to grow third nipples (or get sick in general), you do your research and keep contaminated foods out of your fuckin' pie-hole.

Chapter 22: Don't ever assume consumables are safe; the food industry's toxic roots run deep.

Chapter 23: When making a decision on whether or not to incorporate a controversial product into your diet, do not take the advice of the industry you are questioning. Talk to people *outside* that industry. If you speak to someone *in* the industry about whether or not their product is safe and beneficial, it's like asking a car salesman if they think you look good in a Lamborghini.

Chapter 24: If you don't eat organic, you *will* be giving your insides a chemical-bath. Invest in your health, save yourself, and save your planet by eating as many organically grown foods as you're able.

SECTION IV

Chapter 25: Simply counting calories and eating the right types of foods won't get you in your superhero suit. Add *variety* to the mix, and—SHABAM—you'll be fighting superhero crime in no time.

Chapter 26: Getting the optimal percentages of macronutrients in your diet is key. Your body will respond with health and happiness, and a whole lot of beautiful, submarine-shaped poos.

Chapter 27: Malnutrition causes a million and one diseases and ailments. It's time we start looking to *nutrients* to cure mal*nutrition*. The best way to go about this is to consume a wide variety of whole, untainted foods.

Chapter 28: If you want to improve your health, eat *real* foods. Specifically, *plant* foods full of powerful nutrients that can't be found elsewhere. Don't waste your money by getting fake-ass nutrients out of a bottle. Ya hear?

Chapter 29: If you want to knock malnutrition on its ass, get a head start and take care of your nutritional deficiencies by consuming a juice or smoothie packed with relevant, kick-ass ingredients.

Chapter 30: If you (or someone you know) has cancer, there's a pretty good chance a change in diet can reverse or eliminate it. If you're the lucky bastard that *doesn't* have cancer, it's up to you to make the right nutrition decisions to prevent it.

Chapter 31: Disease sucks. There's overwhelming evidence that a diet high in animal foods and processed foods can increase your risk of disease, while a diet high in plant foods can help inhibit and cure disease. Therefore, in order to promote health, healing, and longevity, cram plant foods in your pie-hole.

SECTION V

Chapter 32: Use your brain not only to assemble a nutrition routine that is full of kick-ass nutrients, but one that is also mentally and physically satisfying.

Chapter 33: Learning how to use your pie-hole is never going to be as simple as "10 Simple Steps," so stop trying to make it such. Find the parts of your nutrition habits you're willing to change first, and begin the extensive journey. Focus on one small change at a time. String a bunch of small changes together. Be consistent. Be *perfectly* consistent. But don't you dare try to be perfect.

Chapter 34: Wherever the fuck you decide to hunt down your edibles, the majority of them should come *without* nutrition labels, and preferably be whole, organically grown, in-season foods.

Chapter 35: Eat some raw plant foods. Past that, try to cook minimally, with little to no oil, on low heat, and consume any resulting liquids along with your meal.

Chapter 36: Take the time **to** chew your food, you gluttonous vacuum! (That may or may not be a direct message for my husband.)

Chapter 37: Eating out is manageable if you know where to go, and what to look for on a menu. First step: start searching your area for restaurants, cafes, diners, or other eateries that may cater to your brilliant, new, healthy eating habits.

Chapter 38: Children won't know what a donut is unless you present them with a donut. They also won't know what broccoli is, unless you present them with broccoli. If you want healthy, optimally-fueled kids, stay away from the fucking donut.

Chapter 39: Once you sort your shit out, have fun fielding nutrition questions. After nutrition, laughter may just be the best medicine.

Chapter 40: Educate yourself and then vote like hell with your pie-hole. Start a fucking FOOD FIGHT.

Chapter 41: Knowledge isn't going to hurdle itself into your head. Get out there, put in some long hours, and educate yourself. Be wise and nutritionize.

Appendix B

Lists of Whole, Healthy, Plant Foods

Experimenting with new foods is like dating. You're probably going to find many of them to be strange and taste funny — but you keep going until you find the right match(es). The last thing you want to do is give up and go back to your last boyfriend who made you feel like shit. Thus, here are several lists of whole, healthy, nutrient-packed, health-promoting plant foods to experiment with — try them all, you little whore!

Let the speed dating begin. Try to find the foods that grow in your area and are in season; long-distance eating never ends well. Hit up the foods you've never eaten, and experiment with them. The more variety, the better! Some foods will taste like shit if you pair them together, and you may find some foods to just taste like shit in general. You'll learn your lesson. Or, maybe you won't if you're the type of person that dates the same, destructive, abusive asshole year after year.

Are the following lists complete? Of course not. There are hundreds of more foods out there, and each food may also have different varieties. Start circling the ones you want to date — I mean *experiment with* — and then search for recipes containing them. Get freaky-naughty and jump out of your comfort zone; I don't want you honing in on tomatoes and cucumbers and calling it a day. Tomatoes and cucumbers are technically fruits, by the way—so get out there and start learning!

Fruits

Fruits are generally the sweet foods that everyone prefers. However, many so-called "savory vegetables" are actually fruits. By definition, if it contains seeds (or a pit), it's a fruit. Surprise, surprise.

acai	fig	peach
acorn squash	goji berry	pear
apple	goldrush squash	persimmon
apricot	gooseberry	pineapple
aronia	grapefruit	plum
avocado	grape	pomegranate
banana	guava	pumpkin
bell pepper	honeydew melon	quince
bilimbi	horned melon	rambutan
black sapote	jackfruit	raspberry
blackberry	kiwi fruit	red kuri squash
blueberry	kumquat	rose hip
butternut squash	kundong	safou
button squash	lemon	sapodilla
cantaloupe	lime	sea buckthorn
cempedak	lychee	sloe
cherry	mandarin	soncoya
chili pepper	mango	spaghetti squash
cranberry	mangosteen	starfruit
cucumber	nectarine	strawberry
dragon fruit	okra	summmer ball zucchini
durian	olive	summer squash
eggplant	orange	tomato
elderberry	papaya	watermelon
feijoa	passion fruit	zucchini

Fungi

First, let's forget about the fact that you just cringed when you read the word "fungi." Second, many of these fantastic fungi come bearing small doses of vitamin D and vitamin B_{12}—two vitamins that are vital and often missing in many diets.

bolete mushroom	cremini mushroom	nutritional yeast
black fungus	enoki mushroom	porcini mushroom
button (white) mushroom	fresh yeast	portabella mushroom
black trumpet mushroom	maitake mushroom	shiitake mushroom
	matsutake mushroom	straw mushroom
	morel mushroom	truffle
chanterelle mushroom	oyster mushroom	

Herbs and Spices

Don't want bland food that tastes like cardboard? Add the following! Just not all at once.

anise	horseradish	perilla (red, green)
basil	kaffir lime	rosemary
bay leaf	lemongrass	sage
cardamom	marjoram	salt wort
cilantro	mint	stevia
cinnamon	mustard	tarragon
cumin	nutmeg	thai basil
curry	oregano	thyme
dill	paprika	turmeric
fennel	parsley	vanilla
fenugreek	pepper	wasabi root
galangal	peppermint	watercress

Legumes

If it grows inside a pod, it's a legume. If it fell to Earth in a pod, it's Superman. Become friends with both.

adzuki bean	groundnut	pinto bean
black bean	kidney bean	red noodle bean
black-eyed pea	lentil	snap pea
borlotti bean	lima bean	snow pea
cannellini bean	moringa	split pea
broad bean	mung bean	soy bean
garbanzo bean	navy bean	tamarind fruit
green bean	pigeonpea	yardlong bean

Nuts

Some of these are actually seeds (like almonds!), but let's pretend.

acorn	chestnut	macadamia nut
almonds	coconut	pine nut
beech nut	ginko nut	pistachio nut
brazil nut	hazelnut	peanut
bread nut	jack nut	pecan
cashew	kola nut	walnut

Seeds

Seeds are confusing in the sense that nuts are technically seeds, legumes are technically seeds, and some grains are technically seeds. But, here are a list of little, tasty, nutrient-dense morsels that are commonly known as "seeds."

cacao bean	fox nut	sesame seed
chia seed	hemp seed	pumpkin seed
coffee bean	lotus seed	sunflower seed
flax seed	poppy seed	

Vegetables

A vegetable is a stem, leaf, bud, or root. Anything that blossoms from a bud or flower and contains seeds is not a vegetable—it's a fruit. You learn something every day!

artichoke	dulse	parsnip
arugula	endive	potatoes
asparagus	fiddlehead ferns	radicchio
bamboo shoot	garlic	radish
beetroot (beet)	ginger	romaine lettuce
bok choy	green onion	romanesco
broccoli	iceberg lettuce	rhubarb
brussels sprouts	jicama	salsify
butter lettuce	kai-lan	samphire
cabbage	kale	silverbeet
carrots	kohlrabi	spinach
cassava	kumara	sunchoke
cauliflower	leek	sweet potato
celeriac	maca	tiger nut
celery	mustard greens	turnip
chard	nopales	water chestnut
chicory	oca	yam
collard greens	onion	yucca
daikon	pak choi	

Whole Grains

Some of these are seeds, but are generally used or cooked as a grain, so for fuck's sake, humor me.

amaranth	farro	rye
barley	freekeh	sorghum
black rice	kamut	spelt
brown rice	millet	teff
buckwheat	oat	wheat
corn	quinoa	wild rice

Appendix C

The Macronutrient Makeup of Foods

When you're confused about how to adjust your macronutrients (in order to more accurately hit the "sweet spot" ratios of fats, carbohydrates, and protein), look no further. Behold: a list of common food options, and the macronutrient percentages that comprise them.[93] I chose to also include water content—because water is awesome, and if you don't want to have a water bottle attached to your hip for the rest of your life, you may as well eat it instead.

All listed foods are raw, wild, and unpeeled unless otherwise noted. The cooked foods (noted with a star) are generally roasted or baked, or when it comes to grains, boiled. None are fried, battered, soaked in oil, covered in sugar, canned, or jarred. These are *foods*. They are not processed, man-made, shit-filled products. When people ask me what the heck I eat, and I say, "food," this is what I'm talking about.

Please remember that as foods are cooked (or cooked with different methods), the nutrients inside them will change, and therefore their macronutrient percentages may also change. Thus, if you take an apple, smother it with caramel and deep-fry it, don't expect it to boast the "apple" percentages listed here. Also, don't smother an apple with caramel and deep-fry it.

As an example of how this works, let's say you log your food and discover that your protein percentage is high and your carbohydrate percentage is low. You would want to reduce some of your high-protein foods, and add some high-carbohydrate foods—which this chart will help you with. Aim for the foods that have the highest percentages of carbohydrate when *compared* to their fat and protein percentages. For instance, carrots are only 10% carbs—but only because they're 88% water. Their fat and protein content is down around 1% each. Thus, carrots will boost your carb percentage, even though they only boast 10% carbs. The macronutrient with the highest percentage in each food has been highlighted for ease of searching.

You'll see I have included some plant foods *and* minimally-processed animal foods (and, of course, no processed foods). However, I will always say that plant foods trump animal foods (when it comes to health-promoting power, anyway). As you can see, the animal foods average around 25% protein. So, knowing what we know now—that our bodies only need around 10% protein—you can see how easily it is to have a high-protein, disease-promoting diet if you live off animal foods. You can also see how ridiculous it is to say that you're going to "cut out carbs."

Table C.1. Macronutrient percentages in common foods

Food	% Fat	%Carbs	% Protein	% Water
almonds	50%	22%	21%	4%
amaranth*	2%	19%	4%	75%
apple	<1%	14%	<1%	86%
artichoke (globe)*	<1%	12%	3%	84%
asparagus	<1%	4%	2%	93%
avocado	15%	9%	2%	73%
banana	<1%	23%	1%	75%
barley*	<1%	28%	2%	69%
beans* (black)	<1%	24%	9%	66%
beans* (kidney)	1%	23%	9%	67%
beef* (top sirloin steak)	6%	0%	29%	64%
beet	<1%	10%	2%	88%
blackberries	<1%	10%	1%	88%
blueberries	<1%	14%	1%	84%
broccoli	<1%	7%	3%	89%
brussels sprouts	<1%	9%	3%	86%
cabbage	<1%	6%	1%	92%
carrot	<1%	10%	1%	88%
cashews	44%	30%	18%	5%
cauliflower	<1%	5%	2%	92%
celery	<1%	3%	1%	95%
chard (swiss)	<1%	4%	2%	93%
cherries	<1%	8%	<1%	91%
chicken breast* (no skin)	4%	0%	31%	65%
chickpeas	6%	63%	20%	8%
clams*	2%	5%	26%	64%
corn*	1%	19%	3%	77%
crab (Alaska king)*	2%	0%	19%	78%
cranberries	<1%	12%	<1%	87%
cucumber	<1%	4%	1%	95%
currants (black)	<1%	15%	1%	82%
egg* (chicken)	11%	2%	12%	75%
eggplant*	<1%	9%	1%	90%
garlic	1%	33%	6%	59%
grapefruit	<1%	8%	1%	91%
grapes	<1%	18%	<1%	81%
jicama	<1%	9%	<1%	90%

Table C.1. (*continued*)

Food	% Fat	%Carbs	% Protein	% Water
kale	1%	9%	4%	84%
lamb* (shoulder chop)	15%	0%	31%	55%
lentils*	<1%	20%	9%	70%
lettuce (cos or romaine)	<1%	3%	1%	95%
lobster* (northern)	1%	0%	19%	78%
mango	<1%	15%	1%	83%
melon (cantaloupe)	<1%	8%	1%	90%
mushroom (portabella)	<1%	4%	2%	93%
mussels*	4%	7%	24%	61%
onion	<1%	9%	1%	89%
orange	<1%	13%	1%	86%
oysters (eastern)	2%	3%	6%	89%
peach	<1%	10%	1%	89%
pear	<1%	15%	<1%	84%
peas	<1%	8%	3%	89%
pepper (hot chili red)	<1%	9%	2%	88%
pepper (sweet red)	<1%	6%	1%	92%
plum	<1%	11%	1%	87%
pork* (center loin)	14%	0%	28%	58%
potato*	<1%	21%	3%	75%
pumpkin seeds	50%	11%	30%	5%
pumpkin*	<1%	5%	1%	94%
quinoa*	2%	21%	4%	72%
raspberries	1%	12%	1%	86%
salmon* (Atlantic)	8%	0%	25%	60%
seaweed (kelp)	1%	10%	2%	82%
shrimp*	<1%	<1%	24%	74%
spinach	<1%	4%	3%	91%
squash* (acorn)	<1%	15%	1%	83%
strawberries	<1%	8%	1%	91%
sweet potato*	<1%	21%	2%	76%
tomato	<1%	4%	1%	95%
tuna* (bluefin)	6%	0%	30%	60%
walnuts	65%	14%	15%	4%
wild rice*	<1%	21%	4%	74%
zucchini	<1%	3%	1%	95%

*cooked versions

Appendix D

The Micronutrient
Makeup of Foods

Most people focus on the *macro*nutrients of food, forgetting all about these powerful little gems that actually do most of the disease-fighting. Keep in mind, I'm talking about the *real* versions of micronutrients—not the artificial crap that's pumped into every nutrient-depleted box or can on a shelf somewhere. If you're worried that you're deficient in a certain vitamin or mineral, find that nutrient and head down the chart to and see which foods may give you a top up. The five plant foods with the highest amount of each nutrient have been highlighted to make this easier. Of course, this list of foods doesn't represent all foods available on this planet, so you'll have to research further if a food isn't listed here. It also doesn't list all vitamins and minerals, nor smaller nutrients like phytonutrients and antioxidants, because . . . baby steps. You'll find two charts here: one for vitamin content, and one for mineral content. Get to know both.

These are the same common foods listed in the macronutrient charts of Appendix C. Again, all foods are raw, wild, and unpeeled unless otherwise noted. The cooked foods (noted with a star) are generally roasted or baked, or when it comes to grains, boiled. None are fried, battered, soaked in oil, covered in sugar, canned, or jarred. Please remember that as foods are cooked (or cooked with different methods), the nutrients inside them will change, and therefore their micronutrient percentages will most definitely change.

Since these nutrients are the "small" guys, I'm not going to express them in percentages as I did for fats, carbohydrates, and protein (they'd come out like 0.004%, which sounds pretty shitty). Don't be fooled though—just because these nutrients are smaller doesn't mean they don't pack a punch. In fact, this "punch" is what's missing from most people's diets who wind up sick and miserable.

Instead, micronutrients will be expressed in the amount you get from every *one hundred milligrams* (mg) of food you eat. Since that sounds a bit confusing, simply check out which foods have the largest numbers of each nutrient next to them (regardless if that number seems small). For example, check out the vitamin A in carrots. That number is ginormous compared to the vitamin A in other foods. Therefore, if you regularly eat carrots, chances are you don't have a vitamin A deficiency. There's so much you can learn from these charts if you spend some time with them. How about the vitamin K in chard! Or the fact that oranges don't even make the top five cut for vitamin C. See what else you can discover—like asparagus having more iron than steak. Crazy. And, if you don't want to eat almonds, chickpeas, pumpkin seeds, and spinach after perusing these charts, you're wrong. You do want to eat them.

Table D.1. Vitamin amounts in 100g of common foods (expressed in mg unless otherwise noted)[93]

Food	A (IU)	B₁	B₂	B₃	B₆	B₉ (µg)	B₁₂ (µg)	C	E	K (µg)
almonds	2	0.21	1.14	3.62	0.14	44	0.00	0.00	25.63	0.00
amaranth*	--	0.02	0.02	0.24	0.11	--	--	--	0.19	--
apple	54	0.02	0.03	0.09	0.04	3	0.00	4.60	0.18	2.20
artichoke (globe)*	13	0.05	0.09	1.11	0.08	89	0.00	7.40	0.19	14.80
asparagus	756	0.14	0.14	0.98	0.09	52	0.00	5.60	1.13	41.60
avocado	146	0.07	0.13	1.74	0.26	81	0.00	10.00	2.07	21.00
banana	64	0.03	0.07	0.67	0.37	20	0.00	8.70	0.10	0.50
barley*	7	0.08	0.06	2.06	0.12	16	0.00	0.00	0.01	0.80
beans* (black)	6	0.24	0.06	0.51	0.07	149	0.00	0.00	--	--
beans* (kidney)	0	0.16	0.06	0.58	0.12	130	0.00	1.20	0.03	8.40
beef* (top sirloin steak)	0	0.08	0.15	8.42	0.63	11	1.68	0.00	0.38	1.40
beet	2	0.03	0.04	0.33	0.07	109	0.00	4.90	0.04	0.20
blackberries	214	0.02	0.03	0.65	0.03	25	0.00	21.00	1.17	19.80
blueberries	80	0.06	0.06	0.62	0.08	9	0.00	14.40	0.84	28.60
broccoli	623	0.07	0.12	0.64	0.18	63	0.00	89.20	0.78	101.60
brussels sprouts	754	0.14	0.90	0.75	0.22	61	0.00	85.00	0.88	177.00
cabbage	98	0.06	0.04	0.23	0.12	43	0.00	36.60	0.15	76.00
carrot	16,706	0.07	0.06	0.98	0.14	19	0.00	5.90	0.66	13.20
cashews	0.00	0.42	0.06	1.06	0.42	25	0.00	0.50	0.90	34.10
cauliflower	0.00	0.05	0.06	0.51	0.18	57	0.00	48.20	0.08	15.50
celery	449	0.02	0.06	0.32	0.07	36	0.00	3.10	0.27	29.30

Table D.1. (*continued*)

Food	A (IU)	B₁	B₂	B₃	B₆	B₉ (µg)	B₁₂ (µg)	C	E	K (µg)
chard (swiss)	6,116	0.04	0.09	0.40	0.10	14	0.00	30.00	1.89	830.00
cherries	64	0.03	0.03	0.15	0.05	4	0.00	7.00	0.07	2.10
chicken breast*(no skin)	93	0.07	0.12	12.71	0.56	4	0.32	0.00	0.27	0.30
chickpeas	67	0.48	0.21	1.54	0.54	557	0.00	4.00	0.82	9.00
clams*	570	0.15	0.43	3.35	0.11	29	98.89	22.10	--	--
corn*	199	0.03	0.06	1.31	0.10	35	0.00	3.50	0.07	0.30
crab (Alaska king)*	29	0.05	0.06	1.34	0.18	51	11.50	7.60	--	5.10
cranberries	60	0.01	0.02	0.10	0.06	1	0.00	13.30	1.20	
cucumber	105	0.03	0.03	0.10	0.04	7	0.00	2.80	0.03	16.40
currants (black)	230	0.05	0.05	0.30	0.07	--	0.00	181.00	1.00	
egg* (chicken)	520	0.07	0.51	0.06	0.12	44	1.11	0.00	1.03	0.30
eggplant*	37	0.08	0.02	0.60	0.09	14	0.00	1.30	0.41	2.90
garlic	9	0.20	0.11	0.70	1.24	3	0.00	31.20	0.08	1.70
grapefruit	927	0.04	0.02	0.25	0.04	10	0.00	46.00	34.40	0.00
grapes	100	0.09	0.06	0.30	0.11	4	0.00	4.00	0.19	14.60
jicama	21	0.02	0.03	0.20	0.04	12	0.00	20.20	0.46	0.30
kale	9,990	0.11	0.13	1.00	0.27	141	0.00	120.00	1.54	704.80
lamb* (shoulder chop)	49	0.05	0.19	2.67	0.10	--	2.11	0.00	0.69	--
lentils*	8	0.17	0.07	1.06	0.18	181	0.00	1.50	0.11	1.70
lettuce (cos or romaine)	8,710	0.07	0.07	0.31	0.07	136	0.00	4.00	0.13	102.50
lobster* (northern)	4	0.02	0.02	1.83	0.12	11	1.43	0.00	1.00	0.00
mango	1,082	0.03	0.04	0.67	0.12	43	0.00	36.40	0.90	4.20

melon (cantaloupe)	3,382	0.04	0.02	0.73	0.07	21	0.00	36.70	0.05	2.50
melon (watermelon)	569	0.03	0.02	0.18	0.05	3	0.00	8.10	0.05	0.10
mushroom (portabella)	0	0.06	0.13	4.49	0.15	28	0.05	0.00	0.02	0.00
mussels*	304	0.30	0.42	3.00	0.10	76	24.0	33.00	--	--
onion	2	0.05	0.03	0.15	0.12	19	0.00	7.40	0.02	0.40
orange	225	0.10	0.04	0.40	0.05	17	0.00	45.00	0.18	0.00
oysters (eastern)	44	0.02	0.09	0.93	0.03	7	8.75	0.00	0.85	1.00
peach	326	0.02	0.03	0.81	0.03	4	0.00	6.60	0.73	2.60
pear	25	0.01	0.03	0.16	0.03	7	0.00	4.30	0.12	4.40
peas	765	0.27	0.13	2.09	0.17	65	0.00	40.00	0.13	24.80
pepper (hot chili red)	952	0.07	0.09	1.24	0.51	23	0.00	143.70	0.69	14.00
pepper (sweet red)	3,131	0.05	0.09	0.98	0.29	46	0.00	127.70	1.58	4.90
plum	345	0.03	0.03	0.42	0.03	5	0.00	9.50	0.26	6.40
pork* (center loin)	14	0.52	0.34	7.87	0.52	0	0.66	0.00	0.19	0.00
potato*	10	0.05	0.04	1.53	0.21	38	0.00	12.60	0.04	2.70
pumpkin seeds	16	0.23	0.15	4.99	0.14	58	0.00	1.90	2.18	7.30
pumpkin*	288	0.03	0.08	0.41	0.04	9	0.00	4.70	0.80	0.80
quinoa*	5	0.11	0.11	0.41	0.12	42	0.00	0.00	0.63	0.00
raspberries	33	0.03	0.04	0.60	0.06	21	0.00	26.20	0.87	7.80
salmon* (Atlantic)	44	0.28	0.49	10.07	0.94	29	3.05	0.00	--	--
seaweed (kelp)	116	0.05	0.15	0.47	0.00	180	0.00	3.00	0.87	66.00
shrimp*	301	0.03	0.02	2.68	0.24	24	1.66	0.00	2.20	0.40
spinach	9,377	0.08	0.19	0.72	0.20	194	0.00	28.10	2.03	482.90
squash* (acorn)	428	0.17	0.01	0.88	0.19	19	0.00	10.80	--	--

Table D.1. (*continued*)

Food	A (IU)	B₁	B₂	B₃	B₆	B₉ (µg)	B₁₂ (µg)	C	E	K (µg)
strawberries	12	0.02	0.02	0.39	0.05	24	0.00	58.80	0.29	2.20
sweet potato*	19,218	0.11	0.11	1.49	0.29	6	0.00	19.60	0.71	2.30
tomato	833	0.04	0.02	0.59	0.08	15	0.00	13.70	0.54	7.90
tuna* (bluefin)	2,520	0.28	0.31	10.54	0.53	2	10.88	0.00	--	--
walnuts	20	0.34	0.15	1.13	0.54	98	0.00	1.30	0.70	2.70
wild rice*	3	0.05	0.09	1.29	0.14	26	0.00	0.00	0.24	0.50
zucchini	200	0.05	0.09	0.45	0.16	24	0.00	17.90	0.12	4.30

*cooked versions, IU = International Units, µg = micrograms

Table D.2. Mineral amounts in 100 grams of common foods (expressed in mg unless otherwise noted)[93]

Food	calcium	iron	magnesium	phosphorus	potassium	sodium	zinc
almonds	269	3.71	270	481	733	1	3.12
amaranth*	47	2.10	65	148	135	6	0.86
apple	6	0.12	5	11	107	1	0.04
artichoke (globe)*	21	0.61	42	73	286	60	0.40
asparagus	24	2.14	14	52	202	2	0.54
avocado	12	0.55	29	52	485	7	0.64
banana	5	0.26	27	22	358	1	0.15
barley*	11	1.33	22	54	93	3	0.82
beans* (black)	27	2.10	70	140	355	1	1.12
beans* (kidney)	35	2.22	42	138	405	1	1.00
beef* (top sirloin steak)	19	1.87	25	233	376	61	5.46
beet	16	0.80	23	40	325	78	0.35
blackberries	29	0.62	20	22	162	1	0.53
blueberries	9	0.41	9	18	114	1	0.24
broccoli	47	0.73	21	66	316	33	0.41
brussels sprouts	42	1.40	23	69	389	25	0.42
cabbage	40	0.47	12	26	170	18	0.18
carrot	33	0.30	12	35	320	69	0.24
cashews	37	6.68	292	593	660	12	5.78
cauliflower	22	0.42	15	44	299	30	0.27
celery	40	0.20	11	24	260	80	0.13

Table D.2. (*continued*)

Food	calcium	iron	magnesium	phosphorus	potassium	sodium	zinc
chard (swiss)	51	1.80	81	46	379	213	0.36
cherries	13	0.36	11	21	222	0	0.07
chicken breast* (no skin)	14	1.07	27	214	245	71	1.02
chickpeas	57	4.31	79	252	718	24	2.76
clams*	92	2.81	18	338	628	1,202	2.73
corn*	3	0.47	28	79	233	1	0.63
crab (Alaska king)*	59	0.76	63	280	262	1,072	7.62
cranberries	8	0.25	6	13	85	2	0.10
cucumber	16	0.28	13	24	147	2	0.20
currants (black)	55	1.54	24	59	322	2	0.27
egg* (chicken)	50	1.19	10	172	126	124	1.05
eggplant*	6	0.25	11	15	123	1	0.12
garlic	181	1.70	25	153	401	17	1.16
grapefruit	12	0.09	8	8	139	0	0.07
grapes	14	0.29	5	10	191	2	0.04
jicama	12	0.60	12	18	150	4	0.16
kale	150	1.47	47	92	491	38	0.56
lamb* (shoulder chop)	34	1.74	20	162	207	57	5.35
lentils*	19	3.33	36	180	369	2	1.27
lettuce (cos or romaine)	33	0.97	14	30	247	8	0.23
lobster* (northern)	96	0.29	43	185	230	486	4.05
mango	11	0.16	10	14	168	1	0.09

melon (cantaloupe)	9	0.21	12	15	267	16	0.18
melon (watermelon)	7	0.24	10	11	112	1	0.10
mushroom (portabella)	3	0.31	--	108	364	9	0.53
mussels*	33	6.72	37	285	268	369	2.67
onion	23	0.21	10	29	146	4	0.17
orange	43	0.09	10	12	169	0	0.08
oysters (eastern)	59	4.61	18	97	156	85	39.30
peach	6	0.25	9	20	190	0	0.17
pear	9	0.18	7	12	116	1	0.10
peas	25	1.47	33	108	244	5	1.24
pepper (hot chili red)	14	1.03	23	43	322	9	0.26
pepper (sweet red)	7	0.43	12	26	211	4	0.25
plum	6	0.17	7	16	157	0	0.10
pork* (center loin)	55	0.86	20	225	273	73	3.28
potato*	10	0.64	27	75	544	7	0.35
pumpkin seeds	46	8.82	592	1,233	809	7	7.81
pumpkin*	15	0.57	9	30	230	1	0.23
quinoa*	17	1.49	64	152	172	7	1.09
raspberries	25	0.69	22	29	151	1	0.42
salmon* (Atlantic)	15	1.03	37	256	628	56	0.82
seaweed (kelp)	168	2.85	121	42	89	233	1.23
shrimp*	91	0.32	37	306	170	947	1.63
spinach	99	2.71	79	49	558	79	0.53
squash* (acorn)	44	0.93	43	45	437	4	0.17

Table D.2. (*continued*)

Food	calcium	iron	magnesium	phosphorus	potassium	sodium	zinc
strawberries	16	0.41	13	24	153	1	0.14
sweet potato*	38	0.69	27	54	475	36	0.32
tomato	10	0.27	11	24	237	5	0.17
tuna* (bluefin)	10	1.31	64	326	323	500	0.77
walnuts	98	2.91	158	346	441	2	3.09
wild rice*	3	0.60	32	82	101	3	1.34
zucchini	16	0.37	18	38	261	8	0.32

*cooked versions, IU = International Units, μg = micrograms

Appendix E

Should I Eat It?

I don't know. *Should* you eat it? Ultimately, that's up to you. However, on the following page you'll find an intricate flow chart that will help you answer that very question. This flow chart represents the process my brain goes through prior to consuming something. I'm not joking. Thankfully, I'm skilled in the art of eating, so the whole process only takes a fraction of a second. For you, it may take longer until you get the hang of it.

Truly though, if you're going to train your brain to make smart decisions about what your choosing to fill your pie-hole with, and you don't want to feel like shit for eternity, you must ask yourself some valid questions. Maybe there are more that will go through your head than are presented here. Any way you look at it, if you're firing up that brain before you throw something down the chute, you're headed in the right direction. Give it a whirl!

Side note: this flow chart only works for foods and beverages. I'll leave you to your own devices if you're about to chomp down on some toothpaste, cigarettes, pills, oral contraceptives, etc.

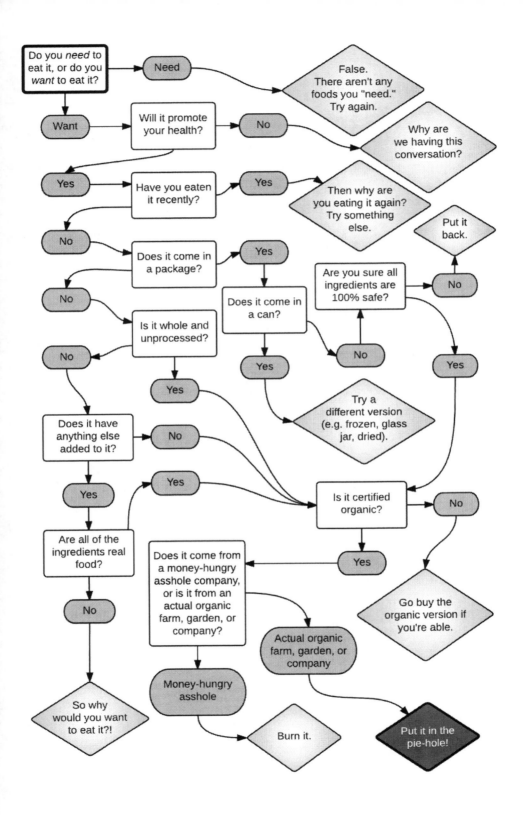

References

1. *Randomised trial of cholesterol lowering in 4444 patients with coronary heart disease: the Scandinavian Simvastatin Survival Study (4S)*. Lancet, 1994. **344**(8934): p. 1383-9.
2. Downs, J.R., et al., *Primary prevention of acute coronary events with lovastatin in men and women with average cholesterol levels: Results of afcaps/texcaps*. JAMA, 1998. **279**(20): p. 1615-1622.
3. Plehn, J.F., et al., *Reduction of stroke incidence after myocardial infarction with pravastatin: the Cholesterol and Recurrent Events (CARE) study. The Care Investigators*. Circulation, 1999. **99**(2): p. 216-23.
4. *MRC/BHF Heart Protection Study of cholesterol lowering with simvastatin in 20,536 high-risk individuals: a randomised placebo-controlled trial*. Lancet, 2002. **360**(9326): p. 7-22.
5. Kulbertus, H. and A.J. Scheen, *The PROSPER Study (PROspective study of pravastatin in the elderly at risk)*. Rev Med Liege, 2002. **57**(12): p. 809-13.
6. Colhoun, H.M., et al., *Primary prevention of cardiovascular disease with atorvastatin in type 2 diabetes in the Collaborative Atorvastatin Diabetes Study (CARDS): multicentre randomised placebo-controlled trial*. Lancet, 2004. **364**(9435): p. 685-96.
7. Tonkin, A.M., et al., *Cost-effectiveness of cholesterol-lowering therapy with pravastatin in patients with previous acute coronary syndromes aged 65 to 74 years compared with younger patients: results from the LIPID study*. Am Heart J, 2006. **151**(6): p. 1305-12.
8. Ford, I., et al., *Long Term Safety and Efficacy of Lowering LDL Cholesterol With Statin Therapy: 20-Year Follow-Up of West of Scotland Coronary Prevention Study*. Circulation, 2016.
9. Dahlof, B., et al., *Prevention of cardiovascular events with an antihypertensive regimen of amlodipine adding perindopril as required versus atenolol adding bendroflumethiazide as required, in the Anglo-*

Scandinavian Cardiac Outcomes Trial-Blood Pressure Lowering Arm (ASCOT-BPLA): a multicentre randomised controlled trial. Lancet, 2005. **366**(9489): p. 895-906.

10. Whitmer, R.W., et al., *A wake-up call for corporate America.* J Occup Environ Med, 2003. **45**(9): p. 916-25.

11. Kris-Etherton, P., et al., *AHA Science Advisory: Lyon Diet Heart Study. Benefits of a Mediterranean-style, National Cholesterol Education Program/American Heart Association Step I Dietary Pattern on Cardiovascular Disease.* Circulation, 2001. **103**(13): p. 1823-5.

12. Macknin, M., et al., *Plant-based, no-added-fat or American Heart Association diets: impact on cardiovascular risk in obese children with hypercholesterolemia and their parents.* J Pediatr, 2015. **166**(4): p. 953-9.e1-3.

13. Plotnick, G.D., M.C. Corretti, and R.A. Vogel, *Effect of antioxidant vitamins on the transient impairment of endothelium-dependent brachial artery vasoactivity following a single high-fat meal.* Jama, 1997. **278**(20): p. 1682-6.

14. Krogsboll, L.T., et al., *General health checks in adults for reducing morbidity and mortality from disease: Cochrane systematic review and meta-analysis.* Bmj, 2012. **345**: p. e7191.

15. Casselman, A. *Identical Twins' Genes Are Not Identical.* Scientific American 2008; Available from: http://www.scientificamerican.com/article/identical-twins-genes-are-not-identical/.

16. World Health Organization, Nutrition for Health and Development, and Sustainable Development and Healthy Environments. *Nutrition for Health and Development: A Global Agenda for Combating Malnutrition.* 2000; Available from: file:///C:/Users/office/Documents/WHIM/Book/References/WHO_NHD_00.6.pdf.

17. Wolters Kluwer Health, *Wolters Kluwer Health 2011 Point-of-Care Survey,* in *Featured Finding: Physicians Challenged By Lack of Time with Patients.* 2011.

18. Dunaif, G.E. and T.C. Campbell, *Dietary protein level and aflatoxin B1-induced preneoplastic hepatic lesions in the rat.* J Nutr, 1987. **117**(7): p. 1298-302.

19. Appleton, B.S. and T.C. Campbell, *Effect of high and low dietary protein on the dosing and postdosing periods of aflatoxin B1-induced hepatic*

preneoplastic lesion development in the rat. Cancer Res, 1983. **43**(5): p. 2150-4.

20. Dunaif, G.E. and T.C. Campbell, *Relative contribution of dietary protein level and aflatoxin B1 dose in generation of presumptive preneoplastic foci in rat liver.* J Natl Cancer Inst, 1987. **78**(2): p. 365-9.

21. Horio, F., et al., *Thermogenesis, low-protein diets, and decreased development of AFB1-induced preneoplastic foci in rat liver.* Nutr Cancer, 1991. **16**(1): p. 31-41.

22. Youngman, L.D. and T.C. Campbell, *The sustained development of preneoplastic lesions depends on high protein intake.* Nutr Cancer, 1992. **18**(2): p. 131-42.

23. Minute Maid. *Minute Maid® Enhanced Pomegranate Blueberry Flavored 100% Juice Blend of 5 juices - 59 fl oz Bottle.* 2012 [cited 2012; Available from: http://www.minutemaid.com/enhanced-juice-drinks/pomegranate-blueberry-flavor-59-fl-oz-bottle.

24. Liptak, A., *Coke Can Be Sued by Rival Over Juice Claim, Court Says*, in *New York Times.* 2014: Business Day.

25. Doctor's Associates Inc. and Subway Sandwiches, *Student Guide*, in *Welcome To The Student And Educator Resource Guide.* 2010.

26. Kindy, K. *Food additives on the rise as FDA scrutiny wanes.* 2014 17 August, 2014; Available from: http://www.washingtonpost.com/national/food-additives-on-the-rise-as-fda-scrutiny-wanes/2014/08/17/828e9bf8-1cb2-11e4-ab7b-696c295ddfd1_story.html.

27. Herman, R., *Following the Government's Food Pyramid Has Limited Effect on Risk of Major Chronic Disease.* 2000, Harvard School of Public Health.

28. McCullough, M.L., et al., *Adherence to the Dietary Guidelines for Americans and risk of major chronic disease in men.* Am J Clin Nutr, 2000. **72**(5): p. 1223-1231.

29. McCullough, M.L., et al., *Adherence to the Dietary Guidelines for Americans and risk of major chronic disease in women.* Am J Clin Nutr, 2000. **72**(5): p. 1214-1222.

30. U.S. Department of Agriculture and U.S. Department of Health and Human Services, *Dietary Guidelines for Americans 2010.* 2010: Washington, D.C.

31. McVey, J.S., *Court Rules Against USDA's Secrecy and Failure to Disclose Conflict of Interest in Setting Nutrition Policies.* 2000, The Physicians Committee Washington, DC.

32. Dolinsky, V.W., et al., *Improvements in skeletal muscle strength and cardiac function induced by resveratrol during exercise training contribute to enhanced exercise performance in rats.* J Physiol, 2012. **590**(Pt 11): p. 2783-99.

33. Goodson, W.H., 3rd, et al., *Assessing the carcinogenic potential of low-dose exposures to chemical mixtures in the environment: the challenge ahead.* Carcinogenesis, 2015. **36 Suppl 1**: p. S254-96.

34. Barbash, F. *Major publisher retracts 43 scientific papers amid wider fake peer-review scandal.* 2015; Available from: http://www.washingtonpost.com/news/morning-mix/wp/2015/03/27/fabricated-peer-reviews-prompt-scientific-journal-to-retract-43-papers-systematic-scheme-may-affect-other-journals/?postshare=4081427725759269.

35. Institue of Medicine, *Crossing The Quality Chasm: A New Health System For The 21st Century*, in *Shaping the Future for Health*, N.A. Press, Editor. 2001, National Academy of Sciences: Washington, D.C.

36. Basow, D., *The Physician's Conundrum: Too Much Information, Too Little Time*, in *Medical Practice Insider: Business & Technology Intelligence For Physician Practices.* 2013.

37. Adams, K.M., M. Kohlmeier, and S.H. Zeisel, *Nutrition Education in U.S. Medical Schools: Latest Update of a National Survey.* Academic Medicine, 2010. **85**(9): p. 1537-1542.

38. Kraschnewski, J.L., et al., *A Silent Response to the Obesity Epidemic: Decline in US Physician Weight Counseling.* Medical Care, 2013. **51**(2): p. 186–192.

39. Parker, W.A., et al., *They think they know but do they? Misalignment of perceptions of lifestyle modification knowledge among health professionals.* Public Health Nutr, 2011. **14**(8): p. 1429-38.

40. Greger, M. *Medical Associations Oppose Bill to Mandate Nutrition Training.* Nutrition Videos 2011 14 November, 2011]; Available from: http://nutritionfacts.org/video/medical-associations-oppose-bill-to-mandate-nutrition-training/.

41. The California Academy of Preventive Medicine, *Senate Committee On Business, Professions And Economic Development: SB 380.* 2011.

42. Lazarou, J., B.H. Pomeranz, and P.N. Corey, *Incidence of adverse drug reactions in hospitalized patients: a meta-analysis of prospective studies.* Jama, 1998. **279**(15): p. 1200-5.

43. Kleinrock, M., *The Use of Medicines in the United States: Review of 2010.* 2001, IMS Institute for Healthcare Informatics.

44. Mayo Clinic. *Simvastatin (Oral Route)*. Drugs and Supplements 2014; Available from: http://www.mayoclinic.org/drugs-supplements/simvastatin-oral-route/side-effects/drg-20069006.

45. Merck & Co., *ZOCOR (simvastatin) Tablets*. 1991, Merck Sharp & Dohme LTD: Whitehouse Station, NJ.

46. Gray, S.L., et al., *Cumulative use of strong anticholinergics and incident dementia: A prospective cohort study*. JAMA Internal Medicine, 2015. **175**(3): p. 401-407.

47. Ornish, D., et al., *Can lifestyle changes reverse coronary heart disease?: The Lifestyle Heart Trial*. The Lancet, 1990. **336**(8708): p. 129-133.

48. World Health Organization. *Fact Sheet: Cardiovascular diseases (CVDs)*. 2013; N 317:[Available from: http://www.who.int/mediacentre/factsheets/fs317/en/.

49. eCornell: T. Colin Campbell Center for Nutrition Studies, *Plant-Based Nutrition: Principles in Practice - Module 3 (TCC503)*. 2014.

50. Carey, J. and A. Barrett. *Is Heart Surgery Worth It?* 2005; Available from: http://www.bloomberg.com/bw/stories/2005-07-06/is-heart-surgery-worth-it.

51. PBS. *Health Costs: How the U.S. Compares With Other Countries*. PBS Newshour 2012 [cited 2012; Available from: http://www.pbs.org/newshour/rundown/health-costs-how-the-us-compares-with-other-countries/.

52. Munro, D. *Annual U.S. Healthcare Spending Hits $3.8 Trillion*. Parma & Healthcare 2014; Available from: http://www.forbes.com/sites/danmunro/2014/02/02/annual-u-s-healthcare-spending-hits-3-8-trillion/.

53. World Health Organization, *The World Health Report 2000: Health Systems: Improving Performance*. 2000: France.

54. Ford, E.S., L.M. Maynard, and C. Li, *Trends in mean waist circumference and abdominal obesity among US adults, 1999-2012*. Jama, 2014. **312**(11): p. 1151-3.

55. Centers for Disease Control and Prevention, *CDC estimates 1 in 88 children in United States has been identified as having an autism spectrum disorder*. 2012.

56. Autism Science Foundation. *How Common is Autism?* 2015; Available from: http://www.autismsciencefoundation.org/what-is-autism/how-common-is-autism.

57. Centers for Disease Control and Prevention, *Prevalence of Autism Spectrum Disorder Among Children Aged 8 Years — Autism and*

Developmental Disabilities Monitoring Network, 11 Sites, United States, 2010, in *Morbidity and Mortality Weekly Report*. 2014, US Department of Health and Human Services: Atlanta, GA.

58. Landrigan, P., L. Lambertini, and L. Birnbaum, *A Research Strategy to Discover the Environmental Causes of Autism and Neurodevelopmental Disabilities*. Environmental Health Perspectives, 2012. **120**(7).

59. Lavelle, T.A., et al., *Economic burden of childhood autism spectrum disorders*. Pediatrics, 2014. **133**(3): p. e520-e529.

60. Jackson, K.D., L.D. Howie, and L.J. Akinbami, *Trends in Allergic Conditions Among Children: United States, 1997–2011*, in *NCHS data brief, no 121*. 2013, National Center for Health Statistics: Hyattsville, MD.

61. U.S. Department of Health and Human Services, *Food Allergy: An Overview*. 2012, National Institutes of Health: National Institute of Allergy and Infectious Diseases. p. 14-15.

62. Graham, F., et al., *Risk of allergic reaction and sensitization to antibiotics in foods*. Ann Allergy Asthma Immunol, 2014. **113**(3): p. 329-30.

63. Gupta, R., et al., *The Economic Impact of Childhood Food Allergy in the United States*. JAMA Pediatr, 2013. **167**(11): p. 1026-1031.

64. U.S. Department of Health and Human Services, Centers for Disease Control and Prevention, and National Center for Health Statistics, *Health, United States, 2012: With Special Feature on Emergency Care*. 2013: Hyattsville, MD.

65. Centers for Disease Control and Prevention. *Heart Disease Facts*. 2014; Available from: http://www.cdc.gov/heartdisease/facts.htm.

66. Finkelstein, E.A., et al., *Annual Medical Spending Attributable To Obesity: Payer-And Service-Specific Estimates*. Health Affairs, 2009. **28**(5): p. w822-831.

67. Anderson, J.W., W.J. Chen, and B. Sieling, *Hypolipidemic effects of high-carbohydrate, high-fiber diets*. Metabolism, 1980. **29**(6): p. 551-8.

68. Barnard, R.J., et al., *Response of non-insulin-dependent diabetic patients to an intensive program of diet and exercise*. Diabetes Care, 1982. **5**(4): p. 370-4.

69. Fraser, G.E., *Associations between diet and cancer, ischemic heart disease, and all-cause mortality in non-Hispanic white California Seventh-day Adventists*. Am J Clin Nutr, 1999. **70**(3 Suppl): p. 532s-538s.

70. Snowdon, D.A. and R.L. Phillips, *Does a vegetarian diet reduce the occurrence of diabetes?* Am J Public Health, 1985. **75**(5): p. 507-12.

71. Story, L., et al., *Adherence to high-carbohydrate, high-fiber diets: long-term studies of non-obese diabetic men.* J Am Diet Assoc, 1985. **85**(9): p. 1105-10.

72. West, K.M. and J.M. Kalbfleisch, *Influence of nutritional factors on prevalence of diabetes.* Diabetes, 1971. **20**(2): p. 99-108.

73. Centers for Disease Control and Prevention, *National diabetes fact sheet: national estimates and general information on diabetes and prediabetes in the United States, 2011.* 2011, U.S. Department of Health and Human Services, Centers for Disease Control and Prevention: Atlanta, GA.

74. Livingstone, B.E. and A.E. Black, *Biomarkers of Nutritional Exposure and Nutritional Status.* J Nutr, 2003. **133**(3): p. 895S-920S.

75. Campbell, T.C. and J. Chen, *Energy balance: interpretation of data from rural China.* Toxicol Sci, 1999. **52**(2 Suppl): p. 87-94.

76. Appleby, P.N., et al., *Low body mass index in non-meat eaters: the possible roles of animal fat, dietary fibre and alcohol.* Int J Obes Relat Metab Disord, 1998. **22**(5): p. 454-60.

77. Levin, N., J. Rattan, and T. Gilat, *Energy intake and body weight in ovo-lacto vegetarians.* J Clin Gastroenterol, 1986. **8**(4): p. 451-3.

78. Poehlman, E.T., et al., *Resting metabolic rate and postprandial thermogenesis in vegetarians and nonvegetarians.* Am J Clin Nutr, 1988. **48**(2): p. 209-13.

79. Valtin, H., *"Drink at least eight glasses of water a day." Really? Is there scientific evidence for "8 x 8"?* Am J Physiol Regul Integr Comp Physiol, 2002. **283**(5): p. R993-1004.

80. Grandjean, P. and P.J. Landrigan, *Neurobehavioural effects of developmental toxicity.* The Lancet Neurology, 2014. **13**(3): p. 330-338.

81. Harvard School of Public Health, *A Silent Pandemic: Industrial Chemicals Are Impairing the Brain Development of Children Worldwide.* 2006.

82. Walia, A. *"Fluoridated Water Is Public Murder On A Grand Scale" – Dr. Dean Burk.* 2013; Available from: http://www.collective-evolution.com/2013/08/30/fluoridated-water-is-public-murder-on-a-grand-scale-dr-dean-burk/.

83. British Fluoridation Society, *One in a Million: The facts about water fluoridation.* 2012.

84. US Department of Health and Human Services, *U.S. Public Health Service Recommendation for Fluoride Concentration in Drinking Water for the Prevention of Dental Caries,* in *Reports and Recommendations.* 2015.

85. Rao, M., et al., *Do healthier foods and diet patterns cost more than less healthy options? A systematic review and meta-analysis.* BMJ Open, 2013. **3**(12).

86. Katz, D.L., et al., *A cost comparison of more and less nutritious food choices in US supermarkets.* Public Health Nutr, 2011. **14**(9): p. 1693-9.

87. Physicians Committee for Responsible Medicine. *Beens vs. Beef.* 2015; Available from: http://www.pcrm.org/media/infographics/beans-vs-beef-infographic.

88. Londoño, E. *Rising number of soldiers being dismissed for failing fitness tests.* National Security 2012; Available from: https://www.washingtonpost.com/world/national-security/2012/12/08/13d2e444-40b8-11e2-ae43-cf491b837f7b_story.html.

89. Bursi, F., et al., *Systolic and diastolic heart failure in the community.* Jama, 2006. **296**(18): p. 2209-16.

90. Kruse, M., et al., *Insulin induces an Inflammatory Cytokine Response in human and murine Adipocytes in vitro via the PI3Kinase/Akt-pathway.* Exp Clin Endocrinol Diabetes, 2013. **121**(03): p. P37.

91. Perkins, J.M., et al., *Acute effects of hyperinsulinemia and hyperglycemia on vascular inflammatory biomarkers and endothelial function in overweight and obese humans.* Am J Physiol Endocrinol Metab, 2015. **309**(2): p. E168-76.

92. Fishel, M.A., et al., *Hyperinsulinemia provokes synchronous increases in central inflammation and beta-amyloid in normal adults.* Arch Neurol, 2005. **62**(10): p. 1539-44.

93. U.S. Department of Agriculture. *National Nutrient Database for Standard Reference Release 27.* Available from: http://ndb.nal.usda.gov/ndb/.

94. The National Academies Press: Institute of Medicine, *Dietary Reference Intakes: The Essential Guide to Nutrient Requirements,* J.J. Otten, J.P. Hellwig, and Linda D. Meyers, Editors. 2006: Washington, D.C.

95. Chardigny, J.M., et al., *Do trans fatty acids from industrially produced sources and from natural sources have the same effect on cardiovascular disease risk factors in healthy subjects? Results of the trans Fatty Acids Collaboration (TRANSFACT) study.* Am J Clin Nutr, 2008. **87**(3): p. 558-66.

96. Motard-Belanger, A., et al., *Study of the effect of trans fatty acids from ruminants on blood lipids and other risk factors for cardiovascular disease.* Am J Clin Nutr, 2008. **87**(3): p. 593-9.

97. Willett, W. and D. Mozaffarian, *Ruminant or industrial sources of trans fatty acids: public health issue or food label skirmish?* Am J Clin Nutr, 2008. **87**(3): p. 515-6.

98. Stendera, S., et al., *A trans world journey,* in *First International Symposium on Trans Fatty Acids and Health.* 2006, Atherosclerosis Supplements: Rungstedgaard, Rungsted Kyst, Denmark. p. 47-52.

99. Food and Drug Administration, *FDA Targets Trans Fat in Processed Foods,* in *Consumer Health Information.* 2013. p. 1-2.

100. U.S. Department of Health and Human Services, *Tentative Determination Regarding Partially Hydrogenated Oils; Request for Comments and for Scientific Data and Information* in *Federal Register.* 2013. p. 67169-67175.

101. Simopoulos, A.P., *The importance of the ratio of omega-6/omega-3 essential fatty acids.* Biomed Pharmacother, 2002. **56**(8): p. 365-79.

102. Simopoulos, A.P., *Evolutionary aspects of diet: the omega-6/omega-3 ratio and the brain.* Mol Neurobiol, 2011. **44**(2): p. 203-15.

103. Marquis, D.M. *How Inflammation Affects Every Aspect of Your Health.* Health Articles 2013; Available from: http://articles.mercola.com/sites/articles/archive/2013/03/07/inflamm ation-triggers-disease-symptoms.aspx.

104. University of Maryland Medical Center. *Omega-3 fatty acids.* Complementary and Alternative Medicine Guide: Supplement 2011 24 June, 2013; Available from: http://umm.edu/health/medical/altmed/supplement/omega3-fatty-acids.

105. Campbell, T.C. *Evaluating the Need for Supplementation.* Treatments and Supplements 2012 1st November, 2012]; Available from: http://nutritionstudies.org/evaluating-need-supplementation/.

106. Rizos, E.C., et al., *Association between omega-3 fatty acid supplementation and risk of major cardiovascular disease events: a systematic review and meta-analysis.* Jama, 2012. **308**(10): p. 1024-33.

107. Chew, E.Y., et al., *Effect of omega-3 fatty acids, lutein/zeaxanthin, or other nutrient supplementation on cognitive function: The areds2 randomized clinical trial.* JAMA, 2015. **314**(8): p. 791-801.

108. Kwak, S.M., et al., *Efficacy of omega-3 fatty acid supplements (eicosapentaenoic acid and docosahexaenoic acid) in the secondary*

prevention of cardiovascular disease: a meta-analysis of randomized,
double-blind, placebo-controlled trials. Arch Intern Med, 2012. **172**(9): p.
686-94.

109. Roncaglioni, M.C., et al., *n-3 fatty acids in patients with multiple*
cardiovascular risk factors. N Engl J Med, 2013. **368**(19): p. 1800-8.

110. Northstone, K., et al., *Are dietary patterns in childhood associated with*
IQ at 8 years of age? A population-based cohort study, in *J Epidemiol*
Community Health. 2011.

111. Farvid, M.S., et al., *Dietary Fiber Intake in Young Adults and Breast*
Cancer Risk. Pediatrics, 2016. **137**(3).

112. Harnden, K.K. and K.L. Blackwell, *Increased Fiber Intake Decreases*
Premenopausal Breast Cancer Risk. Pediatrics, 2016. **137**(3).

113. Sansbury, L.B., et al., *The Effect of Strict Adherence to a High-Fiber,*
High-Fruit and -Vegetable, and Low-Fat Eating Pattern on Adenoma
Recurrence. American Journal of Epidemiology, 2009. **170**(5): p. 576-
584.

114. U.S. Department of Agriculture and U.S. Department of Health and
Human Services, *Dietary Guidelines for Americans.* 2010, Government
Printing Office: Washington, D.C.

115. Institute of Medicine of the National Academies: Food and Nutrition
Board, *Dietary Reference Intakes for Energy, Carbohydrate, Fiber, Fat,*
Fatty Acids, Cholesterol, Protein, and Amino Acids. 2005: Washington,
DC.

116. Fotiadis, C.I., et al., *Role of probiotics, prebiotics and synbiotics in*
chemoprevention for colorectal cancer. World Journal of
Gastroenterology, 2008. **14**(42): p. 6453-6457.

117. Beulens, J.W., et al., *High dietary glycemic load and glycemic index*
increase risk of cardiovascular disease among middle-aged women: a
population-based follow-up study. J Am Coll Cardiol, 2007. **50**(1): p. 14-
21.

118. Bhupathiraju, S.N., et al., *Glycemic index, glycemic load, and risk of type*
2 diabetes: results from 3 large US cohorts and an updated meta-analysis.
Am J Clin Nutr, 2014. **100**(1): p. 218-232.

119. Chavarro, J.E., et al., *A prospective study of dietary carbohydrate quantity*
and quality in relation to risk of ovulatory infertility. Eur J Clin Nutr,
2009. **63**(1): p. 78-86.

120. Chiu, C.J., et al., *Association between dietary glycemic index and age-*
related macular degeneration in nondiabetic participants in the Age-Related
Eye Disease Study. Am J Clin Nutr, 2007. **86**(1): p. 180-8.

121.Choi, Y., E. Giovannucci, and J.E. Lee, *Glycaemic index and glycaemic load in relation to risk of diabetes-related cancers: a meta-analysis.* Br J Nutr, 2012. **108**(11): p. 1934-47.

122.Higginbotham, S., et al., *Dietary glycemic load and risk of colorectal cancer in the Women's Health Study.* J Natl Cancer Inst, 2004. **96**(3): p. 229-33.

123.de Munter, J.S., et al., *Whole grain, bran, and germ intake and risk of type 2 diabetes: a prospective cohort study and systematic review.* PLoS Med, 2007. **4**(8): p. e261.

124.Atkinson, F.S., K. Foster-Powell, and J.C. Brand-Miller, *International Tables of Glycemic Index and Glycemic Load Values.* Diabetic Care, 2008. **31**(12).

125.Geiling, N. *The Science Behind Honey's Eternal Shelf Life.* 2013; Available from: http://www.smithsonianmag.com/science-nature/the-science-behind-honeys-eternal-shelf-life-1218690/?no-ist.

126.Campbell, T.C., *The China study : the most comprehensive study of nutrition ever conducted and the startling implications for diet, weight loss and long-term health / T. Colin Campbell and Thomas M. Campbell II,* ed. T.M. Campbell. 2007, Kent Town, S. Aust: Wakefield Press.

127.World Health Organization, Food and Agriculture Organization of the United Nations, and United Nations University. *Protein and amino acid requirements in human nutrition.* Nutrition publications: Dietary recommendations/Nutritional requirements list of publications 2007; 125]. Available from: http://www.who.int/nutrition/publications/nutrientrequirements/WHO_TRS_935/en/.

128.Muntoni, S., et al., *High meat consumption is associated with type 1 diabetes mellitus in a Sardinian case–control study.* Acta Diabetologica, 2013. **50**(5): p. 713-719.

129.Institute of Medicine: Food and Nutrition Board, *Dietary Reference Intakes for Energy, Carbohydrate, Fiber, Fat, Fatty Acids, Cholesterol, Protein, and Amino Acids.* 2002, National Academy Press: Washington, DC.

130.eCornell: T. Colin Campbell Center for Nutrition Studies, *Plant-Based Nutrition: Nutrition Fundimentals II: An Overemphasis on Protein - Chapter 3 (TCC501M5),* in *Chapter 3: Protein RDA.* 2014.

131.U.S. Environmental Protection Agency. *Global Greenhouse Gas Emissions Data.* Climate Change 2013; Available from: http://www.epa.gov/climatechange/ghgemissions/global.html#two.

132. Scarborough, P., et al., *Dietary greenhouse gas emissions of meat-eaters, fish-eaters, vegetarians and vegans in the UK*. Climatic Change, 2014. **125**: p. 179-192.

133. Gerber, P.J., et al., *Tackling climate change through livestock – A global assessment of emissions and mitigation opportunities*, in *Food and Agriculture Organization of the United Nations (FAO)*. 2013: Rome.

134. Ripple, W.J., et al., *Ruminants, climate change and climate policy*. Nature Climate Change, 2013. **4**: p. 2-5.

135. Willlmott, D. *Feeding 11 Billion People*. 2015; Available from: http://www.huffingtonpost.com/x-prize-foundation/feeding-11-billion-people_b_7208590.html.

136. Hoekstra, A.Y. and A.K. Chapagain, *Water footprints of nations: water use by people as a function of their consumption pattern*. Water Resources Management, 2007. **21**(1): p. 35-48.

137. Pimentel, D. and M. Pimentel, *Sustainability of meat-based and plant-based diets and the environment*. Am J Clin Nutr, 2003. **78**(3 Suppl): p. 660s-663s.

138. Lonnerdal, B., *Nutritional and physiologic significance of human milk proteins*. Am J Clin Nutr, 2003. **77**(6): p. 1537s-1543s.

139. Outram, S.M. and B. Stewart, *Should nutritional supplements and sports drinks companies sponsor sport? A short review of the ethical concerns*. J Med Ethics, 2014.

140. ScienceDaily and BMJ. *Sporting events should ditch nutritional supps, sports drinks sponsorship, experts urge*. 2014 22 September, 2014]; Available from: www.sciencedaily.com/releases/2014/09/140922205642.htm.

141. O'Keefe, J.H., et al., *Effects of Habitual Coffee Consumption on Cardiometabolic Disease, Cardiovascular Health, and All-Cause Mortality*. J Am Coll Cardiol, 2013. **62**(12): p. 1043-1051.

142. Dörner, J., et al., *Cardiac MRI Reveals Energy Drinks Alter Heart Function*. 2013, Radiological Society of North America.

143. Sanchis-Gomar, F., et al., *Energy Drink Overconsumption in Adolescents: Implications for Arrhythmias and Other Cardiovascular Events*. Canadian Journal of Cardiology.

144. Center for Science in the Public Interest, *Coke Loses Again as Vitaminwater Case Moves Forward*, in *Federal Magistrate Recommends Certification of Class Action*. 2013.

145. Food and Drug Administration, *FDA Advances Effort Against Marketed Unapproved Drugs*, in *FDA Orders Unapproved Quinine Drugs*

from the Market and Cautions Consumers About "Off-Label" Use of Quinine to Treat Leg Cramps, U.S.F.a.D. Administration, Editor. 2006.

146. Halfdanarson, T.R., et al., *Severe adverse effects of quinine: Report of seven cases.* Laeknabladid, 2002. **88**(10): p. 717-722.

147. Smale, W. *What exactly is in your beer?* . 2006; Available from: http://news.bbc.co.uk/2/hi/business/4942262.stm.

148. Hari, V. *The Shoking Ingredients in Beer.* 2013; Available from: http://foodbabe.com/2013/07/17/the-shocking-ingredients-in-beer/.

149. Nelson, S.S. *Is A 500-Year-Old German Beer Law Heritage Worth Honoring?* The Salt: What's on your Plate 2013; Available from: http://www.npr.org/blogs/thesalt/2013/12/17/251959392/is-a-500-year-old-german-beer-law-heritage-worth-honoring.

150. Asimov, E., *If Only the Grapes Were the Whole Stroy*, in *The New York Times.* 2013: Dining & Wine.

151. Semba, R.D., et al., *Resveratrol levels and all-cause mortality in older community-dwelling adults.* JAMA Internal Medicine, 2014.

152. Hamajima, N., et al., *Alcohol, tobacco and breast cancer--collaborative reanalysis of individual data from 53 epidemiological studies, including 58,515 women with breast cancer and 95,067 women without the disease.* Br J Cancer, 2002. **87**(11): p. 1234-45.

153. Smith-Warner, S.A., et al., *Alcohol and breast cancer in women: a pooled analysis of cohort studies.* Jama, 1998. **279**(7): p. 535-40.

154. Allen, N.E., et al., *Moderate alcohol intake and cancer incidence in women.* J Natl Cancer Inst, 2009. **101**(5): p. 296-305.

155. Cho, E., et al., *Alcohol intake and colorectal cancer: a pooled analysis of 8 cohort studies.* Ann Intern Med, 2004. **140**(8): p. 603-13.

156. Gonzales, J.F., et al., *Applying the Precautionary Principle to Nutrition and Cancer.* J Am Coll Nutr, 2014: p. 1-8.

157. Research and Markets: The Worlds Largest Market Research Store, *Food Additives: The U.S. Market.* 2013: United States. p. 174.

158. CODEX: International Food Standards, *Class names and the international numbering system for food additives.* 2013.

159. CODEX: International Food Standards, *Codex General Standard for Food Additives.* 2013.

160. Food and Drug Administration. *Food Additive Status List.* 2014; Available from: http://www.fda.gov/food/ingredientspackaginglabeling/foodadditivesingredients/ucm091048.htm#ftnC.

161. Food and Drug Administration. *Everything Added to Food in the United States (EAFUS)*. 2014; Available from: http://www.accessdata.fda.gov/scripts/fcn/fcnNavigation.cfm?rpt=ea fusListing&displayAll=true.

162. Food and Drug Administration. *Color Additive Status List*. 2014; Available from: http://www.fda.gov/ForIndustry/ColorAdditives/ColorAdditiveInve ntories/ucm106626.htm.

163. King, A. *Antimicrobial resistance will kill 300 million by 2050 without action*. 2014; Available from: http://www.rsc.org/chemistryworld/2014/12/antimicrobial-resistance-will-kill-300-million-2050-without-action.

164. Bravo, K. *Today's Outrageous Fact*. 2014; Available from: http://www.takepart.com/photos/shocking-stats-gallery/land-of-the-sick-meat-eaters?cmpid=foodinc-fb.

165. Nadimpalli, M., et al., *Persistence of livestock-associated antibiotic-resistant Staphylococcus aureus among industrial hog operation workers in North Carolina over 14 days*. Occup Environ Med, 2014.

166. Cowan, S. *Meat Kills, and Going Vegan Won't Help*. 2014; Available from: http://www.takepart.com/video/2014/07/02/meat-kills-and-going-vegan-wont-help?cmpid=foodinc-fb.

167. The Organic Report. *Organic is Good for Cows*. Organic, It's Worth It 2009; Available from: http://www.organicitsworthit.org/learn/organic-good-cows.

168. *Health Canada restricts use of growth-promoting antibiotics in livestock*, in *The Canadian Press*. 2014: Saskatoon.

169. Food and Drug Administration. *Phasing Out Certain Antibiotic Use in Farm Animals*. Consumer Updates 2013; Available from: http://www.fda.gov/forconsumers/consumerupdates/ucm378100.ht m.

170. Crocker, C. and G. Totheroh. *Aspartame (Nutrasweet and Equal)*. 2012 4 February, 2012]; Available from: http://www.aitse.org/aspartame-nutrasweet-and-equal/.

171. European Food Safety Authority, *EFSA completes full risk assessment on aspartame and concludes it is safe at current levels of exposure*. 2013.

172. Bradsiock, M.K., et al., *Evaluation of reactions to food additives: the aspartame experience*. Am J Clin Nutr, 1986. **43**: p. 464-469.

173. Geib, A. *More aspartame side effects revealed - headaches, blurred vision, neurological symptoms and more*. Natural Health News & Scientific

Discoveries 2012; Available from:
http://www.naturalnews.com/035382_aspartame_side_effects_heada
ches.html.

174. Connealy, L.E. *Aspartame: Is the sweet taste worth the harm?* 2013;
Available from: http://www.foodmatters.tv/articles-1/aspartame-is-
the-sweet-taste-worth-the-harm.

175. Maher, T.J. and R.J. Wurtmant, *Possible Neurologic Effects of
Aspartame, a Widely Used Food Additive.* Environ. Health Perspect,
1987. **75**: p. 53-57.

176. Vyas, A., et al., *Diet drink consumption and the risk of cardiovascular
events: a report from the Women's Health Initiative.* J Gen Intern Med,
2015. **30**(4): p. 462-8.

177. Lin, J. and G.C. Curhan, *Associations of sugar and artificially sweetened
soda with albuminuria and kidney function decline in women.* Clin J Am
Soc Nephrol, 2011. **6**(1): p. 160-6.

178. Schernhammer, E.S., et al., *Consumption of artificial sweetener- and
sugar-containing soda and risk of lymphoma and leukemia in men and
women.* Am J Clin Nutr, 2012. **96**(6): p. 1419-28.

179. Abhilash, M., et al., *Long-term consumption of aspartame and brain
antioxidant defense status.* Drug Chem Toxicol, 2013. **36**(2): p. 135-40.

180. Olney, J.W., et al., *Increasing brain tumor rates: is there a link to
aspartame?* J Neuropathol Exp Neurol, 1996. **55**(11): p. 1115-23.

181. Walton, R.G., *Seizure and mania after high intake of aspartame.*
Psychosomatics, 1986. **27**(3): p. 218, 220.

182. Wurtman, R.J., *Aspartame: possible effect on seizure susceptibility.*
Lancet, 1985. **2**(8463): p. 1060.

183. Drake, M., *Panic attacks and excessive aspartame ingestion.* The Lancet,
1986. **328**(8507): p. 631.

184. Magnuson, B.A., et al., *Aspartame: a safety evaluation based on current
use levels, regulations, and toxicological and epidemiological studies.* Crit
Rev Toxicol, 2007. **37**(8): p. 629-727.

185. Thirteenth Congress of the Republic of the Philippines, *Prohibiting
the use of aspartame on food, beverages, and drugs: Bill 2147,* Senator
Miriam Defensor Santiago, Editor. 2008.

186. Patton, D. *Indonesia consults on aspartame, sweetener use in food.* 2007;
Available from: http://www.foodnavigator-
asia.com/Formulation/Indonesia-consults-on-aspartame-sweetener-
use-in-food.

187. UK News and The Telegraph. *M&S and Asda to axe E-numbers.* 2007; Available from: http://www.telegraph.co.uk/news/uknews/1551684/MandS-and-Asda-to-axe-E-numbers.html.

188. *Sainsbury's takes the chemicals out of cola.* Mail Online 2007 23 April]; Available from: http://www.dailymail.co.uk/news/article-450254/Sainsburys-takes-chemicals-cola.html.

189. European Food Safety Authority, *Aspartame: EFSA consults on its first full risk assessment.* 2013: News & Events.

190. Mercola, J. *Subway to Remove Shoe Leather Chemical from Their Bread.* 2014 19 February, 2014]; Available from: http://articles.mercola.com/sites/articles/archive/2014/02/19/azodicarbonamide-subway-sandwich.aspx.

191. Cary, R., S. Dobson, and E. Ball, *Azodicarbonamide.* 1999, World Health Organization: Geneva.

192. *Commission Directive 2004/1/EC: amending directive 2002/72/EC as regards to the suspension of the use of azodicarbonamide as blowing agent.* Official Journal of the European Union, 2004. **L7**(45).

193. Chicago Tribune News, *A look at food additives that are legal in the U.S.: Find out what they are -- and where they're banned.* 2013.

194. United Nations Environment Programme and The Organisation for Economic Co-operation and Development, *2,6-di-tert-butyl-p-cresol (BHT) Screening Information Data Set: Initial Assessment Report.* 2002: Paris, France. p. 4-5.

195. World Health Organization: International Agency for Research on Cancer. *Sorne Naturally Occurring and Synthetic Food Cornponents, Furocournarins and Ultraviolet Radiation.* in *IARC Monographs on the Evaluation of the Carcinogenic Risk of Chemicals to Humans.* 1985. Lyon, France: Secretariat of the World Health Organization.

196. Calton, J. and M. Calton. *8 Additives From The Us That Are Banned In Other Countries.* You are what you eat 2013; Available from: http://foodmatters.tv/articles-1/8-additives-from-the-us-that-are-banned-in-other-countries.

197. Vogel, S.A., *The Politics of Plastics: The Making and Unmaking of Bisphenol A "Safety".* Am J Public Health, 2009. **99**(Suppl 3): p. S559–S566.

198. Taylor, P., *BPA being absorbed from canned food,* in *The Globe and Mail.* 2011: Canada.

199. Raja, R., et al., *Bisphenol A and human chronic diseases: Current evidences, possible mechanisms, and future perspectives.* Environment International 2014. **64**: p. 83-90.

200. Panzica, G.C., et al., *Effects of xenoestrogens on the differentiation of behaviorally-relevant neural circuits.* Frontiers in neuroendocrinology 2007. **28**(4): p. 179-200.

201. Kashiwagi, K., et al., *Disruption of Thyroid Hormone Function by Environmental Pollutants.* Journal of Health Science 2009. **55**(2): p. 147-160.

202. Soto, A.M. and C. Sonnenschein, *Environmental causes of cancer: Endocrine disruptors as carcinogens.* Nature Reviews Endocrinology, 2010. **6**(7): p. 363-370.

203. Benachour, N. and A. Aris, *Toxic effects of low doses of Bisphenol-A on human placental cells.* Toxicology and Applied Pharmacology 2009. **241**(3): p. 322-328.

204. Schöpel, M., et al., *Bisphenol A Binds to Ras Proteins and Competes with Guanine Nucleotide Exchange: Implications for GTPase-Selective Antagonists.* Journal of Medicinal Chemistry, 2013. **56**(23): p. 9664-9672.

205. Penn State. *Chemical in plastic, BPA, exposure may be associated with wheezing in children.* 2011; Available from: www.sciencedaily.com/releases/2011/05/110501183817.htm.

206. Melzer, D., et al., *Association of Urinary Bisphenol A Concentration with Heart Disease: Evidence from NHANES 2003/06.* PLoS ONE, 2010. **5**(1): p. e8673.

207. Rogers, J.A., L. Metz, and V.W. Yong, *Review: Endocrine disrupting chemicals and immune responses: A focus on bisphenol-A and its potential mechanisms.* Molecular Immunology, 2013. **53**(4): p. 421-430.

208. Calafat, A.M., et al., *Exposure of the U.S. population to bisphenol A and 4-tertiary-octylphenol: 2003–2004.* Environ. Health Perspect, 2008. **116**(1): p. 39-44.

209. Raloff, J. *FDA bans BPA in baby bottles, cups.* Science & The Public 2012; 17 July, 2012:[Available from: https://www.sciencenews.org/blog/science-public/fda-bans-bpa-baby-bottles-cups.

210. Hartle, J.C., M.A. Fox, and R.S. Lawrence, *Probabilistic modeling of school meals for potential bisphenol A (BPA) exposure.* J Expos Sci Environ Epidemiol, 2015.

211.Bromer, J.G., et al., *Bisphenol-A exposure in utero leads to epigenetic alterations in the developmental programming of uterine estrogen response.* The FASEB Journal, 2010. **24**(7): p. 2273-2280.

212.Geller, S. *BPA in Canned Food: Behind the brand curtain.* 2015; Available from: http://www.ewg.org/research/bpa-canned-food.

213.Food and Drug Administration. *Questions & Answers on Bisphenol A (BPA) Use in Food Contact Applications.* Protecting and Promoting Your Health 2013; Available from: http://www.fda.gov/Food/IngredientsPackagingLabeling/FoodAddit ivesIngredients/ucm355155.htm.

214.FDA, *2014 Updated safety assessment of Bisphenol A (BPA) for use in food contact applications.* 2014, Department of Health & Human Services.

215.European Information Centre on Bisphenol A. *European Union and Member States.* 2014; Available from: http://www.bisphenol-a-europe.org/en_GB/legislation/eu-states.

216.Schlanger, Z., *Coke to Remove Flame-Retardant Chemical From All its Drinks.* 2014, Newsweek.

217.Hart, J.R., *Ethylenediaminetetraacetic Acid and Related Chelating Agents.* Ullmann's Encyclopedia of Industrial Chemistry, 2011.

218.WebMD. *EDTA.* 2014; Available from: http://www.webmd.com/vitamins-supplements/ingredientmono-1032-EDTA.aspx?activeIngredientId=1032&activeIngredientName=EDTA.

219.ConsumerReports.Org. *Caramel color: The health risk that may be in your soda.* 2014; It's the most common coloring in foods and drinks— and it can contain a potential carcinogen. Here's what Consumer Reports found when it tested soft drinks that have caramel color.]. Available from: http://www.consumerreports.org/cro/news/2014/01/caramel-color-the-health-risk-that-may-be-in-your-soda/index.htm.

220.Borthakur, A., et al., *Carrageenan induces interleukin-8 production through distinct Bcl10 pathway in normal human colonic epithelial cells.* Am J Physiol Gastrointest Liver Physiol, 2007. **292**: p. G829 –G838.

221.Watanabe, K., et al., *Effect of Dietary Undegraded Carrageenan on Colon Carcinogenesis in F344 Rats Treated with Azoxymethane or Methylnitrosourea.* Cancer Res, 1978. **38**: p. 4427-4430.

222.Tobacman, J.K., *Review of Harmful Gastrointestinal Effects of Carrageenan in Animal Experiments.* Environmental Health Perspectives, 2001. **109**(10): p. 983-994.

223. Bhattacharyya, S., et al., *Exposure to common food additive carrageenan alone leads to fasting hyperglycemia and in combination with high fat diet exacerbates glucose intolerance and hyperlipidemia without effect on weight.* J Diabetes Res, 2015. **2015**: p. 513429.

224. Bhattacharyya, S., et al., *Toll-like receptor 4 mediates induction of the Bcl10-NFkappaB-interleukin-8 inflammatory pathway by carrageenan in human intestinal epithelial cells.* J Biol Chem, 2008. **283**(16): p. 10550-8.

225. Delwiche, J., *The impact of perceptual interactions on perceived flavor.* Food Quality and Preference, 2004. **15**(2): p. 137-146.

226. Potera, C., *The artificial food dye blues.* Environ. Health Perspect, 2010. **118**(10): p. A428.

227. Kobylewski, S. and M.F. Jacobson, *Food Dyes, a Rainbow of Risks.* 2010, Center for Science in the Public Interest.

228. Stevens, L.J., et al., *Amounts of Artificial Food Dyes and Added Sugars in Foods and Sweets Commonly Consumed by Children.* Clin Pediatr (Phila), 2014.

229. China Research & Intelligence Co, Ltd.,, *Research Report on Global and China Glyphosate Industry, 2013-2017*, in *Agricultural Chemicals.* 2013. p. 50.

230. Benbrook, C.M., *Trends in glyphosate herbicide use in the United States and globally.* Environmental Sciences Europe, 2016. **28**(1): p. 1-15.

231. Honeycutt, Z. and H. Rowlands, *Glyphosate Testing Report: Findings in American Mothers' Breast Milk, Urine and Water.* 2014, Moms Across America.

232. Brandli, D. and S. Reinacher, *Herbicides found in Human Urine.* Ithaka Journal, 2012. **1**: p. 270–272

233. Samsel, A. and S. Seneff, *Glyphosate's Suppression of Cytochrome P450 Enzymes and Amino Acid Biosynthesis by the Gut Microbiome: Pathways to Modern Diseases.* Entropy, 2013. **15**(4): p. 1416-1463.

234. Thongprakaisang, S., et al., *Glyphosate induces human breast cancer cells growth via estrogen receptors.* Food Chem Toxicol, 2013. **59**: p. 129-36.

235. Guyton, K.Z., et al., *Carcinogenicity of tetrachlorvinphos, parathion, malathion, diazinon, and glyphosate.* The Lancet Oncology.

236. World Health Organization, *IARC Monographs Volume 112: evaluation of five organophosphate insecticides and herbicides.* 2015, International Agency for Research on Cancer.

237. Ho, M.-W. *Roundup Listed Carcinogen by Danish Authority.* 2015; Available from: http://www.i-sis.org.uk/Roundup_Listed_Carcinogen_by_Danish_Authority.php.

238.Schinasi, L. and M.E. Leon, *Non-Hodgkin lymphoma and occupational exposure to agricultural pesticide chemical groups and active ingredients: a systematic review and meta-analysis.* Int J Environ Res Public Health, 2014. **11**(4): p. 4449-527.

239.Roberts, E.M., et al., *Maternal Residence Near Agricultural Pesticide Applications And Autism Spectrum Disorders Among Children In The Californa Central Valley.* Environ Health Perspect, 2007. **115**(10): p. 1482-1489.

240.O'Brien, R. *Allergy Kids Foundation.* 2014; Available from: http://www.robynobrien.com/Allergy-kids-foundation.

241.Heyes, J.D. *Monsanto's Glyphosate Herbicide Should Be Banned, Brazil's Public Prosecutor Says.* 2014; Available from: http://www.globalresearch.ca/monsantos-glyphosate-herbicide-should-be-banned-brazils-public-prosecutor-says/5377443.

242.Gammon, C., *Weed-Whacking Herbicide Proves Deadly to Human Cells,* in *Scientific American.* 2009, Environmental Health News.

243.Hyman, M. *5 Reasons High Fructose Corn Syrup Will Kill You.* 2013; Available from: http://drhyman.com/blog/2011/05/13/5-reasons-high-fructose-corn-syrup-will-kill-you/#close.

244.Mercola, J. *MSG: Is This Silent Killer Lurking in Your Kitchen Cabinets.* 2009; Available from: http://articles.mercola.com/sites/articles/archive/2009/04/21/msg-is-this-silent-killer-lurking-in-your-kitchen-cabinets.aspx.

245.Minton, B.L. *The Dangers of MSG.* 2013; Available from: http://foodmatters.tv/articles-1/the-dangers-of-msg.

246.Food And Drug Administration and Department Of Health And Human Services, *Section 101.22 - Foods; labeling of spices, flavorings, colorings and chemical preservatives.,* in *Code of Federal Regulations.* 2010.

247.U.S. Environmental Protection Agency, *Nitrates and Nitrites,* in *TEACH Chemical Summary.* 2007.

248.Kurokawa, Y., et al., *Toxicity and Carcinogenicity of Potassium Bromate - A New Renal Carcinogen.* Environ. Health Perspect, 1990. **87**: p. 309-335.

249.Cefic: European Chemical Industry Association, *Propylene glycol – the safe enabler* P.O.P.G.s.g. Cefic, Editor. 2008: Brussels.

250.Rosenberg, M. *If You Liked Bovine Growth Hormone, You'll Love Beta Agonists.* 2010 25 Jan, 2010]; Available from: http://www.foodconsumer.org/newsite/Opinion/bovine_growth_hormone_love_beta_agonists_2501100529.html.

251. Center for Veterinary Medicine, *CVM ADE Comprehensive Clinical Detail Report Listing*, in *Drug Listing: N;O;P;Q;R;S*. 2013. p. 276-287.

252. Liu, X., D.K. Grandy, and A. Janowsky, *Ractopamine, a livestock feed additive, is a full agonist at trace amine-associated receptor 1*. J Pharmacol Exp Ther, 2014. **350**(1): p. 124-9.

253. Poletto, R., et al., *Aggressiveness and brain amine concentration in dominant and subordinate finishing pigs fed the beta-adrenoreceptor agonist ractopamine*. J Anim Sci, 2010. **88**(9): p. 3107-20.

254. Mersmann, H.J., *Overview of the effects of beta-adrenergic receptor agonists on animal growth including mechanisms of action*. J Anim Sci, 1998. **76**(1): p. 160-72.

255. O'Brien, R., *Meet Ractopamine: The Drug in Your Meat that Is Banned in 100 Countries*. 2015.

256. Mercola, J. *Ractopamine: The Meat Additive Banned Almost Everywhere But America*. 2013 24 Dec, 2013]; Available from: http://articles.mercola.com/sites/articles/archive/2013/12/24/ractopam ine-beta-agonist-drug.aspx.

257. Center for Food Safety, *Public Interest Groups Sue FDA Demanding Records on Controversial Animal Growth Drugs Under Freedom of Information Act*, in *Challenges to Industry Use of Ractopamine and Zilpaterol in Light of Animal Welfare, Food Safety Concerns*. 2013: News Room.

258. Epstein, S.S. *Milk: America's Health Problem*. 2010; Available from: http://americannutritionassociation.org/toolsandresources/milk-america%C3%A2%E2%82%AC%E2%84%A2s-health-problem.

259. Epstein, S.S., *Warning from European Commission on IGF-1*. 1999, Cancer Prevention Coalition: University of Illinois School of Public Health: Chicago.

260. Epstein, S.S., *Unlabeled milk from cows treated with biosynthetic growth hormones: a case of regulatory abdication*. Int J Health Serv, 1996. **26**(1): p. 173-85.

261. Epstein, S.S., *Potential public health hazards of biosynthetic milk hormones*. Int J Health Serv, 1990. **20**(1): p. 73-84.

262. Biro, F.M., et al., *Pubertal assessment method and baseline characteristics in a mixed longitudinal study of girls*. Pediatrics, 2010. **126**(3): p. e583-90.

263. Epstein, S.S., *Monsanto's Genetically Modified Milk Ruled Unsafe by The United Nations*. 1999, Cancer Prevention Coalition: University of Illinois School of Public Health: Chicago.

264. Vally, H., N.L. Misso, and V. Madan, *Clinical effects of sulphite additives.* Clin Exp Allergy, 2009. **39**(11): p. 1643-51.

265. Gunnison, A.F. and D.W. Jacobsen, *Sulfite hypersensitivity. A critical review.* CRC Crit Rev Toxicol, 1987. **17**(3): p. 185-214.

266. Lester, M.R., *Sulfite sensitivity: significance in human health.* J Am Coll Nutr, 1995. **14**(3): p. 229-32.

267. Montano Garcia, M.L., *Adverse reactions induced by food additives: sulfites.* Rev Alerg Mex, 1989. **36**(3): p. 107-9.

268. Przybilla, B. and J. Ring, *[Sulfite hypersensitivity].* Hautarzt, 1987. **38**(8): p. 445-8.

269. Willett, W.C. and A. Ascherio, *Trans fatty acids: are the effects only marginal?* Am J Public Health, 1994. **84**(5): p. 722-4.

270. Zaloga, G.P., et al., *Trans fatty acids and coronary heart disease.* Nutr Clin Pract, 2006. **21**(5): p. 505-12.

271. *Position paper on trans fatty acids. ASCN/AIN Task Force on Trans Fatty Acids. American Society for Clinical Nutrition and American Institute of Nutrition.* Am J Clin Nutr, 1996. **63**(5): p. 663-70.

272. Food and Drug Administration, *Talking About Trans Fat: What You Need to Know,* in *Food Facts.* 2012, The U.S. Food and Drug Administration Center for Food Safety   p. 2.

273. Kiage, J.N., et al., *Intake of trans fat and all-cause mortality in the Reasons for Geographical and Racial Differences in Stroke (REGARDS) cohort.* Am J Clin Nutr, 2013. **97**(5): p. 1121-8.

274. Kummerow, F.A., *The negative effects of hydrogenated trans fats and what to do about them.* Atherosclerosis, 2009. **205**(2): p. 458-65.

275. Girl Scouts. *Statement from GSUSA CEO Kathy Cloninger: Girl Scout Cookies Now Have Zero Trans Fats.* 2006; Available from: http://www.girlscouts.org/news/news_releases/2006/gs_cookies_no w_have_zero_trans_fats.asp.

276. Wilson, T.A., M. McIntyre, and R.J. Nicolosi, *Trans fatty acids and cardiovascular risk.* J Nutr Health Aging, 2001. **5**(3): p. 184-7.

277. The Coca-Cola Company. *Coca-Cola Sponsorships: London 2012 Olympic Games.* 2012 1 January, 2012]; Available from: http://www.coca-colacompany.com/stories/coca-cola-sponsorships-london-2012-olympic-games.

278. U.S. Department of Health and Human Services, et al., *The Health Consequences of Smoking —50 Years of Progress. A Report of the Surgeon General.* 2014: Atlanta, GA.

279. Philip Morris USA. *Marlboro Gold Pack 25's Box*. Ingredients by Brand 2014; Available from: http://www.philipmorrisusa.com/en/cms/Products/Cigarettes/Ingredients/Ingredients_by_Brand/Marlboro/Marlboro_Gold_Pack_25s_Box.aspx.

280. Ortho-Mcneil Pharmaceutical, Inc.,, *Physicians' Package Insert: Ortho Tri-Cyclen® Tablets, Ortho-Cyclen® Tablets (Norgestimate/Ethinyl Estradiol)*, I. Ortho-Mcneil Pharmaceutical, Editor. 2014: Raritan, New Jersey.

281. Burkman, R., J.J. Schlesselman, and M. Zieman, *Safety concerns and health benefits associated with oral contraception*. Am J Obstet Gynecol, 2004. **190**(4 Suppl): p. S5-22.

282. Grossman-Barr, N., *Managing Adverse Effects of Hormonal Contraceptives*. Am Fam Physician, 2010. **82**(12): p. 1499-1506.

283. Pletzer, B., M. Kronbichler, and H. Kerschbaum, *Differential effects of androgenic and anti-androgenic progestins on fusiform and frontal gray matter volume and face recognition performance*. Brain Research, 2014(0).

284. Coca-Cola Amatil. *L&P*. 2013; Available from: http://ccamatil.co.nz/brands/lp/.

285. O'Brien, R. *Pigs: A Feeding Trial Exposes Problems and "He Said, She Said" Science*. 2013 13 June, 2013]; Available from: http://www.robynobrien.com/_blog/Inspiring_Ideas/tag/food_allergies/.

286. Carman, J.A., et al., *A long-term toxicology study on pigs fed a combined genetically modified (GM) soy and GM maize diet*. Journal of Organic Systems, 2013. **8**(1): p. 38-54.

287. Pederson, I.B. *Changing from GMO to Non-GMO Natural Soy, Experiences from Denmark*. 2014; Available from: http://www.i-sis.org.uk/Changing_from_GMO_to_non-GMO_soy.php.

288. Ho, M.-W. *Lab Study Establishes Glyphosate Link to Birth Defects*. 2010; Available from: http://www.i-sis.org.uk/glyphosateCausesBirthDefects.php.

289. Warren, M. and N. Pisarenko. *Birth defects, cancer in Argentina linked to agrochemicals: AP investigation*. myHealth 2013; Available from: http://www.ctvnews.ca/health/birth-defects-cancer-in-argentina-linked-to-agrochemicals-ap-investigation-1.1505096.

290. Paganelli, A., et al., *Glyphosate-based herbicides produce teratogenic effects on vertebrates by impairing retinoic acid signaling*. Chem Res Toxicol, 2010. **23**(10): p. 1586-95.

291. Ho, M.-W. *GM Soya Fed Rats: Stunted, Dead, or Sterile.* 2006; Available from: http://www.i-sis.org.uk/GM_Soya_Fed_Rats.php.

292. Robinson, C. and Institue of Sciene in Society. *Argentina's Roundup Human Tragedy.* 2010; Available from: http://www.i-sis.org.uk/argentinasRoundupHumanTragedy.php.

293. Lovejoy, G.M. *Local farmer turns to non-GMO seeds.* 2015; Available from: http://www.bluffcountrynews.com/Content/Default/Homepage-Rotator/Article/Local-farmer-turns-to-non-GMO-seeds/-3/548/60533.

294. GM Watch. *Chaco government report confirms link between glyphosate/agrochemicals and cancer/birth defects in Argentina.* 2014; Available from: http://www.gmwatch.eu/index.php?option=com_content&view=article&id=12481:reports-official-report-confirms-correlation.

295. Center for Food Safety. *GE Food Labeling Laws.* Protecting Our Food, Our Farms & Our Environment 2014; Available from: http://www.centerforfoodsafety.org/ge-map/.

296. Sarich, C. *El Salvador Farmers Beat Monsanto's Monopoly: Refusing GMO and Outperforming with Record Crop Yields.* 2015; Available from: http://www.globalresearch.ca/el-salvador-farmers-beat-monsantos-monopoly-refusing-gmo-and-outperforming-with-record-crop-yields/5442783.

297. Mellman, M. *Majority want more labels on food.* 2012; April 17, 2012:[Available from: http://mellmangroup.com/majority_want_more_labels_on_food/.

298. Non-GMO Project. *GMO Facts.* Working together to ensure the sustained availability of non-GMO food & products 2014; Available from: http://www.nongmoproject.org/learn-more/.

299. Gillam, C. *U.S. GMO labeling foes triple spending in first half of this year over 2013.* U.S. 2014 3 September, 2014; Available from: http://www.reuters.com/article/2014/09/03/us-usa-gmo-labeling-idUSKBN0GY09O20140903.

300. Institute for Responsible Technology. *Non-GMO Shopping Guide: Invisible GM Ingredients.* Avoiding GMOs 2010; Available from: http://www.nongmoshoppingguide.com/brands/invisible-gm-ingredients.html.

301. Non-GMO Project. *What is GMO? Agricultural Crops That Have a Risk of Being GMO.* Working together to ensure the sustained availability

of non-GMO food & products 2014; Available from: http://www.nongmoproject.org/learn-more/what-is-gmo/.

302. Messina, M., *Soy foods, isoflavones, and the health of postmenopausal women.* Am J Clin Nutr, 2014.

303. Liu, X.O., et al., *Association between dietary factors and breast cancer risk among Chinese females: systematic review and meta-analysis.* Asian Pac J Cancer Prev, 2014. **15**(3): p. 1291-8.

304. Nagata, C., et al., *Soy intake and breast cancer risk: an evaluation based on a systematic review of epidemiologic evidence among the Japanese population.* Jpn J Clin Oncol, 2014. **44**(3): p. 282-95.

305. D'Adamo, C.R. and A. Sahin, *Soy foods and supplementation: a review of commonly perceived health benefits and risks.* Altern Ther Health Med, 2014. **20 Suppl 1**: p. 39-51.

306. Messina, M. and G. Redmond, *Effects of soy protein and soybean isoflavones on thyroid function in healthy adults and hypothyroid patients: a review of the relevant literature.* Thyroid, 2006. **16**(3): p. 249-58.

307. Teas, J., et al., *Seaweed and soy: companion foods in Asian cuisine and their effects on thyroid function in American women.* J Med Food, 2007. **10**(1): p. 90-100.

308. Brink, E., et al., *Long-term consumption of isoflavone-enriched foods does not affect bone mineral density, bone metabolism, or hormonal status in early postmenopausal women: a randomized, double-blind, placebo controlled study.* Am J Clin Nutr, 2008. **87**(3): p. 761-70.

309. Ma, D.F., et al., *Soy isoflavone intake increases bone mineral density in the spine of menopausal women: meta-analysis of randomized controlled trials.* Clin Nutr, 2008. **27**(1): p. 57-64.

310. Messina, M., S. Ho, and D.L. Alekel, *Skeletal benefits of soy isoflavones: a review of the clinical trial and epidemiologic data.* Curr Opin Clin Nutr Metab Care, 2004. **7**(6): p. 649-58.

311. Biesiekierski, J.R., et al., *No effects of gluten in patients with self-reported non-celiac gluten sensitivity after dietary reduction of fermentable, poorly absorbed, short-chain carbohydrates.* Gastroenterology, 2013. **145**(2): p. 320-8.e1-3.

312. Welsh, J., *Researchers Who Provided Key Evidence For Gluten Sensitivity Have Thoroughly Shown That It Doesn't Exist*, in *Briefing*. 2014, Business Insider Australia.

313. Brouns, F.J.P.H., V.J. van Buul, and P.R. Shewry, *Does wheat make us fat and sick?* Journal of Cereal Science, 2013. **58**(2): p. 209-215.

314. McKeown, N.M., et al., *Whole- and refined-grain intakes are differentially associated with abdominal visceral and subcutaneous adiposity in healthy adults: the Framingham Heart Study.* Am J Clin Nutr, 2010. **92**(5): p. 1165-71.

315. Bazzano, L.A., et al., *Dietary intake of whole and refined grain breakfast cereals and weight gain in men.* Obes Res, 2005. **13**(11): p. 1952-60.

316. Liu, S., et al., *Relation between changes in intakes of dietary fiber and grain products and changes in weight and development of obesity among middle-aged women.* Am J Clin Nutr, 2003. **78**(5): p. 920-7.

317. Murtaugh, M.A., et al., *Epidemiological support for the protection of whole grains against diabetes.* Proc Nutr Soc, 2003. **62**(1): p. 143-9.

318. Samsel, A. and S. Seneff, *Glyphosate, pathways to modern diseases II: Celiac sprue and gluten intolerance.* Interdiscip Toxicol, 2013. **6**(4): p. 159-184.

319. Trasande, L., P.J. Landrigan, and C. Schechter, *Public health and economic consequences of methyl mercury toxicity to the developing brain.* Environ Health Perspect, 2005. **113**(5): p. 590-6.

320. Sheehan, M.C., et al., *Global methylmercury exposure from seafood consumption and risk of developmental neurotoxicity: a systematic review.* Bull World Health Organ, 2014. **92**(4): p. 254-269f.

321. Food and Drug Administration. *Mercury Concentrations in Fish: FDA Monitoring Program (1990-2010).* 2013; Available from: http://www.fda.gov/Food/FoodborneIllnessContaminants/Metals/ucm191007.htm.

322. Adams, M. *Mercury Capturing Effect of Common Foods.* Forensic Food Lab 2014; Available from: http://labs.naturalnews.com/Mercury-Capturing-Effect-of-Common-Foods.html.

323. Hites, R.A., et al., *Global Assessment of Polybrominated Diphenyl Ethers in Farmed and Wild Salmon.* Environmental Science & Technology, 2004. **38**(19): p. 4945-4949.

324. World Health Organization. *Dioxins and their effects on human health.* 2010 May 2010]; Available from: http://www.who.int/mediacentre/factsheets/fs225/en/.

325. U.S. Environmental Protection Agency. *Polychlorinated Biphenyls (PCBs).* 2013; Available from: http://www.epa.gov/epawaste/hazard/tsd/pcbs/about.htm.

326. Malisch, R. and A. Kotz, *Dioxins and PCBs in feed and food - Review from European perspective.* Sci Total Environ, 2014.

327. Schantz, S.L., et al., *Impairments of memory and learning in older adults exposed to polychlorinated biphenyls via consumption of Great Lakes fish.* Environ Health Perspect, 2001. **109**(6): p. 605-11.

328. Monterey Bay Aquarium. *Select a Seafood Watch Pocket Guide.* 2014; Available from: http://www.seafoodwatch.org/cr/cr_seafoodwatch/download.aspx.

329. Vince, G. *How the world's oceans could be running out of fish.* Science & Environment 2012 21 September, 2012]; Global fish stocks are exploited or depleted to such an extent that without urgent measures we may be the last generation to catch food from the oceans.]. Available from: http://www.bbc.com/future/story/20120920-are-we-running-out-of-fish.

330. Food and Agriculture Orginization of the United Nations and Fisheries and Aquaculture Department. *Fishery Statistics: reliability and Policy Implications.* Available from: http://www.fao.org/docrep/FIELD/006/Y3354M/y3354m00.htm.

331. Rong, Y., et al., *Egg consumption and risk of coronary heart disease and stroke: dose-response meta-analysis of prospective cohort studies.* Bmj, 2013. **346**: p. e8539.

332. Hu, F.B., et al., *A prospective study of egg consumption and risk of cardiovascular disease in men and women.* Jama, 1999. **281**(15): p. 1387-94.

333. Qureshi, A.I., et al., *Regular egg consumption does not increase the risk of stroke and cardiovascular diseases.* Med Sci Monit, 2007. **13**(1): p. Cr1-8.

334. Djousse, L., et al., *Egg consumption and risk of type 2 diabetes in older adults.* Am J Clin Nutr, 2010. **92**(2): p. 422-7.

335. Krauss, R.M., et al., *AHA Dietary Guidelines: revision 2000: A statement for healthcare professionals from the Nutrition Committee of the American Heart Association.* Circulation, 2000. **102**(18): p. 2284-99.

336. Djousse, L., et al., *Egg consumption and risk of type 2 diabetes in men and women.* Diabetes Care, 2009. **32**(2): p. 295-300.

337. Djousse, L. and J.M. Gaziano, *Egg consumption and risk of heart failure in the Physicians' Health Study.* Circulation, 2008. **117**(4): p. 512-6.

338. Djousse, L. and J.M. Gaziano, *Egg consumption in relation to cardiovascular disease and mortality: the Physicians' Health Study.* Am J Clin Nutr, 2008. **87**(4): p. 964-9.

339. Houston, D.K., et al., *Dietary fat and cholesterol and risk of cardiovascular disease in older adults: the Health ABC Study.* Nutr Metab Cardiovasc Dis, 2011. **21**(6): p. 430-7.

340. Tanasescu, M., et al., *Dietary fat and cholesterol and the risk of cardiovascular disease among women with type 2 diabetes.* Am J Clin Nutr, 2004. **79**(6): p. 999-1005.

341. Spence, J.D., D.J. Jenkins, and J. Davignon, *Dietary cholesterol and egg yolks: not for patients at risk of vascular disease.* Can J Cardiol, 2010. **26**(9): p. e336-9.

342. Kayikcioglu, M. and I. Soydan, *[Egg consumption and cardiovascular health].* Turk Kardiyol Dern Ars, 2009. **37**(5): p. 353-7.

343. Physicians Committee for Responsible Medicine. *The Physicians Committee Sues USDA and DHHS, Exposing Industry Corruption in Dietary Guidelines Decision on Cholesterol: Egg Industry Board Paid Millions in Grants Seeking to Remove Lifesaving Cholesterol Limits.* 2016; Available from: https://www.pcrm.org/media/news/physicians-committee-sues-usda-and-dhhs.

344. Physicians Committee for Responsible Medicine, *The Physicians Committee Praises New Dietary Guidelines for Strengthening Cholesterol Warnings, But Demands Investigation into Cholesterol Money Trail: Doctors Applaud Lifesaving Decision Affecting Millions of Americans at Risk for Heart Disease, Obesity.* 2016.

345. Clarkson, S. and L.H. Newburgh, *The relation between atherosclerosis and ingested cholesterol in the rabbit.* J Exp Med, 1926. **43**(5): p. 595-612.

346. Meeker, D.R. and H.D. Kesten, *Effect of high protein diets on experimental atherosclerosis of rabbits.* Arch. Pathology, 1941. **31**: p. 147-162.

347. Newburgh, L.H. and S. Clarkson, *PRoduction of arteriosclerosis in rabbits by diets rich in animal proteins.* Journal of the American Medical Association, 1922. **79**(14): p. 1106-1108.

348. Newburgh, L.H. and S. Clarkson, *THe production of atherosclerosis in rabbits by feeding diets rich in meat.* Archives of Internal Medicine, 1923. **31**(5): p. 653-676.

349. Meeker, D.R. and H.D. Kesten, *Experimental atherosclerosis and high protein diets.* Exp Biol Med, 1940. **45**(2): p. 543-545.

350. Sirtori, C.R., G. Noseda, and G.C. Descovich, *Current Topics in Nutrition and Disease, Volume 8: Animal and Vegetable Proteins in Lipid Metabolism and Atherosclerosis,* ed. M.J. Gibney and D. Kritchevsky. 1983: Alan R. Liss, Inc.

351. American Heart Association. *Know your fats.* 2014; Available from: http://www.heart.org/HEARTORG/Conditions/Cholesterol/Preventi

onTreatmentofHighCholesterol/Know-Your-Fats_UCM_305628_Article.jsp.

352. Richman, E.L., et al., *Choline intake and risk of lethal prostate cancer: incidence and survival.* Am J Clin Nutr, 2012. **96**(4): p. 855-63.

353. Richman, E.L., et al., *Egg, red meat, and poultry intake and risk of lethal prostate cancer in the prostate-specific antigen-era: incidence and survival.* Cancer Prev Res (Phila), 2011. **4**(12): p. 2110-21.

354. Iscovich, J.M., et al., *Colon cancer in Argentina. I: Risk from intake of dietary items.* Int J Cancer, 1992. **51**(6): p. 851-7.

355. Radosavljevic, V., et al., *Diet and bladder cancer: a case-control study.* Int Urol Nephrol, 2005. **37**(2): p. 283-9.

356. Zhang, J., Z. Zhao, and H.J. Berkel, *Egg consumption and mortality from colon and rectal cancers: an ecological study.* Nutr Cancer, 2003. **46**(2): p. 158-65.

357. Li, Y., et al., *Egg consumption and risk of cardiovascular diseases and diabetes: a meta-analysis.* Atherosclerosis, 2013. **229**(2): p. 524-30.

358. Qiu, C., et al., *Risk of gestational diabetes mellitus in relation to maternal egg and cholesterol intake.* Am J Epidemiol, 2011. **173**(6): p. 649-58.

359. Anderson, K.E., *Comparison of fatty acid, cholesterol, and vitamin A and E composition in eggs from hens housed in conventional cage and range production facilities.* Poult Sci, 2011. **90**(7): p. 1600-8.

360. Samman, S., et al., *Fatty acid composition of certified organic, conventional and omega-3 eggs.* Food Chemistry, 2009. **116**(4): p. 911-914.

361. Küçükyılmaz, K., et al., *Effect of an organic and conventional rearing system on the mineral content of hen eggs.* Food Chemistry, 2012. **132**(2): p. 989-992.

362. Torde, R.G., et al., *Multiplexed analysis of cage and cage free chicken egg fatty acids using stable isotope labeling and mass spectrometry.* Molecules, 2013. **18**(12): p. 14977-88.

363. Health TV. *Helping Kiwis and their whānau get the most out of their medical appointments.* 2011; Available from: http://www.htv.co.nz/.

364. Frassetto, L.A., et al., *Worldwide incidence of hip fracture in elderly women: relation to consumption of animal and vegetable foods.* J Gerontol A Biol Sci Med Sci, 2000. **55**(10): p. M585-92.

365. Abelow, B.J., T.R. Holford, and K.L. Insogna, *Cross-cultural association between dietary animal protein and hip fracture: a hypothesis.* Calcif Tissue Int, 1992. **50**(1): p. 14-8.

366.Hegsted, D.M., *Calcium and osteoporosis.* J Nutr, 1986. **116**(11): p. 2316-9.

367.Sellmeyer, D.E., et al., *A high ratio of dietary animal to vegetable protein increases the rate of bone loss and the risk of fracture in postmenopausal women. Study of Osteoporotic Fractures Research Group.* Am J Clin Nutr, 2001. **73**(1): p. 118-22.

368.Barzel, U.S., *Acid loading and osteoporosis.* J Am Geriatr Soc, 1982. **30**(9): p. 613.

369.Brosnan, J.T. and M.E. Brosnan, *Dietary protein, metabolic acidosis, and calcium balance.* Adv Nutr Res, 1982. **4**: p. 77-105.

370.Wachsman, A. and D. Bernstein, *Diet and Osteoporosis.* Lancet, 1968. **May 4, 1968**: p. 958-959.

371.Frassetto, L.A., et al., *Estimation of net endogenous noncarbonic acid production in humans from diet potassium and protein contents.* Am J Clin Nutr, 1998. **68**(3): p. 576-83.

372.Sherman, H., *Calcium requirement for maintenance in man.* J. Biol. Chem, 1920. **39**: p. 21-27.

373.Kerstetter, J.E. and L.H. Allen, *Dietary protein increases urinary calcium.* J Nutr, 1990. **120**(1): p. 134-6.

374.Hegsted, M., et al., *Urinary calcium and calcium balance in young men as affected by level of protein and phosphorus intake.* J Nutr, 1981. **111**(3): p. 553-62.

375.Margen, S., et al., *Studies in calcium metabolism. I. The calciuretic effect of dietary protein.* Am J Clin Nutr, 1974. **27**(6): p. 584-9.

376.Westman, E.C., et al., *Effect of 6-month adherence to a very low carbohydrate diet program.* Am J Med, 2002. **113**(1): p. 30-6.

377.Pollan, M., *In Defense of Food: An Eaters Manifesto.* 2008: Penquin Group.

378.Harvard School of Public Health. *Food Pyramids and Plates: What Should You Really Eat?* The Nutrition Source 2012; Available from: http://www.hsph.harvard.edu/nutritionsource/pyramid-full-story/.

379.Ahn, J., et al., *Dairy products, calcium intake, and risk of prostate cancer in the prostate, lung, colorectal, and ovarian cancer screening trial.* Cancer Epidemiol Biomarkers Prev, 2007. **16**(12): p. 2623-30.

380.Chan, J.M., et al., *Dairy products, calcium, phosphorous, vitamin D, and risk of prostate cancer (Sweden).* Cancer Causes Control, 1998. **9**(6): p. 559-66.

381. Rodriguez, C., et al., *Calcium, dairy products, and risk of prostate cancer in a prospective cohort of United States men.* Cancer Epidemiol Biomarkers Prev, 2003. **12**(7): p. 597-603.

382. Tseng, M., et al., *Dairy, calcium, and vitamin D intakes and prostate cancer risk in the National Health and Nutrition Examination Epidemiologic Follow-up Study cohort.* Am J Clin Nutr, 2005. **81**(5): p. 1147-54.

383. Feskanich, D., et al., *Milk consumption during teenage years and risk of hip fractures in older adults.* JAMA Pediatr, 2014. **168**(1): p. 54-60.

384. Michaelsson, K., et al., *Milk intake and risk of mortality and fractures in women and men: cohort studies.* Bmj, 2014. **349**: p. g6015.

385. Schooling, C.M., *Milk and mortality.* Bmj, 2014. **349**: p. g6205.

386. Walker, N.W., *Become Younger.* 2 ed. 1995, Summertown, TN: Norwalk Press.

387. Environmental Working Group. *EWG's 2014 Shopper's Guide to Pesticides in Produce: Executive Summary.* 2014; Available from: http://www.ewg.org/foodnews/summary.php.

388. Bouchard, M.F., et al., *Prenatal exposure to organophosphate pesticides and IQ in 7-year-old children.* Environ Health Perspect, 2011. **119**(8): p. 1189-95.

389. Engel, S.M., et al., *Prenatal exposure to organophosphates, paraoxonase 1, and cognitive development in childhood.* Environ Health Perspect, 2011. **119**(8): p. 1182-8.

390. Rauh, V., et al., *Seven-year neurodevelopmental scores and prenatal exposure to chlorpyrifos, a common agricultural pesticide.* Environ Health Perspect, 2011. **119**(8): p. 1196-201.

391. Baranski, M., et al., *Higher antioxidant and lower cadmium concentrations and lower incidence of pesticide residues in organically grown crops: a systematic literature review and meta-analyses.* Br J Nutr, 2014: p. 1-18.

392. Chiu, Y.H., et al., *Fruit and vegetable intake and their pesticide residues in relation to semen quality among men from a fertility clinic.* Hum Reprod, 2015.

393. U.S. Department of Agriculture, *Pesticide Data Program: Annual Summary, Calendar Year 2012,* in *Science and Technology Program.* 2014, United States Department of Agriculture.

394. American Academy of Pediatrics, *Pesticide exposure in children.* Pediatrics, 2012. **130**(6).

395. Pesticide Action Network. *What's on my food? Potatoes.* 2014; Available from: http://www.whatsonmyfood.org/food.jsp?food=PO.

396. Howard, P. *Who Owns Organic.* Promoting Economic Justice for Family Scale Farming 2014; Available from: http://www.cornucopia.org/who-owns-organic/.

397. Lagos, J.E., et al., *China - Peoples Republic of: Organics Report.* 2010, USDA Foreign Agricultural Service.

398. Laux, M. *Organic Food Trends Profile.* 2013 Nov 2013; Available from: http://www.agmrc.org/markets__industries/food/organic-food-trends-profile/.

399. Partos, L. *Organic Opportunities Open Up in France as Growth Marks 'Historic' Levels.* 2010; Available from: http://www.foodnavigator.com/Market-Trends/Organic-opportunities-open-up-in-France-as-growth-marks-historic-levels.

400. USDA Foreign Agricultrual Service, *Organic Foods Find Growing Niche in Mexico.* 2011.

401. Farm Futures. *Organic Foods Enjoying Recession Rebound.* 2013 6 November, 2013]; Available from: http://farmfutures.com/story-organic-foods-enjoying-recession-rebound-0-104390.

402. Gattingera, A., et al., *Enhanced top soil carbon stocks under organic farming.* PNAS, 2012. **109**(44): p. 18226–18231.

403. Zahn, J., et al., *World Investment Report 2013: Global Value Chains: Investment and Trade for Development.* 2013, United Nations: Switzerland.

404. Schwingshackl, L. and G. Hoffmann, *Low-carbohydrate diets impair flow-mediated dilatation: evidence from a systematic review and meta-analysis.* Br J Nutr, 2013. **110**(5): p. 969-70.

405. Rao, T.S.S., et al., *Understanding nutrition, depression and mental illnesses.* Indian Journal of Psychiatry, 2008. **50**(2): p. 77-82.

406. Briani, C., et al., *Cobalamin Deficiency: Clinical Picture and Radiological Findings.* Nutrients, 2013. **5**(11): p. 4521-4539.

407. Fitzpatrick, T.B., et al., *Vitamin Deficiencies in Humans: Can Plant Science Help?* The Plant Cell, 2012. **24**(2): p. 395-414.

408. Hossein-nezhad, A. and M.F. Holick, *Vitamin D for Health: A Global Perspective.* Mayo Clinic proceedings. Mayo Clinic, 2013. **88**(7): p. 720-755.

409. Pierce, M.R., et al., *Combined Vitamin C & E deficiency induces motor defects in gulo(−/−)/SVCT2(+/−) mice.* Nutritional neuroscience, 2013. **16**(4): p. 10.1179/1476830512Y.0000000042.

410. Venu, M., et al., *High Prevalence of Vitamin A and D Deficiency in Patients Evaluated for Liver Transplantation*. Liver transplantation : official publication of the American Association for the Study of Liver Diseases and the International Liver Transplantation Society, 2013. **19**(6): p. 627-633.

411. Wacker, M. and M.F. Holick, *Vitamin D—Effects on Skeletal and Extraskeletal Health and the Need for Supplementation*. Nutrients, 2013. **5**(1): p. 111-148.

412. Dauncey, M.J., *Genomic and Epigenomic Insights into Nutrition and Brain Disorders*. Nutrients, 2013. **5**(3): p. 887-914.

413. Holick, M.F., *Sunlight and vitamin D for bone health and prevention of autoimmune diseases, cancers, and cardiovascular disease*. Am J Clin Nutr, 2004. **80**(6 Suppl): p. 1678s-88s.

414. Mercola, J. *Magnesium: An Invisible Deficiency That Could Be Harming Your Health*. 2015; Available from: http://articles.mercola.com/sites/articles/archive/2015/01/19/magnesium-deficiency.aspx?x_cid=20150217_ranart_magnesium-deficiency_facebookdoc.

415. Chariot, P. and O. Bignani, *Skeletal muscle disorders associated with selenium deficiency in humans*. Muscle & Nerve, 2003. **27**(6): p. 662-668.

416. Montefiore Hospital. *Cardiac Wellness Program: Reversing Heart Disease with a Whole Food/Plant-based Diet*. 2015; Available from: http://www.montefiore.org/cardiacwellnessprogram.

417. Brannon, K. *Tulane University School of Medicine to open first-of-its-kind teaching kitchen*. 2013; Available from: http://tulane.edu/news/releases/pr05012013.cfm.

418. Ginde, A.A., M.C. Liu, and C.A.J. Camargo, *Demographic differences and trends of vitamin d insufficiency in the us population, 1988-2004*. Archives of Internal Medicine, 2009. **169**(6): p. 626-632.

419. Forrest, K.Y. and W.L. Stuhldreher, *Prevalence and correlates of vitamin D deficiency in US adults*. Nutr Res, 2011. **31**(1): p. 48-54.

420. Gorham, E.D., et al., *Optimal vitamin D status for colorectal cancer prevention: a quantitative meta analysis*. Am J Prev Med, 2007. **32**(3): p. 210-6.

421. Melamed, M.L., et al., *25-hydroxyvitamin D levels and the risk of mortality in the general population*. Arch Intern Med, 2008. **168**(15): p. 1629-37.

422. Plotnikoff, G.A. and J.M. Quigley, *Prevalence of severe hypovitaminosis D in patients with persistent, nonspecific musculoskeletal pain.* Mayo Clin Proc, 2003. **78**(12): p. 1463-70.

423. Wang, T.J., et al., *Vitamin D deficiency and risk of cardiovascular disease.* Circulation, 2008. **117**(4): p. 503-11.

424. Holick, M.F., *The vitamin D epidemic and its health consequences.* J Nutr, 2005. **135**(11): p. 2739s-48s.

425. Holick, M.F. and T.C. Chen, *Vitamin D deficiency: a worldwide problem with health consequences.* Am J Clin Nutr, 2008. **87**(4): p. 1080s-6s.

426. Campbell, T.C., *Vitamin D (Part 1)* M.R.o.S. 503: Principles in Practice, Editor. 2014, eCornell: T. Colin Campbell's Center for Nutrition Studies.

427. Breslau, N.A., et al., *Relationship of animal protein-rich diet to kidney stone formation and calcium metabolism.* J Clin Endocrinol Metab, 1988. **66**(1): p. 140-6.

428. Woodside, J.V., et al., *Micronutrients: dietary intake v. supplement use.* Proc Nutr Soc, 2005. **64**(4): p. 543-53.

429. Thiel, R.J., *Natural vitamins may be superior to synthetic ones.* Med Hypotheses, 2000. **55**(6): p. 461-9.

430. Bjelakovic, G., et al., *Mortality in randomized trials of antioxidant supplements for primary and secondary prevention: systematic review and meta-analysis.* Jama, 2007. **297**(8): p. 842-57.

431. Carlsen, M.H., et al., *The total antioxidant content of more than 3100 foods, beverages, spices, herbs and supplements used worldwide.* Nutr J, 2010. **9**: p. 3.

432. Brody, J.E., *A Body's Bacterial Companions,* in *The New York Times.* 2014, The New York Times.

433. Kalghatgi, S., et al., *Bactericidal antibiotics induce mitochondrial dysfunction and oxidative damage in Mammalian cells.* Sci Transl Med, 2013. **5**(192): p. 192ra85.

434. Harnly, J.M., et al., *Flavonoid content of U.S. fruits, vegetables, and nuts.* J Agric Food Chem, 2006. **54**(26): p. 9966-77.

435. Cazarolli, L.H., et al., *Flavonoids: prospective drug candidates.* Mini Rev Med Chem, 2008. **8**(13): p. 1429-40.

436. Cushnie, T.P. and A.J. Lamb, *Recent advances in understanding the antibacterial properties of flavonoids.* Int J Antimicrob Agents, 2011. **38**(2): p. 99-107.

437. Cushnie, T.P. and A.J. Lamb, *Antimicrobial activity of flavonoids.* Int J Antimicrob Agents, 2005. **26**(5): p. 343-56.

REFERENCES 521

438. de Sousa, R.R., et al., *Phosphoprotein levels, MAPK activities and NFkappaB expression are affected by fisetin.* J Enzyme Inhib Med Chem, 2007. **22**(4): p. 439-44.

439. Friedman, M., *Overview of antibacterial, antitoxin, antiviral, and antifungal activities of tea flavonoids and teas.* Mol Nutr Food Res, 2007. **51**(1): p. 116-34.

440. Kyle, J.A., et al., *Dietary flavonoid intake and colorectal cancer: a case-control study.* Br J Nutr, 2010. **103**(3): p. 429-36.

441. Manner, S., et al., *Systematic exploration of natural and synthetic flavonoids for the inhibition of Staphylococcus aureus biofilms.* Int J Mol Sci, 2013. **14**(10): p. 19434-51.

442. Parhiz, H., et al., *Antioxidant and Anti-Inflammatory Properties of the Citrus Flavonoids Hesperidin and Hesperetin: An Updated Review of their Molecular Mechanisms and Experimental Models.* Phytother Res, 2014.

443. Schuier, M., et al., *Cocoa-related flavonoids inhibit CFTR-mediated chloride transport across T84 human colon epithelia.* J Nutr, 2005. **135**(10): p. 2320-5.

444. Theodoratou, E., et al., *Dietary flavonoids and the risk of colorectal cancer.* Cancer Epidemiol Biomarkers Prev, 2007. **16**(4): p. 684-93.

445. Woo, H.D. and J. Kim, *Dietary flavonoid intake and smoking-related cancer risk: a meta-analysis.* PLoS One, 2013. **8**(9): p. e75604.

446. Woo, H.D., et al., *Dietary flavonoids and gastric cancer risk in a korean population.* Nutrients, 2014. **6**(11): p. 4961-73.

447. Gaziano, J.M., et al., *A prospective study of consumption of carotenoids in fruits and vegetables and decreased cardiovascular mortality in the elderly.* Ann Epidemiol, 1995. **5**(4): p. 255-60.

448. Johnson, E.J., *The role of carotenoids in human health.* Nutr Clin Care, 2002. **5**(2): p. 56-65.

449. Khachik, F., G.R. Beecher, and J.C. Smith, Jr., *Lutein, lycopene, and their oxidative metabolites in chemoprevention of cancer.* J Cell Biochem Suppl, 1995. **22**: p. 236-46.

450. Krinsky, N.I. and E.J. Johnson, *Carotenoid actions and their relation to health and disease.* Mol Aspects Med, 2005. **26**(6): p. 459-516.

451. Paiva, S.A. and R.M. Russell, *Beta-carotene and other carotenoids as antioxidants.* J Am Coll Nutr, 1999. **18**(5): p. 426-33.

452. National Cancer Institute. *SEER Cancer Statistics Review 1975-2010.* 2013; Available from: http://seer.cancer.gov/archive/csr/1975_2010/results_merged/topic_lifetime_risk_diagnosis.pdf.

453. Ward, E., et al., *Childhood and adolescent cancer statistics, 2014.* CA Cancer J Clin, 2014. **62**(2): p. 83-103.

454. World Health Organization and International Agency for Research on Cancer. *World Cancer Incidence.* 2012; Available from: http://publications.cancerresearchuk.org/downloads/Product/CS_IN FOG_WORLD_INC.PDF.

455. International Network for Cancer Treatment and Research. *Cancer in Developing Countries: Cancer – A Neglected Health Problem in Developing Countries.* 2014; Available from: http://www.inctr.org/about-inctr/cancer-in-developing-countries/.

456. Frank, J. and Harvard School of Public Health. *Cancer is on the rise in developing countries.* 2009; Available from: http://www.hsph.harvard.edu/news/magazine/shadow-epidemic/.

457. Pulitzer Center on Crisis Reporting. *Cancer's Global Footprint: Global Cancer Incidence.* 2008; Available from: www.globalcancermap.com.

458. Jemal, A., et al., *Global cancer statistics.* CA Cancer J Clin, 2011. **61**(2): p. 69-90.

459. Cancer Research UK. *About genes, cancer and family history.* About Cancer 2013; Available from: http://www.cancerresearchuk.org/cancer-help/about-cancer/causes-symptoms/genes-and-inherited-cancer-risk/about-genes-cancer-and-family-history.

460. Campbell, T.C. *Genetic Seeds of Disease: How to Beat the Odds.* Oncology 1995 1st November, 1995]; Available from: http://nutritionstudies.org/genetic-seeds-disease-beat-odds/.

461. Doll, R. and R. Peto, *The causes of cancer: quantitative estimates of avoidable risks of cancer in the United States today.* J Natl Cancer Inst, 1981. **66**(6): p. 1191-308.

462. Anand, P., et al., *Cancer is a preventable disease that requires major lifestyle changes.* Pharm Res, 2008. **25**(9): p. 2097-116.

463. Campbell, T.C. *Animal vs. Plant Protein.* Healthy Lifestyle 2013; Available from: http://nutritionstudies.org/animal-vs-plant-protein/.

464. World Cancer Research Fund / American Institute for Cancer Research, *Food, Nutrition, Physical Activity, and the Prevention of Cancer: a Global Perspective.* 2007, American Institute for Cancer Research/World Cancer Research Fund: Washington, DC.

465. Nestle, M., *Animal v. plant foods in human diets and health: is the historical record unequivocal?* Proc Nutr Soc, 1999. **58**(2): p. 211-8.

466. Lewis, C., P. Xun, and K. He, *Effects of adjuvant chemotherapy on recurrence, survival, and quality of life in stage II colon cancer patients: a 24-month follow-up.* Supportive Care in Cancer, 2015: p. 1-9.

467. The Gerson Institute. *Your Stories.* 2014; Available from: http://gerson.org/gerpress/category/your-stories/.

468. Gerson, M., *The cure of advanced cancer by diet therapy: a summary of 30 years of clinical experimentation.* Physiol Chem Phys, 1978. **10**(5): p. 449-64.

469. Hildenbrand, G.L., et al., *Five-year survival rates of melanoma patients treated by diet therapy after the manner of Gerson: a retrospective review.* Altern Ther Health Med, 1995. **1**(4): p. 29-37.

470. Jacob, R. and A. Schloz, *[Gerson therapy of malignant tumors].* Med Klin (Munich), 1955. **50**(44): p. 1866-9.

471. MacLean, S., *The Gerson therapy. Interview by Pamela Holmes.* Nurs Times, 1988. **84**(14): p. 41-2.

472. Cope, F.W., *A medical application of the Ling association-induction hypothesis: the high potassium, low sodium diet of the Gerson cancer therapy.* Physiol Chem Phys, 1978. **10**(5): p. 465-8.

473. Molassiotis, A. and P. Peat, *Surviving against all odds: analysis of 6 case studies of patients with cancer who followed the Gerson therapy.* Integr Cancer Ther, 2007. **6**(1): p. 80-8.

474. Spain, J. *Book review: The Dublin doctor who is beating cancer.* 2014; Available from: http://www.independent.ie/entertainment/books/book-reviews/book-review-the-dublin-doctor-who-is-beating-cancer-30796329.html.

475. Lavie, O., et al., *The risk of developing uterine sarcoma after tamoxifen use.* International Journal of Gynecological Cancer, 2008. **18**(2): p. 352-356.

476. Kolata, G. *Forty Years' War: Advances Elusive in the Drive to Cure Cancer.* Money & Policy 2009 23 April, 2009]; Available from: http://www.nytimes.com/2009/04/24/health/policy/24cancer.html?pagewanted=all&_r=0.

477. Simpson, S., Jr., et al., *Latitude is significantly associated with the prevalence of multiple sclerosis: a meta-analysis.* J Neurol Neurosurg Psychiatry, 2011. **82**(10): p. 1132-41.

478. Mackay, I.R., *Tolerance and autoimmunity.* Vol. 321. 2000. 93-96.

479. D'Andrea, M.R., *Add Alzheimer's disease to the list of autoimmune diseases.* Med Hypotheses, 2005. **64**(3): p. 458-63.

480. Karjalainen, J., et al., *A bovine albumin peptide as a possible trigger of insulin-dependent diabetes mellitus.* N Engl J Med, 1992. **327**(5): p. 302-7.

481. Knip, M., et al., *Environmental triggers and determinants of type 1 diabetes.* Diabetes, 2005. **54 Suppl 2**: p. S125-36.

482. Saukkonen, T., et al., *Significance of cow's milk protein antibodies as risk factor for childhood IDDM: interactions with dietary cow's milk intake and HLA-DQB1 genotype. Childhood Diabetes in Finland Study Group.* Diabetologia, 1998. **41**(1): p. 72-8.

483. Thorsdottir, I., et al., *Different beta-casein fractions in Icelandic versus Scandinavian cow's milk may influence diabetogenicity of cow's milk in infancy and explain low incidence of insulin-dependent diabetes mellitus in Iceland.* Pediatrics, 2000. **106**(4): p. 719-24.

484. Virtanen, S.M., et al., *Cow's milk consumption, disease-associated autoantibodies and type 1 diabetes mellitus: a follow-up study in siblings of diabetic children. Childhood Diabetes in Finland Study Group.* Diabet Med, 1998. **15**(9): p. 730-8.

485. Birgisdottir, B.E., et al., *Lower Consumption of Cow Milk Protein A1 β-Casein at 2 Years of Age, Rather than Consumption among 11- to 14-Year-Old Adolescents, May Explain the Lower Incidence of Type 1 Diabetes in Iceland than in Scandinavia.* Ann Nutr Metab, 2006. **50**: p. 177-183.

486. Rosenbauer, J., P. Herzig, and G. Giani, *Early infant feeding and risk of type 1 diabetes mellitus—a nationwide population-based case–control study in pre-school children.* Diabetes Metab, 2007. **24**(3): p. 211-222.

487. Sadauskaitė-Kuehne, V., et al., *Longer breastfeeding is an independent protective factor against development of type 1 diabetes mellitus in childhood.* Diabetes Metab, 2004. **20**(2): p. 150-157.

488. U.S. Department of Health and Human Services, *Healthy People 2010.* 2000, CDC: Washington DC: US Department of Health and Human Services.

489. Mimura, G., K. Murakami, and M. Gushiken, *Nutritional factors for longevity in Okinawa--present and future.* Nutr Health, 1992. **8**(2-3): p. 159-63.

490. Wilcox, B., M. Suzuki, and C. Wilcox, *The Okinawa Program.* 2002: Harmony.

491. Willcox, D.C., et al., *The Okinawan diet: health implications of a low-calorie, nutrient-dense, antioxidant-rich dietary pattern low in glycemic load.* J Am Coll Nutr, 2009. **28 Suppl**: p. 500s-516s.

492.Miyagi, S., et al., *Longevity and diet in Okinawa, Japan: the past, present and future.* Asia Pac J Public Health, 2003. **15 Suppl**: p. S3-9.

493.Buettner, D., *The Blue Zones, Second Edition: 9 Lessons for Living Longer From the People Who've Lived the Longest.* Vol. 2nd Edition. 2012, Washington, D. C. : National Geographic.

494.National Public Radio. *Eating To Break 100: Longevity Diet Tips From The Blue Zones.* The Salt: What's on Your Plate 2015; Available from: http://www.npr.org/sections/thesalt/2015/04/11/398325030/eating-to-break-100-longevity-diet-tips-from-the-blue-zones.

495.Tuso, P.J., et al., *Nutritional update for physicians: plant-based diets.* Perm J, 2013. **17**(2): p. 61-6.

496.Traka, M.H. and R.F. Mithen, *Plant science and human nutrition: challenges in assessing health-promoting properties of phytochemicals.* Plant Cell, 2011. **23**(7): p. 2483-97.

497.Martin, C., et al., *Plants, diet, and health.* Annu Rev Plant Biol, 2013. **64**: p. 19-46.

498.Esselstyn, C.B., Jr., *Resolving the Coronary Artery Disease Epidemic Through Plant-Based Nutrition.* Prev Cardiol, 2001. **4**(4): p. 171-177.

499.Esselstyn, C.B., Jr., et al., *A way to reverse CAD?* J Fam Pract, 2014. **63**(7): p. 356-364, 364a, 364b.

500.McDougall, J., et al., *Effects of 7 days on an ad libitum low-fat vegan diet: the McDougall Program cohort.* Nutr J, 2014. **13**(1): p. 99.

501.Turner-McGrievy, G.M., et al., *Comparative effectiveness of plant-based diets for weight loss: A randomized controlled trial of five different diets.* Nutrition.

502.Orlich, M.J., et al., *Vegetarian dietary patterns and mortality in Adventist Health Study 2.* JAMA Intern Med, 2013. **173**(13): p. 1230-8.

503.Bodai, B.I. and P. Tuso, *Breast cancer survivorship: a comprehensive review of long-term medical issues and lifestyle recommendations.* Perm J, 2015. **19**(2): p. 48-79.

504.O'Connor, A., *Advice From a Vegan Cardiologist*, in *The New York Times*. 2014.

505.Obama, M., *Remarks by the First Lady on a Nutrition Facts Label Announcement.* 2014, The White House: Office of the First Lady.

506.International Federation for Produce Standards, *Produce PLU Codes: A User's Guide - 2012.* 2012.

507.Krol, W.J., et al., *Reduction of pesticide residues on produce by rinsing.* J Agric Food Chem, 2000. **48**(10): p. 4666-70.

508.Pimentel, D., et al., *Reducing Energy Inputs in the US Food System.* Human Ecology, 2008. **36**(4): p. 459-471.

509.Miglio, C., et al., *Effects of Different Cooking Methods on Nutritional and Physicochemical Characteristics of Selected Vegetables.* Journal of Agricultural and Food Chemistry, 2007. **56**(1): p. 139-147.

510.Yuan, G.F., et al., *Effects of different cooking methods on health-promoting compounds of broccoli.* J Zhejiang Univ Sci B, 2009. **10**(8): p. 580-8.

511.U.S. Department of Agriculture, *USDA Table of Nutrient Retention Factors,* N.D. Laboratory, et al., Editors. 2007, U.S. Department of Agriculture, Agricultural Research Service: Beltsville, Maryland.

512.Hasnol, N.D., S. Jinap, and M. Sanny, *Effect of different types of sugars in a marinating formulation on the formation of heterocyclic amines in grilled chicken.* Food Chem, 2014. **145**: p. 514-21.

513.Helmus, D.S., et al., *Red meat-derived heterocyclic amines increase risk of colon cancer: a population-based case-control study.* Nutr Cancer, 2013. **65**(8): p. 1141-50.

514.Jamin, E.L., et al., *Combined genotoxic effects of a polycyclic aromatic hydrocarbon (B(a)P) and an heterocyclic amine (PhIP) in relation to colorectal carcinogenesis.* PLoS One, 2013. **8**(3): p. e58591.

515.Yao, Y., et al., *Effects of frying and boiling on the formation of heterocyclic amines in braised chicken.* Poult Sci, 2013. **92**(11): p. 3017-25.

516.Friedman, M., *Nutritional consequences of food processing.* Forum Nutr, 2003. **56**: p. 350-2.

517.Cross, G.A., D.Y.C. Fung, and R.V. Decareau, *The effect of microwaves on nutrient value of foods.* C R C Critical Reviews in Food Science and Nutrition, 1982. **16**(4): p. 355-381.

518.Lassen, A. and L. Ovesen, *Nutritional effects of microwave cooking.* Nutrition & Food Science, 1995. **95**(4): p. 8-10.

519.*Case of Hertel vs. Switzerland* in *Cour Européenne Des Droits De L'homme (European Court Of Human Rights).* 1998: Strasbourg, Switzerland. p. 1-41.

520.Bittner, G.D., C.Z. Yang, and M.A. Stoner, *Estrogenic chemicals often leach from BPA-free plastic products that are replacements for BPA-containing polycarbonate products.* Environ Health, 2014. **13**(1): p. 41.

521.Cassady, B.A., et al., *Mastication of almonds: effects of lipid bioaccessibility, appetite, and hormone response.* Am J Clin Nutr, 2009. **89**(3): p. 794-800.

522.Andrade, A.M., G.W. Greene, and K.J. Melanson, *Eating slowly led to decreases in energy intake within meals in healthy women.* J Am Diet Assoc, 2008. **108**(7): p. 1186-91.

523.Galsziou, P., et al., *Pre-meal water consumption for weight loss.* Aust Fam Physician, 2013. **42**(7): p. 478.

524.Davy, B.M., et al., *Water consumption reduces energy intake at a breakfast meal in obese older adults.* J Am Diet Assoc, 2008. **108**(7): p. 1236-9.

525.ScienceDaily and Johns Hopkins University Bloomberg School of Public Health. *Home cooking a main ingredient in healthier diet, study shows.* 2014 17 November 2014]; Available from: http://www.sciencedaily.com/releases/2014/11/141117084711.htm.

526.Wolfson, J.A. and S.N. Bleich, *Is cooking at home associated with better diet quality or weight-loss intention?* Public Health Nutr, 2014: p. 1-10.

527.Kolodinsky, J.M. and A.B. Goldstein, *Time use and food pattern influences on obesity.* Obesity (Silver Spring), 2011. **19**(12): p. 2327-35.

528.Doctor's Associates, Inc., and Subway Sandwiches. *US Product Ingredients.* 2014; Available from: https://www.subway.com/Nutrition/Files/usProdIngredients.pdf.

529.Nguyen, D., B. Kit, and M. Carroll, *Abnormal Cholesterol Among Children and Adolescents in the United States, 2011–2014.* 2015, National Center for Health Statistics, Centers for Disease Control and Prevention: Hyattsville, MD.

530.Silverberg, J. *Eat Yourself Well.* 2015; Available from: http://eatyourselfwell.com/about/.

531.Wabitsch, M., A. Moss, and K. Kromeyer-Hauschild, *Unexpected plateauing of childhood obesity rates in developed countries.* BMC Med, 2014. **12**: p. 17.

532.Organisation for Economic Co-operation and Development, *Obestiy Update.* 2014, OECD.

533.Allergy Kids Foundation. *So What Has Changed?* 2014; Available from: http://www.allergykids.com/defining-food-allergies/so-what-has-changed/.

534.BBC News, *Offer vegetables early and often to fussy toddlers, study says,* in *Health.* 2014.

535.Caton, S.J., et al., *Learning to Eat Vegetables in Early Life: The Role of Timing, Age and Individual Eating Traits.* PLoS ONE, 2014. **9**(5): p. e97609.

536.Nicklaus, S., et al., *A prospective study of food variety seeking in childhood, adolescence and early adult life.* Appetite, 2005. **44**(3): p. 289-97.

537.Bayer HealthCare, *Flintsones (TM) Complete,* B.H. LLC, Editor. 2011. p. 2.

538.Iyyaswamy, A. and S. Rathinasamy, *Effect of chronic exposure to aspartame on oxidative stress in the brain of albino rats.* J Biosci, 2012. **37**(4): p. 679-88.

539.Soffritti, M., et al., *First experimental demonstration of the multipotential carcinogenic effects of aspartame administered in the feed to Sprague-Dawley rats.* Environ Health Perspect, 2006. **114**(3): p. 379-85.

540.Lambrot, R., et al., *Low paternal dietary folate alters the mouse sperm epigenome and is associated with negative pregnancy outcomes.* Nat Commun, 2013. **4**.

541.Maslova, E., et al., *Maternal protein intake during pregnancy and offspring overweight 20 y later.* Am J Clin Nutr, 2014. **100**(4): p. 1139-48.

542.Villar, J., et al., *The likeness of fetal growth and newborn size across non-isolated populations in the INTERGROWTH-21st Project: the Fetal Growth Longitudinal Study and Newborn Cross-Sectional Study.* The Lancet Diabetes & Endocrinology, 2014.

543.Miese-Looy, G., J. Rollings-Scattergood, and A. Yeung, *Long-term health consequences of poor nutrition during pregnancy.* Studies by Undergraduate Researchers at Guelph, 2008. **1**(2): p. 73-81.

544.Bennis-Taleb, N., et al., *A Low-Protein Isocaloric Diet During Gestation Affects Brain Development and Alters Permanently Cerebral Cortex Blood Vessels in Rat Offspring.* J. Nutr, 1999. **129**(8): p. 1613-1619.

545.Reilly, J.J., et al., *Early life risk factors for obesity in childhood: cohort study.* BMJ 2005. **330**(1357): p. 1-7.

546.Oken, E., et al., *Gestational weight gain and child adiposity at age 3 years.* American Journal of Obstetrics & Gynecology, 2007. **196**(4): p. 322.e1-322.e8.

547.Bayol, S.A., et al., *Offspring from mothers fed a 'junk food' diet in pregnancy and lactation exhibit exacerbated adiposity that is more pronounced in females.* J Phsyiol, 2008. **586**(13): p. 3219-3230.

548.Napoli, C., et al., *Fatty streak formation occurs in human fetal aortas and is greatly enhanced by maternal hypercholesterolemia. Intimal accumulation of low density lipoprotein and its oxidation precede monocyte recruitment into early atherosclerotic lesions.* J Clin Invest, 1997. **100**(11): p. 2680-90.

549. Nakhai-Pour, H.R., et al., *Use of nonaspirin nonsteroidal anti-inflammatory drugs during pregnancy and the risk of spontaneous abortion.* CMAJ, 2011. **183**(15): p. 1713-1720.

550. Liew, Z., et al., *Acetaminophen Use During Pregnancy, Behavioral Problems, and Hyperkinetic Disorders.* JAMA Pediatr, 2014. **168**(4): p. 313-320.

551. Daniel, S., et al., *Fetal exposure to nonsteroidal anti-inflammatory drugs and spontaneous abortions.* CMAJ, 2014. **186**(5): p. E177-E182.

552. EasyDex, *Oral Glucose Tolerance Beverage: Orange.* 2014.

553. Andres, A., et al., *Developmental status of 1-year-old infants fed breast milk, cow's milk formula, or soy formula.* Pediatrics, 2012. **129**(6): p. 1134-40.

554. Belfield, C.R. and I.R. Kelly, *The Benefits Of Breastfeeding Across The Early Years Of Childhood.* Journal of Human Capital, 2012. **6**(3): p. 251-277.

555. Gale, C., et al., *Effect of breastfeeding compared with formula feeding on infant body composition: a systematic review and meta-analysis.* Am J Clin Nutr, 2012. **95**(3): p. 656-69.

556. Ip, S., et al., *Breastfeeding and maternal and infant health outcomes in developed countries.* Evid Rep Technol Assess (Full Rep), 2007(153): p. 1-186.

557. Ortega-Garcia, J.A., et al., *Full breastfeeding and paediatric cancer.* J Paediatr Child Health, 2008. **44**(1-2): p. 10-3.

558. Stuebe, A., *The risks of not breastfeeding for mothers and infants.* Rev Obstet Gynecol, 2009. **2**(4): p. 222-31.

559. Yum, J., *The Effects of Breast Milk Versus Infant Formulae on Cognitive Development.* Journal On Developmental Disabilities, 2007. **13**(1): p. 135-164.

560. Chase, H.P. and H.P. Martin, *Undernutrition and Child Development.* New England Journal of Medicine, 1970. **282**(17): p. 933-939.

561. Greenberg, J. *Unstable emotions of children tied to poor diet.* Science 1981 18 August, 1981; Available from: http://www.nytimes.com/1981/08/18/science/unstable-emotions-of-children-tied-to-poor-diet.html.

562. Korenman, S., J.E. Miller, and J.E. Sjaastad, *Long-term poverty and child development in the United States: Results from the NLSY.* Children and Youth Services Review, 1995. **17**(1–2): p. 127-155.

563. Martorell, R., et al., *Weight gain in the first two years of life is an important predictor of schooling outcomes in pooled analyses from five birth*

cohorts from low- and middle-income countries. J Nutr, 2010. **140**(2): p. 348-54.

Index